Emergency Medicine: Clinical Practice

Emergency Medicine: Clinical Practice

Editor: Vincent Mitchell

FOSTER ACADEMICS

www.fosteracademics.com

www.fosteracademics.com

FOSTER ACADEMICS

Cataloging-in-Publication Data

Emergency medicine : clinical practice / edited by Vincent Mitchell.
p. cm.
Includes bibliographical references and index.
ISBN 978-1-63242-876-9
1. Emergency medicine. 2. Critical care medicine. 3. Disaster medicine. 4. Medical emergencies. I. Mitchell, Vincent.
RC86.7 .E44 2020
616.025--dc23

Foster Academics,
118-35 Queens Blvd., Suite 400,
Forest Hills, NY 11375, USA

ISBN 978-1-63242-876-9 (Hardback)

Contents

Preface

The purpose of the book is to provide a glimpse into the dynamics and to present opinions and studies of some of the scientists engaged in the development of new ideas in the field from very different standpoints. This book will prove useful to students and researchers owing to its high content quality.

Emergency medicine is the medical specialty that is concerned with the care of injuries and medical conditions that require urgent medical attention. The chief dimensions of focus in this area of medicine are life-saving operations such as resuscitation and stabilization, and the diagnosis and treatment of illnesses in the acute phase. The sub-specializations of emergency medicine are medical toxicology, critical care medicine, disaster medicine, hyperbaric medicine, etc. Some of the medical situations that require emergency medical care include heart attack, stroke, fracture, pregnancy related emergencies and complications, manic episode, airway obstruction, etc. This book elucidates the concepts and innovative models around prospective developments with respect to emergency medicine. While understanding the long-term perspectives of the topics, the book makes an effort in highlighting their impact as a modern tool for the growth of the discipline. It attempts to assist those with a goal of delving into this field.

At the end, I would like to appreciate all the efforts made by the authors in completing their chapters professionally. I express my deepest gratitude to all of them for contributing to this book by sharing their valuable works. A special thanks to my family and friends for their constant support in this journey.

Editor

1

Implementing blended learning in emergency airway management training

Madeleine Huei Tze Kho[1], Keng Sheng Chew[2*], Muhaimin Noor Azhar[3], Mohd Lotfi Hamzah[4], Kee Man Chuah[5], Aida Bustam[3] and Hiang Chuan Chan[1]

Abstract

Background: While emergency airway management training is conventionally conducted via face-to-face learning (F2FL) workshops, there are inherent cost, time, place and manpower limitations in running such workshops. Blended learning (BL) refers to the systematic integration of online and face-to-face learning aimed to facilitate complex thinking skills and flexible participation at a reduced financial, time and manpower cost. This study was conducted to evaluate its effectiveness in emergency airway management training.

Methods: A single-center prospective randomised controlled trial involving 30 doctors from Sarawak General Hospital, Malaysia was conducted from September 2016 to February 2017 to compare the effectiveness of BL versus F2FL for emergency airway management training. Participants in the BL arm were given a period of 12 days to go through the online materials in a learning management system while those in the F2FL arm attended a-day of face-to-face lectures (8 h). Participants from both arms then attended a day of hands-on session consisting of simulation skills training with airway manikins. Pre- and post-tests in knowledge and practical skills were administered. E-learning experience and the perception towards BL among participants in the BL arm were also assessed.

Results: Significant improvements in post-test scores as compared to pre-test scores were noted for participants in both BL and F2FL arms for knowledge, practical, and total scores. The degree of increment between the BL group and the F2FL arms for all categories were not significantly different (total scores: 35 marks, inter-quartile range (IQR) 15.0 – 41.0 vs. 31 marks, IQR 24.0 – 41.0, $p = 0.690$; theory scores: 18 marks, IQR 9 – 24 vs. 19 marks, IQR 15 – 20, $p = 0.992$; practical scores: 11 marks, IQR 5 -18 vs. 10 marks, IQR 9 – 20, $p = 0.461$ respectively). The overall perception towards BL was positive.

Conclusions: Blended learning is as effective as face-to-face learning for emergency airway management training of junior doctors, suggesting that blended learning may be a feasible alternative to face-to-face learning for such skill training in emergency departments.

Keywords: Emergency airway management, Blended learning, Online learning, E-learning

* Correspondence: kschew@unimas.my
[2]Faculty of Medicine and Health Sciences, Universiti Malaysia Sarawak, Kota Samarahan 94300, Sarawak, Malaysia
Full list of author information is available at the end of the article

Background

One essential skill every emergency doctor needs to have is the skill of emergency airway management. Conventionally, emergency airway management training is carried out via face-to-face learning workshops. Unfortunately, these workshops can only admit a limited number of participants per course and the participants are required to be there in person throughout the entire workshop. There are inherent cost, time, place and manpower limitations in running such conventional face-to-face workshops. Hence, it is useful to explore the feasibility of using the blended learning approach in overcoming the aforementioned limitations.

Blended learning (BL) refers to the systematic integration of online and face-to-face learning (F2FL) in order to facilitate critical, creative and complex thinking skills [1]. As poignantly alluded by Garrison and Kanuka (2004), while internet and technology is certainly involved, BL is not just about delivering or uploading old contents in a new medium [1]. Rather, it involves a fundamental reconceptualization and restructuring of the entire learning process [1]. In other words, the focus is not on the technological tools [2], but on how best to combine certain aspects for online learning (e.g. topics that require extensive theoretical discussion) and other aspects (e.g. skills training) for F2FL [3]. A well-blended course, therefore, should translate into better learning outcomes at a reduced long-term cost, time and manpower while at the same time enable flexible participation from any location at any time [2, 4]. Essentially, instead of bringing the people to learning, BL is about bringing learning to the people [5] without compromising on the quality of instructional and content delivery.

A closely related learning approach known as the flipped learning (also called "the inverted classroom"), is a pedagogical model which reverses what typically occurs in classes [6]. Students are first exposed to the material outside of class, typically in the form of video-based lectures, and then class time is transformed into an interactive learning environment where students engage in activities for active learning such as problem solving, discussion, and analysis [6]. In this study, BL rather flipped learning was chosen as emergency airway management training still requires the instructor to take a central role during practical skills learning.

In a systematic review on the role of BL in clinical education, Rowe et al. (2012) emphasized that as clinical education is highly context-dependent, generalization across disciplines can be challenging, because the success of implementing BL in one clinical domain does not necessarily mean that it will have similar value in another domain [2]. With that in mind, we embarked on a study with the primary outcome of evaluating the effectiveness of implementing BL in emergency airway management workshop for junior doctors as compared to F2FL. It is hypothesized that BL is at least as effective as F2FL workshop for emergency airway management training. Secondary outcomes of this study are 1) the participants' subjective perception of BL; and since it has been shown in literature that the lack of information and communication technology (ICT) skills is a concern in BL [4], 2) subgroup analyses of the influence of the participants' prior ICT skills on their test performance.

Methods

This was a single center, single blinded, prospective randomised controlled trial (from September 2016 to February 2017) aimed to compare the efficacy of BL versus F2FL in emergency airway management workshop for junior doctors. In the F2FL arm, the participants attended an 8-h one-day F2FL lectures on emergency airway management and discussion followed by a day of hands-on session consisting of simulation skill training with airway manikins.

For the BL arm, course materials consisting of videos, manuals and quizzes were first developed and made available to participants through an online learning management system (openlearning.com). Course contents were standardized with those delivered in the F2FL arm. Social networking services were utilized to enhance discussions among participants and the instructors. Participants were given a period of 12 days (estimated at 40 min per day) to go through the materials during their own personal time, followed by a day of hands-on session consisting of simulation skill training with airway manikins (similar to that in F2FL arm).

Ethical approval was obtained from the Medical Research and Ethics Committee, Ministry Of Health Malaysia and the study was registered under the Malaysian National Medical Research Register (NMRR, website URL: https://tinyurl.com/y9mhztog) with the research number of NMRR1669630190 prior to the commencement of the study.

Participants

Junior doctors working in the emergency department of Sarawak General Hospital, Malaysia were invited to participate in this study. We define a "junior doctor" as a doctor in his or her second and third year of clinical service. The reason for choosing junior doctors in their second or third year of clinical service (rather than those in their first year of service) is because these doctors have had at least 1 year of basic clinical experience which we believe enables them to better comprehend the contents of this training and to actively participate in the discussions with critical thinking skills. Any junior doctor who had participated in any prior airway training course was excluded from the study. Informed consents were obtained from all participants prior to their participation in this study. The detailed descriptions of the participants are given in Table 1.

The sample size estimation was calculated based on the 2-mean formula on the G*Power software version 3.1.9.2 [7] based on a study by Lancester et al. in 2012 which compared examination scores of nursing degree students who went through either traditional or blended methods of lecture delivery on pharmacotherapeutics [8]. In that study, it was found that the mean scores were 92.7 +/− 3.8 and 96.6 +/− 1.9 for traditional learning and blended learning respectively [7]. Therefore, using a priori analysis with a 95% power of study with an alpha of 0.05, a total sample size of 28 with 14 in each group was determined. This sample size was further inflated by 10% to compensate for potential drop out, thus making our sample size 30 participants in total, or 15 participants in each arm.

Table 1 Baseline characteristics of participants

Variable	Face-to-face Group (*N* = 15)	Blended Group (N = 15)
Age (year)		
Median	27	27
Interquartile range	2	2
Sex – n (%)		
Male	8 (53.3)	10 (66.7)
Female	7 (46.7)	5 (33.3)
Years of service – n (%)		
Second	8 (53.3)	10 (66.7)
Third	7 (46.7)	5 (33.3)
Current position – n (%)		
Houseman	8 (53.3)	8 (53.3)
Medical Officer	7 (46.7)	7 (46.7)
Prior related training courses – n (%)		
Basic Life Support	9 (60.0)	8 (53.3)
Neonatal Resuscitation Programme	12 (80.0)	13 (86.7)
Pediatric Life Support	1 (6.7)	1 (6.7)
Advanced Pediatric Life Support (APLS)	0 (0.0)	0 (0.0)
Pediatric Advanced Life Support (PALS)	3 (20.0)	2 (13.3)
Advanced Cardiovascular Life Support (ACLS)	4 (26.7)	4 (26.7)
Advanced Life Support (ALS)	0 (0.0)	2 (13.3)
Advanced Trauma Life Support (ATLS)	1 (6.7)	0 (0.0)
Malaysian Trauma Life Support (MTLS)	0 (0.0)	0 (0.0)
Amount of prior training courses per person - n (%)		
One	3 (20.0)	6 (40.0)
Two	10 (66.7)	4 (26.7)
Three	1 (6.7)	4 (26.7)
Four	1 (6.7)	1 (6.7)

Materials

Besides training the participants in the fundamentals of airway management, this workshop also aimed to address the safety gaps identified in the 4th National Audit Project of The Royal College of Anaesthetists and The Difficult Airway Society (NAP4). The topics for this workshop were first gleaned, selected and compiled from two existing airway management courses in Malaysia, i.e., the East Coast Airway Course (EAST), as well as the airway management course from a postgraduate emergency medicine training program (i.e., the University of Malaya Emergency Medicine Masters' Program curriculum). All materials were internally validated via a modified Delphi method to reach a consensus by a panel of experts in emergency medicine (MHTK, KSC, MNA, MLH, AB) with one of them having a special interest in emergency airway management (MLH). These module topics and skill stations were as listed in Additional file 1: Table S1.

Procedure

The study was divided into two stages. The first stage was the development of teaching contents and assessment questions using a modified Delphi method in three rounds of online discussion. As the experts are based in different locations within Malaysia, a video conferencing discussion was carried as the first round of discussion. In this round, the overarching aims and objectives of the workshop were clarified among the experts. The experts then listed out the probable topics for the workshop as well as the assessment questions. Topics of interest were then emailed by the experts to author MHTK who was responsible in compiling them. In the second round of online discussion, the list of topics were then emailed out by author MHTK to all experts who then scrutinized and gave their suggestions to these topics. The agreed topics were then compiled by author MHTK and emailed out again to all experts for a third round of online discussion. In this round, specific tasks of preparing the lecture notes, presentation slides and video lectures were assigned to specific experts. Experts also contributed the pre-test and post-test assessment questions (comprising of four sections: 1) one best answer (OBA) 2) true/false section (T/F) 3) "fill-in-the-blanks" and 4) practical skills stations) (see Additional file 1: Table S1 for the detailed descriptions). These questions were then vetted and agreed upon by the experts. Any differences in opinion among the experts were resolved via further discussions and consensus.

For participants in the BL arm, the notes were uploaded in the learning management system (URL: https://www.openlearning.com/courses/emergency-airway-management/HomePage); whereas for participants in the F2FL arm, it was in the form of printed handouts). Online activities in the form of quizzes, "fill in the blanks", and crossword puzzle were created for participants in BL arm. A similar quiz was prepared for those in the F2FL arm as well, but the "fill in the blanks" and crossword puzzle were not administered to the F2FL arm as these are optional enhancing activities in a BL setting.

The learning management system was then checked independently by 2 of the researchers (MNA and KMC); and all errors were rectified before the online course was opened for enrollment. All participants (from both arms of the study) participated in this study without any fee or charges.

The second stage of this study was participant recruitment and randomization as well as the implementation of educational interventions. Junior doctors who consented to this voluntary, anonymous study were first randomized using an online number generator (http://www.graphpad.com/quickcalcs/randMenu/) into either the BL arm or the F2FL arm. Upon registration, all participants completed a pre-test theory & practical assessment by an independent emergency physician who was blinded to the participants' study arms. To assess their information and communication technology (ICT) skills, participants in the BL arm also completed a validated questionnaire on ICT skills using a Likert scale from 0 to 10 where 0 means the participant finds it the easiest to perform the ICT task and 10 means the participant finds it the hardest to perform the ICT task [9]. The information gleaned from these participants' prior ICT skills were then analyzed for any possible correlation between their ICT skill proficiency levels with the scores they obtained. Participants from the BL arm had access to the online learning materials, online quizzes and discussions via an online blended learning classroom for 12 days before they joined participants from the F2FL arm for the one-day hands-on session. A social networking messaging application was utilized to enhance discussions among participants and the instructors. For the F2FL arm, the exact same lecture notes were made available to them for 12 days before the first day of the workshop. They then attended an 8-h one-day of F2FL lectures covering all of the above-mentioned modules on emergency airway management using PowerPoint slides with the same content as that which was used for video lectures. Time was allocated after each lecture for discussion and to answer any questions that the participants had. They also participated in a group quiz and also watched video demonstration of certain procedures relevant to emergency airway management (available also on the online learning system). Participants from the F2FL arm underwent a one-day (or 8 h) training consisting of face-to-face classroom lectures. This was followed by a one-day hands-on session consisting of simulation skill training with airway manikins. All participants then completed a post-test theory and practical assessment by the same emergency physician who conducted the pre-test practical assessment. The assessor was blinded to the participants' arm all throughout the study.

In addition, participants from the BL arm also answered a validated quantitative e-learning experience questionnaire adapted from Ginns & Ellis (2007) [10] and a qualitative questionnaire to gauge their perception towards blended learning, adapted from Larsen (2012) [11]. All the quantitative data that was collected was then analyzed using IBM SPSS Statistics 15.0 for Windows. Thematic analysis was manually performed to code or interpret the qualitative data.

Results

A total of 30 junior doctors participated in this study (with 15 participants in each of the 2 arms). None of these participants dropped out from the study. The median age of each group was 27 with the interquartile range of 2 years. In terms of years of experience, 8 (53.3%) participants and 10 (66.7%) participants in the F2FL and BL arm respectively had 2 years of clinical experience. The rest of the participants had 3 years of clinical experience. The detailed descriptions of the participants are presented in Table 1. Non-parametric tests were used, as the assumptions of normality were not satisfied for the variables of theory, practical and total scores. When analyzed using Wilcoxon Signed Rank Test, the post-test scores for the theory, practical and total scores were significantly higher than the pre-test for both BL and F2FL arms (see Table 2).

However, while there were significantly higher scores in all post-tests compared to the pre-tests, the degree of increment was not significantly more in one arm compared to the other. In particular, while the median increment from pre-test to post-test total score was higher in the BL arm than in the F2FL arm; i.e., 35 marks (inter-quartile range, IQR 15.0 - 41.0; mean rank =14.83; sum of ranks 222.50) in the BL arm compared to 31 marks (IQR 24.0 - 41.0; mean rank = 16.17; sum of ranks 242.50) in the F2FL arm, this was not statistically significant ($U = 102.5$; $z = -0.415$; $p = 0.690$). For the theory score, the median increment from pre-test to post-test was about the same across both arms; with 18 marks (IQR 9 - 24; mean rank = 14.27; sum of ranks = 232) and 19 marks (IQR = 15 - 20; mean rank = 15.53; sum of ranks = 233) in BL arm and F2FL arm ($U = 112$; $z = -0.21$; $p = 0.992$). For the practical score, the median increment from pre-test to post-test was also almost the same across both arms; with 11 marks (IQR 5 -18; mean rank = 15.47; sum of ranks = 214) and 10 marks (IQR = 9 – 20; mean rank = 16.73; sum of ranks = 251) in BL arm and F2FL arm respectively ($U = 94$; $z = -0.769$; $p = 0.461$).

Table 2 Comparison of pre-test vs. post-test scores for theory, practical and total scores

	Group	Pre-test Median IQR (1st, 3rd)	Post-test Median IQR (1st, 3rd)	Wilcoxon Signed Rank Test
Theory score	F2FL	62 (54, 67)	80 (75, 85)	$Z = -3.416$ $P = 0.001$
	BL	58 (56, 64)	79 (72, 82)	$Z = -3.409$ $P = 0.001$
Practical score	F2FL	64 (58, 72)	80 (74, 86)	$Z = -3.079$ $P = 0.002$
	BL	65 (57, 72)	75 (70, 82)	$Z = -3.068$ $P = 0.002$
Total score	F2FL	124 (119, 131)	156 (151, 164)	$Z = -3.409$ $P = 0.001$
	BL	124 (113, 136)	155 (144, 162)	$Z = -3.409$ $P = 0.001$

F2FL means participants in face-to-face learning arm; BL means participants in blended learning arm

For the subgroup analysis of the participants' responses to BL experience, 12 out of 15 participants (80%) were satisfied with the overall quality of the online materials and activities in the BL (Item no. 32). With regards to the participants' interaction and engagement in online postings (Items 7, 16, 18 and 21), while the majority of them agreed that reading other participants' on-line submissions helped to clarify (Item no. 7; 53.3% of the participants), aided in their own "understanding" of some of the contents (Item no. 18; 73.3% of the participants) and appeared to have motivated them to read further (Item no. 21; 60.0% of the participants). However, only 20% of the 15 participants indicated that they had interacted with other students' on-line postings (Item no. 20). For other detailed responses of the participants' BL experience, refer Table 3.

In terms of the level of prior ICT skills of the participants, it was found that most participants did not consider the list of ICT skills in the questionnaire to be difficult, as all items or tasks listed in the questionnaire had responses concentrated in the easy category (> 60.0%). Less than 10% of the participants considered any of the items as difficult (see Additional file 1: Table S2 for the detailed responses). Spearman's correlation was used to determine the correlation between prior ICT skills of the participants and their e-learning experience. There was no significant correlation between these two variables ($r_s = -0.411$, $n = 15$, $p = 0.128$). In other words, the participants' e-learning experience did not seem to be affected by the level of their ICT skills. Besides that, Spearman's correlation was also used to determine the correlation between the ICT skills of the participants and the BL course outcome in terms of the increment of score from pre-test to post-test. It was found that there was no significant correlation between the level of prior ICT skills of participants and the blended learning course outcome (increment of total score among participants in BL group) ($r_s = -0.64$, $n = 15$, $p = 0.822$).

From the qualitative questionnaire on the participants' perspectives towards BL, it was noted that most of the participants responded positively to BL (refer Table 4 for all highlighted responses). For example, when asked to describe the training they received via blended learning (Question 3), two participants mentioned that BL affords the learning flexibility allowing them to go through the materials *"over and over again"*. The course was also described as *"informative"* (4 responses), *"comprehensive"* (1 response), *"concise"* (1 response), *"efficient"* (1 response), *"enjoyable"* (1 response), *"well-organised"* (1 response), *"good"* (3 responses), *"ample time provided"* (1 response), and *"extremely good and valuable training which is hard to learn via textbook only"* (1 response). One person however, remarked that *"learning through the blended program was a little boring"* as the videos were monotonous. In response to the question (question no. 12) on what would improve the participants' involvement in online discussions, one participant mentioned that the online facilitators/instructors should have taken a more active role to pose more questions to the participants because when the participants were not asking questions, it could be because *"we don't know what we don't know"*.

Discussion

This study seems to suggest that BL is not inferior to, but as effective as F2FL in emergency airway management training as evidenced by the fact that there is a significant improvement from pre-test to post-test for theory, practical and total scores in the BL arm as well as in the F2FL, but there is no statistically significant difference in terms of the degree of increment of the scores across the two arms. This finding suggests that blended

Table 3 Responses of participants in BL arm on their e-Learning experience

No	Item	Mean*	S.D.*	Likert scale response [N (%)] **			
				Disagree	Neutral	Agree	Missing data
1	To do well in the on-line quizzes all you really need is a good memory.	3.31	0.263	1 (6.7)	2 (13.3)	12 (80.0)	–
2	The teacher used the on-line environment when appropriate to keep students informed about results.	3.77	0.166	0 (0.0)	4 (26.7)	11 (73.3)	–
3	I received too much feedback on-line from my teacher.	2.62	0.180	4 (26.6)	10 (66.6)	0 (0.0)	1
4	The teacher's responses on-line motivated me to learn more deeply.	3.85	0.191	0 (0.0)	4 (26.6)	10 (66.6)	1
5	The teacher helped to guide on-line discussions between students	4.00	0.160	0 (0.0)	2 (13.3)	13 (86.7)	–
6	The teacher used the on-line environment to regularly update students about relevant unit of study information.	4.08	0.178	0 (0.0)	2 (13.3)	13 (86.7)	–
7	Reading other students' on-line submissions clarified some of my own ideas.	3.46	0.215	1 (6.7)	6 (40.0)	8 (53.3)	–
8	The on-line teaching materials in this unit of study are extremely good at explaining things.	3.92	0.239	1 (6.7)	2 (13.3)	12 (80.0)	–
9	The teacher's interaction with me on-line encouraged me to get the most out of my learning.	4.00	0.160	0 (0.0)	2 (13.3)	13 (86.7)	–
10	On-line quizzes helped me to learn effectively.	4.15	0.154	3 (20.0)	4 (26.7)	8 (53.3)	–
11	The workload for the on-line component of this unit of study is too heavy.	2.54	0.268	6 (40.0)	6 (40.0)	3 (20.0)	–
12	The teacher's on-line responses motivated me to do more on-line learning than I would have done otherwise.	3.85	0.222	0 (0.0)	6 (40.0)	9 (60.0)	–
13	Information needed to understand the purpose and contents of the unit was integrated in one place on-line.	3.77	0.281	2 (13.3)	3 (20.0)	10 (66.7)	–
14	I generally had enough time to understand the things I had to learn on-line.	3.54	0.243	1 (6.7)	6 (40.0)	8 (53.3)	–
15	I didn't receive enough helpful on-line feedback from my teacher.	2.15	0.249	8 (53.3)	7 (46.7)	0 (0.0)	–
16	I interacted with students' on-line postings/submissions even if they weren't assessed.	2.77	0.231	4 (26.7)	8 (53.3)	3 (20.0)	–
17	The on-line activities are designed to get the best out of students.	3.92	0.137	0 (0.0)	3 (20.0)	12 (80.0)	–
18	Other students' on-line submissions helped me understand my ideas from a new perspective.	3.77	0.166	0 (0.0)	4 (26.7)	11 (73.3)	–
19	The guidelines for using on-line discussions were clear to me.	3.92	0.211	0 (0.0)	4 (26.7)	11 (73.3)	–
20	The on-line teaching materials are designed to really try to make topics interesting to students.	3.92	0.239	1 (6.7)	2 (13.3)	12 (80.0)	–
21	Other students' on-line submissions encouraged me to investigate further sources of knowledge.	3.69	0.208	0 (0.0)	6 (40.0)	9 (60.0)	–
22	The sheer volume of work for the on-line component of this unit of study means it can't all be thoroughly comprehended.	2.92	0.348	3 (20.0)	7 (46.7)	5 (33.3)	–
23	The on-line learning materials helped me to learn during the face-to-face situations in this unit of study.	3.62	0.213	1 (6.7)	4 (26.7)	10 (66.7)	–
24	It was clear if on-line resources were related to assessment.	4.23	0.201	0 (0.0)	2 (13.3)	13 (86.7)	–
25	The on-line activities helped me to understand the face-to face activities in this unit of study.	3.85	0.191	0 (0.0)	4 (26.7)	11 (73.3)	–
26	The on-line materials supported some key assessment items in this unit.	4.08	0.178	0 (0.0)	1 (6.7)	14 (93.3)	–
27	The relationship between the on-line resources and the whole unit of study was clarified on the unit's website.	3.69	0.237	1 (6.7)	5 (33.3)	9 (60.0)	–
28	The teacher helped to focus on-line discussions between students.	4.00	0.196	0 (0.0)	3 (20.0)	12 (80.0)	–
29	Information needed for assignments was integrated in the one place on-line.	3.85	0.222	1 (6.7)	3 (20.0)	11 (73.3)	–

Table 3 Responses of participants in BL arm on their e-Learning experience *(Continued)*

No	Item	Mean*	S.D.*	Likert scale response [N (%)] **			
				Disagree	Neutral	Agree	Missing data
30	It was clear to me how the website for this unit related to the whole unit of study	3.92	0.239	1 (6.7)	3 (20.0)	11 (73.3)	–
31	The teacher ensured continuous access to the relevant on-line materials throughout the semester.	4.08	0.239	0 (0.0)	4 (26.7)	11 (73.3)	–
32	Overall, I was satisfied with the quality of the on-line materials and activities of this unit of study.	4.15	0.274	1 (6.7)	2 (13.3)	12 (80)	–

items 3, 4, 5, 9, 12, 15 and 28 represent "quality of teaching in e-learning context"
items 7, 16, 18, 21 = "student interaction and engagement"
items 13, 19, 29 = "clarity of goals and standards for online component"
items 8, 17, 20, 23 = "quality of online resources"
items 1, 10 and 26 = "appropriateness of assessment in e-learning context"
items 11, 14 and 22 = "appropriateness of workload related to online materials & activities"
items 2, 6 and 31 = "issues related to student management"
items 24, 25, 27 and 30 = "degree to which online materials and activities support face-to-face learning"
item 32 = "overall satisfaction with the quality of online materials and activities"

learning can be a feasible alternative to deliver skill-based training materials in a more accessible and affordable manner. The relevance of BL in such emergency medical trainings has also been suggested in other literature [12, 13]. BL has also been shown to be an effective method of training in other medical fields with high levels of student satisfaction [14–16]. A subgroup analysis in this study also suggests that the participants' prior information and communication technology (ICT) skills do not seem to influence their test performance. This seems to suggest that the chosen BL platform is friendly enough to be learned without much technical difficulty, which in turn promotes a positive virtual leaning environment.

Nonetheless, while the implementation of BL as well as the perception of the participants towards BL were apparently positive, these were not be overly so. One might argue that this was because some (6 out of 15) of the participants in the BL arm seemed to prefer to work in a F2FL environment. For example, some participants mentioned that they would prefer to have interaction and discussions with the instructors and with other participants *"there and then"*, so that they would know better what mistakes they might have made. This is known as the theory of instructor immediacy which describes the ability and availability of the instructor to engage in nonverbal and verbal communications with the learners to enhance their learning experience and to increase their learning motivation [17, 18].

Tobin (1998) described a 3-dimensional framework to evaluate participants' perception of an online environment with each dimension covering a number of categories [19]. These three dimensions are 1) "emancipatory activities" dimension (the degree of autonomy afforded to the participants in controlling the pace, place and depth of learning) 2) "co-participatory activities" dimension (the collaboration and interaction among participants and with the instructors) and 3) the "qualia" dimension (the degree of satisfaction, enjoyment as well as frustration of the participants with the online learning). In this study, while the dimension of emancipatory activities seems to be rated rather highly by the participants, the dimension of "co-participatory activities" seems to leave much to be desired. For example, a number of participants felt that the instructors should have played a much more active role in the online community by facilitating more active discussions. As Ellaway and Masters (2008) said, instructors should not be the "absent landlord" [20] but rather, be actively guiding the participants.

The limitations of this study include the small sample size as well as the fact that this study only involved participants from a single center. Only internal validation of the contents has been performed for the contents of this workshop (with no external validation yet when the study was carried out). Combining participants from both arms for the one-day practical session could have been a source of confounder, obscuring any potential differences in outcomes between the two interventions. Furthermore, there was no real patient-based outcome measured in the assessment of this study (e.g. the competency in managing emergency airway in real patients). Furthermore, this emergency airway management training only entails contents equivalent of a 2-day F2FL workshop. As such, its effectiveness may not be generalizable to more extensive or lengthy courses. Lastly, while the participants in the BL arm had been instructed not to reveal their course materials to their peers assigned to the F2FL arm and vice versa, the risk of cross-contamination remains. Similarly, participants in both arms were combined together during the practical training session and their interaction and discussions might have a confounding effect on the post-test performance.

Table 4 Qualitative Questionnaire on Participants' Perspective towards Blended Learning Emergency Airway Management Training

Questions	Highlighted Responses
Why did you take part in this program (emergency airway management training)?	To improve one's knowledge (12 out of 15 participants) and skills (5 responses)
Would you recommend this course (blended learning emergency airway management training) to a friend? Why?	All participants responded "yes" to recommend this course to a friend because it was beneficial (9 responses), informative (9 responses), simple and concise (2 responses), and helped to improve skills (6 responses) and the videos are accessible anytime and at any location (1 response).
How would you describe the training you received via blended learning?	"Informative" (4 responses), "comprehensive" (1 response), "concise" (1 response), "efficient" (1 response), "enjoyable" (1 response), "well-organized" (1 response), "good" (3 responses), "ample time provided" (1 response), "extremely good and valuable training which is hard to learn via textbook only" (1 response), "affords flexibility in learning" (2 responses), "can go through the materials over and again" (1 response), "a little boring" (1 response).
Did you do all the activities in the course? Why or why not?	Yes (13 responses). No (2 responses) because "it was getting boring" (1 response)
Do you feel this course has any advantage(s) for the students? Which?	Yes (15 responses); all of the modules (1 response), airway anatomy (1 response), algorithms (1 response), pharmacology (1 response), difficult intubation (1 response) and rapid sequence induction (1 response).
Do you feel this course has any disadvantages for the students? Which?	Yes (4 responses), as it requires discipline (2 responses), good internet connection (1 response) and more engaging videos as "monotonous presentation had me losing my concentration" (1 response).
In which class, do you think you would work more actively: in a face-to-face classroom or in an online learning? Why?	Online learning (4 responses) because it affords flexibility (2 responses). Face-to-face classroom (6 responses) it is "not easily distracted" in face-to-face classroom (1 response), and it allows for "interaction and discussion there and then" (1 response), and that they would know better what mistakes were made in face-to-face classroom (1 response).
What did you like the most about this course?	Materials and knowledge gained (8 responses) as there "depths in the knowledge and skill that I can acquire regarding airway management" (1 response) and "easy learning with good teaching and guidance" (1 response), Flexibility of time (2 responses), "making it easy to accommodate in a busy schedule" (1 response).
Would you like to take more courses that use blended learning? Why?	Yes (14 responses), because of the flexibility of time and place (3 responses), "being able to re-play the videos to comprehend the important points that I might have missed" (1 response), ability to monitor own progress (1 response), and "for knowledge and self-improvement" (2 responses). No, still prefer traditional lecture-style of learning (1 response).
If you could suggest changes to this course what would you suggest?	Should allocate longer duration for the course so that they would not have to "cram things daily" (1 response), using better quality audio system in the videos (1 response), to put up more interesting videos (1 response).
What would improve your participation in online discussions?	Incentive for active participation (e.g. achievement points or participation rewards) (1 response), "more involvement by all participants, with everyone taking the initiative to discuss the topics" (1 response) and facilitators/instructors should have taken a more active role to pose more questions to the participants because when the participants were not asking questions, it is because "we don't know what we don't know" (1 response).

Future works that could be performed include embarking on developing BL with more technologically-enabled engaging contents. The SAMR model [21, 22] describes four levels of technology integration and engagement in instructional design. These four levels are S = substitution, A = augmentation, M = modification, and R = redefinition. In the first two stages, technology is merely used as an enhancement tool. In the latter two stages, technology is actually used to transform education. In our BL arm, the face-to-face lectures were substituted by video lectures. This was further augmented by utilization of online quizzes and activities such as crossword puzzles and 'fill in the blanks' with instant feedback in the form of answers to help solidify the lessons learnt. One of the ways to advance to "M" or "R" stages of the SAMR model is to create simulation games based on experiential learning theory, flow theory and game design [23], with the aim to further engage students with serious games consisting of challenges appropriate to the skill level that affords immediate feedback. This will likely to result in intense focus and deep learning with high levels of self-satisfaction. Besides that, the effectiveness of BL should also be evaluated on all the four levels of the Kirkpatrick Training Evaluation Model [24]. Based on the Kirkpatrick Training Evaluation Model, we only evaluated Level 1 (reaction towards training) and Level 2 (the degree to which participants acquire the intended knowledge, skills, attitude, confidence and commitment based on their participation in the training). It will be good if further studies can evaluate Level 3 and 4 of Kirkpatrick Training Evaluation Model, i.e., 1) the behaviour change (the degree to which participants apply what they learned during training when they are back on the job) and 2) results (the degree to which the targeted outcomes occur as a result of the training), respectively.

Conclusion

In conclusion, this study suggests that BL may be a feasible alternative to F2FL for skill-based training such as the emergency airway management training as it was shown that the effectiveness of the BL is non-inferior to F2FL.

Abbreviations

BL: Blended learning; EAST: East Coast Airway Course; F2FL: Face-to-face learning; ICT: Information and communication technology; SAMR: Substitution, Augmentation, Modification, and Redefinition model

Funding

Not applicable

Authors' contributions

MHTK and KSC were involved in the initial conception of the study design, conducting the study, analyzing and interpreting the results as well as writing up the draft of the manuscript to be approved by all authors. MNA, MLH and AB were involved in the initial conception of the study design, conducting the study, analyzing and interpreting the results. KMC and HCC were involved in the initial conception of the study design and conducting the study. MHTK, KSC, MNA, MLH, AB were involved in the selection of topics, development of teaching contents and construction of assessment questions for the airway management training workshop. All authors approved of the final draft of this manuscript.

Competing interests

The authors declare that they have no competing interests.

Author details

[1]Emergency Medicine and Trauma Department, Sarawak General Hospital, Jalan Hospital, Kuching 93586, Sarawak, Malaysia. [2]Faculty of Medicine and Health Sciences, Universiti Malaysia Sarawak, Kota Samarahan 94300, Sarawak, Malaysia. [3]Faculty of Medicine, University of Malaya, Kuala Lumpur 50603, Malaysia. [4]Emergency Medicine and Trauma Department, Hospital Sultanah Nur Zahirah, Kuala Terengganu 20400, Trengganu, Malaysia. [5]Faculty of Language Studies and Communication Studies, Universiti Malaysia Sarawak, Kota Samarahan 94300, Sarawak, Malaysia.

References

1. Garrison DR, Kanuka H. Blended learning: uncovering its transformative potential in higher education. Internet High Educ. 2004;7(2):95–105.
2. Rowe M, Frantz J, Bozalek V. The role of blended learning in the clinical education of healthcare students: a systematic review. Med Teach. 2012;34(4):e216–21.
3. Laurillard D. Rethinking university teaching: a conversational framework for the effective use of learning technologies. London: Routledge; 2001.
4. Glogowska M, Young P, Lockyer L, Moule P. How 'blended' is blended learning? Students' perceptions of issues around the integration of online and face-to-face learning in a continuing professional development (CPD) health care context. Nurse Educ Today. 2011;31(8):887–91.
5. Beldarrain Y. Distance education trends: integrating new technologies to foster student interaction and collaboration. Distance Educ. 2006;27(2):139–53.
6. Bergmann J, Sams A. Flip your classroom: reach every student in every class every day. Arlington: International Society for Technology in Education (ISTE); 2012.
7. Faul F, Erdfelder E, Lang AG, Buchner A. G*power 3: a flexible statistical power analysis program for the social, behavioral, and biomedical sciences. Behav Res Methods. 2007;39(2):175–91.
8. Lancaster JW, Wong A, Roberts SJ. 'Tech' versus 'talk': a comparison study of two different lecture styles within a master of science nurse practitioner course. Nurse Educ Today. 2012;32(5):e14–8.
9. Torres AAL, Abbad GS, Bousquet-Santos K. Validation of a Questionnaire on ICTs (Information and Communication Technologies) Skills of Undergraduate Health Students in Brazil. Psychology Research. 2013;3(9). Available online at URL: http://www.davidpublisher.org/index.php/Home/Article/index?id=24241.html Accessed 06 June 2017.
10. Ginns P, Ellis R. Quality in blended learning: exploring the relationships between on-line and face-to-face teaching and learning. Internet High Educ. 2007;10(1):53–64.
11. Larsen LJE. Teacher and student perspectives on a blended learning intensive English program writing course. Iowa State University; 2012. Available online at URL: http://lib.dr.iastate.edu/cgi/viewcontent.cgi?article=3382&context=etd Accessed 6 June 2017.
12. Knox S, Cullen W, Dunne C. Continuous professional competence (CPC) for emergency medical technicians in Ireland: educational needs assessment. BMC Emerg Med. 2013;13:25.
13. Knox S, Cullen W, Dunne C. Continuous professional competence (CPC) for Irish paramedics and advanced paramedics: a national study. BMC Med Educ. 2014;14:41.
14. Makhdoom N, Khoshhal KI, Algaidi S, Heissam K, Zolaly MA. 'Blended learning' as an effective teaching and learning strategy in clinical medicine: a comparative cross-sectional university-based study. J Taibah Univ Med Sci. 2013;8(1):12–7.
15. Howlett D, Vincent T, Watson G, Owens E, Webb R, Gainsborough N, Fairclough J, Taylor N, Miles K, Cohen J, Vincent R. Blending online techniques with traditional face to face teaching methods to deliver final year undergraduate radiology learning content. Eur J Radiol. 2011;78(3):334–41.
16. Wu J-H, Tennyson RD, Hsia T-L. A study of student satisfaction in a blended e-learning system environment. Comput Educ. 2010;55(1):155–64.
17. Christophel DM. The relationships among teacher immediacy behaviors, student motivation, and learning. Commun Educ. 1990;39(4):323–40.
18. Klein HJ, Noe RA, Wang C. Motivation to learn and course outcomes: the impact of delivery mode, learning goal orientation, and perceived barriers and enablers. Pers Psychol. 2006;59(3):665–702.
19. Tobin K. Qualitative perceptions of learning environments on the world wide web. Learn Environ Res. 1998;1(2):139.
20. Ellaway R, Masters K. AMEE guide 32: e-learning in medical education part 1: learning, teaching and assessment. Med Teach. 2008;30(5):455–73.
21. Puentedura R.R. A Matrix Model for Designing and Assessing Network-enhanced courses. 2003. In: Hippasus website. Available at URL: http://www.hippasus.com/resources/matrixmodel/puentedura_model.pdf Accessed 6 June 2017.
22. Romrell D, Kidder LC, Wood E. The SAMR Model as a Framework for Evaluating mLearning. In: Online Learning Journal. Available at URL: https://olj.onlinelearningconsortium.org/index.php/olj/article/view/435. Accessed 12 Jan 2018.
23. Kiili K. Digital game-based learning: towards an experiential gaming model. Internet High Educ. 2005;8(1):13–24.
24. Kirkpatrick JD, Kirkpatrick WK. Kirkpatrick's Four Levels of Training Evaluation. Alexandria: Association for Talent Development; 2016.

2

Frequency of intra-abdominal organ injury is higher in patients with concomitant stab wounds to other anatomical areas

Igor Jeroukhimov[1*†], Itay Wiser[1†], Yehuda Hershkovitz[1], Zahar Shapira[1], Kobi Peleg[2], Ricardo Alfici[3], Adi Givon[2], Israeli Trauma Group and Boris Kessel[4]

Abstract

Background: Management of stable patients with abdominal stab wound remains controversial, particularly for those with no clear indications for explorative laparotomy. We evaluated the risk of intra-abdominal injury in stab wound victims concomitantly stabbed in other anatomical body areas.

Methods: We performed a retrospective cohort study of patients with abdominal stab wounds recorded in the Israeli National Trauma Registry from January 1st, 1997, to December 31st, 2013. Patients with an isolated abdominal stab wound were compared to those with concomitant stab wounds to other anatomical areas. Intra-abdominal organ injury was defined by imaging or surgery findings. Multivariate analysis using a logistic regression model was conducted to assess independent risk for intra-abdominal organ injury.

Results: The study included 3964 patients. After controlling for age, gender and hypotension on arrival, patients with multi-regional stab wounds had an increased risk of intra-abdominal injury (OR = 1.3, CI 95% 1.1–1.6, $p < 0.001$). These patients also had a higher rate of injury to the solid organs than patients with an isolated abdominal stab wound.

Conclusions: Patients with multi-regional stab wounds have an increased risk of intra-abdominal injury. Worldwide accepted "clinical follow up" protocol may not be appropriate in management of patients with multi-regional stab wounds.

Keywords: Stab wound, Penetrating abdominal organ injury, Abdominal trauma

Background

Penetrating abdominal trauma continues to be a major cause of trauma admissions worldwide [1]. Non-operative management is a widely accepted approach for the stable patient with an abdominal stab wound who does not require urgent surgery [2–4].

Clinical observation of stable patients with anterior abdominal stab wounds with no signs of peritonitis has been adopted by most of the trauma centers [5].

Currently, the management approach for patients with multi-regional stab wounds including the abdomen is not distinguished from those with isolated abdominal stab wounds.

We assume that the management approach to the patients with multiple abdominal stab wound may be different from those with isolated abdominal stab wound. That was intuitively based on idea that multiple stab wounds have potentially worse mechanism of injury and higher probability to penetrate peritoneal cavity and cause more damage. We hypothesized that the rate of intra-abdominal injury is higher in patients with multi-regional stab wounds compare to patients with isolated abdominal stab wounds.

* Correspondence: igorjer65@gmail.com
The work was performed at the National Center for Trauma and Emergency Medicine Research, Gertner Institute for Epidemiology and Health Policy Research, Tel Hashomer, Israel
†Igor Jeroukhimov and Itay Wiser contributed equally to this work.
[1]Trauma Unit, Assaf Harofeh Medical Center, Zerifin 7030000, Israel, affiliated with the Sackler Faculty of Medicine, Tel Aviv University, Tel Aviv, Israel
Full list of author information is available at the end of the article

Our aim was to find out whether an association exists between intra-abdominal injury and other anatomical area involvement in stab wound injury.

Methods

Study population

We conducted a retrospective cohort study of trauma patients with abdominal stab wounds admitted to 19 Trauma Centers between the years 1997 and 2013. Data was obtained from the records of the Israeli National Trauma Registry maintained by Israel's National Center for Trauma and Emergency Medicine Research, Gertner Institute for Epidemiology and Health Policy Research. This institute records information concerning trauma patients hospitalized in 19 hospitals of which six are Level I, and 13 are Level II Trauma Centers. Data was obtained from the Israeli National Trauma Registry and included only anonymous information regarding the patients with no possibility of identification for the purposes of quality assessment and research. Ethical approval was obtained from the Helsinki Committee at Sheba Medical Center where the Israeli Trauma Registry located (Approval Number 5138–18-SMC).

The study population was divided into two groups: isolated abdominal stab wounds and abdominal stab wound with concomitant multi-regional stab wounds (defined as one or more concomitant stab wounds located in an anatomic area other than the abdomen). Knife was the only assaulting instrument. Patients with isolated thoraco-abdominal stab wound and patients with multiple abdominal stab wounds were excluded from the study.

Data collected included: age, gender, presence and location of intra-abdominal injury according to ICD-9 diagnosis, Injury Severity Score (ISS), Abbreviated Injury Score (AIS), systolic blood pressure on admission, Glasgow Comma Scale (GCS), hospital length of stay (LOS) and mortality.

Patients with admission systolic blood pressure 90 mmHg or less were defined as hemodynamically unstable. In case of hemodynamic instability, presence of peritoneal signs, or evisceration of abdominal content all the victims were referred directly to operating room. In absence of absolute indications for surgery, the treatment algorithm included observation with serial physical examinations, local wound exploration, computed tomography and diagnostic laparoscopy in selected cases depends of particular hospital protocol.

We compared the presence of abdominal penetration and the other variables between both groups.

Data analysis

Statistical analysis was performed using the SAS statistical software (SAS, Cary, NC, version 9.2). Statistical tests included chi-square tests for categorical data and the Wilcoxon nonparametric test for continuous variables that were not normally distributed. A multivariate analysis was conducted using binary log two-tailed. Univariate and multivariate odds ratios appear for all variables (unadjusted – univariate, adjusted – multivariate).

Results

Participants

We found 438,765 trauma victims in the Israeli National Trauma Registry between the years 1997 to 2013. Of these, 3964 suffered from abdominal stab wounds (0.9%). Baseline characteristics of both groups are presented in Table 1. No significant differences were observed between groups in age and gender. The multi-regional stab wounds group had a significantly higher rate of hypotension on arrival and GCS ≤8 compared to the group with an isolated stab wound (9.3% vs 5.5%, $p < 0.0001$ and 4.1% vs. 1.3%, $p < 0.0001$; respectively). The intra-abdominal injury rate was higher in the multi-regional stab wound group of patients (40% vs. 35%, $p = 0.0004$) (Table 2).

Mortality was significantly higher (2.5% vs. 0.9%, $p = 0.0001$) and mean LOS was longer in patients with multi-regional stab wounds (5.2 ± 6.5 vs. 3.9 ± 5.4 days, $p < 0.0001$). Frequency of injury to the liver, kidney and spleen was higher in the multi-regional stab wound group (13.2% vs. 8.4%, $p < 0.0001$; 5.6% vs. 3.6%, $p = 0.004$; 8.2% vs. 1.2%, $p < 0.0001$; respectively). The small bowel was injured more frequently in the isolated abdominal stab wound group (10.4% vs. 5.4%, $p < 0.001$) (Table 3).

Independent adjusted risk factors for intra-abdominal injury were systolic blood pressure ≤ 90 mmHg (OR = 1.5 (1.1–2.1, $p = 0.02$), GCS < 13 (OR = 3.9 (2.4–6.2, p < 0.001), age ≥ 50 years (OR = 2.2 (1.01–4.6, $p = 0.048$) and multi-regional stab wounds (OR = 1.3 (1.1–1.6, $p < 0.001$) (Table 4).

Key results

Patients with multi-regional stab wounds have a higher rate of intra-abdominal injuries compared with patients with isolated abdominal stab wounds.

Discussion

Until the late twentieth century, operative management was the only accepted standard for penetrating wounds to the abdomen. In 1969, in a study of 600 stabbed patients, Nance et al. [6] reported the advantage of a selective non operative approach compared to mandatory explorative laparotomy. Later, several studies supported evidence that not all penetrating abdominal wounds require surgery. Navsaria et al. [7] in a study on 186 stabbed trauma victims successfully managed 53.8% of

Table 1 Baseline Characteristics, Injury Pattern and Outcomes [a]

	n/n (%)			*p* Value
	Isolated ASW	Multiregional SW	All	
Demographics				
Age ≥ 50	88/1866 (4.7%)	118/2088 (5.7%)	206/3954 (5.2%)	0.19
Male gender	1786/1870 (95%)	1993/2093 (95%)	3779/3963 (95%)	0.67
Injury characteristic				
SBP < 90 mmHg	101/1852 (5.5%)	193/2072 (9,3%)	294/3924 (7.5%)	< 0.0001
GCS ≤8	24/1833 (1.3%)	83/2046 (4.1%)	107/3879 (2.8%)	< 0.0001
Abdomen AIS ≥3	443/1871 (24%)	517/2093 (25%)	960/3964 (24%)	0.45
Intra-abdominal injury	660/1871 (35%)	852/2093 (40%)	1512/3964 (38%)	0.0004
ISS ≥25	19/1871 (1%)	197/2093 (9.4%)	216/3964	< 0.0001
Outcomes				
Mortality	17/1871 (0.9%)	53/2093 (2.5%)	70/3964 (1.8%)	0.0001
LOS, mean (SD)	3.9 ± 5.4 (*n* = 1866)	5.2 ± 6.5 (*n* = 2077)	4.6 ± 6.0 (*n* = 3943)	< 0.0001

SW stab wound, *ASW* abdominal stab wound, *SBP* systolic blood pressure, *GCS* Glasgow Coma Scale, *AIS* Abbreviated Injury Score, *ISS* Injury Severity Score, *LOS* hospital length of stay

[a] Categorical variables were compared using Chi-square test, Continuous variables were compared using Wilcoxon rank test

them non-operatively. Friedmann [8] in a study of 108 victims with abdominal SW found that a policy of mandatory laparotomy would have resulted in a negative laparotomy rate of 70%. Renz and Feliciano [9] in a prospective observational study found a complication rate of 42% in patients who underwent non-therapeutic laparotomy for trauma. Later, a selective non operative approach was extended not only to anterior abdominal wall wounds, but also to flank and back injuries. Ocampo et al. [10] in a study of 473 patients stabbed to the posterior abdomen demonstrated a 76% success rate with conservative management. Increased liberal use of CT in such cases demonstrated a high accuracy for the presence of intra-abdominal injury and even peritoneal violation [11, 12]. In order to avoid missing serious, but initially asymptomatic injuries, several diagnostic algorithms have been suggested. These algorithms take into consideration physical examination, local wound exploration, diagnostic peritoneal lavage and/or imaging. Eastern Association for the Surgery of Trauma guidelines strongly recommend considering abdominal CT in patients with abdominal stab wounds that have been selected for conservative management [5]. Nevertheless, potential risk of exposure to ionized radiation causing by CT should not be ignored [11, 13]. Inaba et al. [14] prospectively compared CT against serial physical examination in the evaluation of 249 patients with a stab wound to the abdomen. In their study, CT findings did not alter clinical decision making. The sensitivity and specificity of physical examination were 100.0 and 98.7%, respectively, while those of CT were 31.3 and 84.2%, respectively. The authors concluded that a physical examination-based diagnostic algorithm is effective and decreased the radiation burden in the management of patients with abdominal stab wounds.

Little is known about the therapeutic approach in the management of patients with multiple stab wounds in different body areas including the abdomen compared with isolated abdominal wounds. We live in a world where crime and the severity of violence consistently worsen over the years. Kessel et al. [15] in a study based on the national trauma database showed a gradual increase in both the absolute rate and the relative incidence of serious stab injuries in Israel. The authors also found that 50% of the victims suffered from multiple stab wounds to different body areas. A similar tendency has been reported in other countries [16, 17].

In the current study, we assumed that the frequency of intra-abdominal organ injury in patients with multi-regional stab wounds may be higher than that reported in the

Table 2 Comparison of Penetration/Penetration with Intra-abdominal Injury Incidence in Patients with Isolated Versus Multiple Anatomical Area Stab Wounds

Type of injury	Abdominal and other area (*n* = 2093)	Abdominal only (*n* = 1871)	Total (*n* = 3964)	*p* Value
No penetration	693 (33.1%)	568 (30.5%)	1261	0.063
Penetration only	548 (26.2%)	643 (34.4%)	1191	< 0.001
Penetration with intra-abdominal injury	852 (40.7%)	660 (35.3%)	1512	0.0004

Table 3 Comparison of Intra-abdominal Injury Abdominal Stab Wound Patients with or without Other Area Involvement

Organ	Abdominal and other area (n = 2093)	Abdominal only (n = 1871)	*p* Value
Vascular	73 (3.5%)	80 (4.3%)	0.2
Liver	276 (13.2%)	158 (8.4%)	< 0.0001
Kidney	117 (5.6%)	68 (3.6%)	0.004
Spleen	171 (8.2%)	36 (1.9%)	< 0.001
Stomach	92 (4.4%)	77 (4.1%)	0.66
Pancreas	16 (0.8%)	24 (1.3%)	0.103
Small bowel	213 (10.1%)	516 (27.5%)	< 0.001
Colon/rectum	97 (4.6%)	109 (5.8%)	0.09

literature for patients with isolated abdominal stab wounds. We hypothesized that multiple stabs reflected increased aggression by the attacker, that would resulted in increased severity of the injuries. About 30% of our study population had no penetration into the abdominal cavity. Two thirds of all stab wounds patients in our study had violation of the abdominal cavity with or without intra-abdominal organ injuries. Similar findings have been reported in other studies [18, 19]. However, the major finding of this work was a significantly higher incidence of most intra-abdominal organ injuries in patients with multiregional stab wounds.

We were unable to find similar studies in the relevant English medical literature According to the literature, the most commonly injured organs in patients with stab wounds are the liver and small bowel. Each of them comprises 30% of all intra-abdominal injuries [20]. In our study, the overall incidence of solid organ injury was lower, but frequency these organs injury was significantly higher in patients with multiple body areas stab wounds.

Clinical observation and serial abdominal examination is a worldwide accepted approach to the patient with isolated abdominal SW [14]. Nevertheless it may not be appropriate in patients with multiple stab wounds due to relatively high probability of missing intra-abdominal injury.

This tendency may have an impact on current acceptable management approach to the patient with abdominal stab wound. Presence of additional to abdomen stab wounds may complicate the patient manage because of various aspects. Other wounds, even superficial, may be the source of significant pain that often requires more pain medications, sedation or in some cases even intubation. Major wounds may draw the physician attention and seem to be of major priority, thereby delay treatment of life-threatening injuries. Moreover, such injuries make the clinical observation and serial examination very limited or even impossible in some cases.

Study limitations

The trauma registry does not include patients discharged from emergency departments. Therefore, the real incidence of non-penetrating abdominal stab wounds is unknown. However, in these mildly injured patients, the presence of other anatomical areas wounds has no impact on the abdominal management protocol.

The second limitation of this study is that we had no complete information regarding injuries aside from the abdomen. Nevertheless, we assume that the variability between the groups should be minimized by the large sample size provided by the registry.

Conclusions

The incidence of almost all intra-abdominal organ injuries in patients with multi-regional stab wounds was significantly higher compared to isolated abdominal stab wounds. These findings may support the development of different diagnostic approaches to patients with multiple body areas stab wounds. Based on the study results we conclude that only clinical observation may not be an appropriate management approach in patients with multi-regional stab wounds. We believe that abdominal

Table 4 Univariate versus Multivariate Analysis of Risk Factors for Intra-abdominal Injury in Patients with Abdominal Stab Wounds

Variable	Unadjusted	*p*-Value	Adjusted [a]	*p* Value
SBP ≤90 mm HG	2.24 (1.7–2.9)	< 0.001	1.5 (1.1–2.1)	0.02
GCS < 13	6.2 (4.2–9.3)	< 0.001	3.9 (2.4–6.2)	< 0.001
Age ≥ 50	3.3 (1.7–6.1)	< 0.001	2.2 (1.01–4.6)	0.048
Female gender	1.24 (0.9–1.7)	0.16	1.16 (0.8–1.7)	0.45
Multiregional stab wounds	1.24 (1.1–1.4)	0.001	1.3 (1.1–1.6)	< 0.001

SBP systolic blood pressure, *GCS* Glasgow Coma Scale

[a] Regression odds ratio compared with: systolic blood pressure 90 mmHg and above, GCS 15, age group 0–14 years, male gender, abdominal-only stab wounds

CT in patients with abdominal and other anatomical body areas stab wounds should be considered. Future prospective studies will assist to develop unique management protocol for these patients.

Abbreviations
AIS: Abbreviated Injury Score; CT: Computerized Tomography; GCS: Glasgow Comma Scale; ISS: Injury Severity Score; LOS: length of stay; SBP: Systolic Blood Pressure; SW: Stab Wound

Acknowledgements
The authors would like to thank the members of Israel Trauma Group for their help in data accumulation.

The Israeli Trauma Group includes
Hany Bahouth, MD
Alexander Becker, MD
Ben Ely Michael, MD
Alexander Braslavsky, MD
Igor Jeroukhimov, MD
Milad Qarawany, MD
Boris Kessel, MD
Yoram Klein, MD
Guy Lin, MD
Ofer Merin, MD
Miklosh Bala, MD
Youri Mnouskin, MD, PhD
Avraham I. Rivkind, MD
Gad Shaked, MD
Dror Soffer, MD
Michael Stein, MD
Michael Weiss, MD.

Affiliations of The Israeli Trauma Group: Trauma and Emergency Surgery Division of General Surgery, Rambam Health Care Campus, Haifa, Israel (Bahouth); Department of Surgery, HaEmek Medical Center, Afula, Ruth and Bruce Rappaport Medical School, Technion, Haifa, Israel (Becker); Wolfson Medical Center, Holon, Israel (Ben Ely); Trauma Unit, Ziv Medical Center, Zfat, Israel (Braslavsky); Assaf Harofeh Medical Center, Tel Aviv University, Tel Aviv, Israel (Jeroukhimov); Trauma Unit, Poriya Medical Center, Tiberias, Israel (Qarawany); Trauma Unit, Hillel Yaffe Medical Center, Hadera, Israel (Kessel); Bruce Rappaport Medical School, Technion, Haifa, Israel, Divison of Acute Care Surgery and Trauma, Chaim Sheba Medical Center, Tel Hashomer, Israel (Klein); Kaplan Medical Center, Rehovot, Israel (Lin); Shaare Zedek Medical Center, Jerusalem, Israel (Merin); Hadassah Medical Center, Jerusalem, Israel (Bala, Rivkind); Surgery Department, Barzilai Medical Center, Ashkelon, Israel (Mnouskin); Trauma Unit, Soroka Medical Center, Beer-Sheva, Israel (Shaked); The Yitzhak Rabin Trauma Division, Division of Surgery, Tel Aviv Sourasky Medical Center, Tel Aviv, Israel (Soffer); Trauma Unit, Rabin Medical Center-Beilinson Hospital, Petah Tikva, Israel (Stein); Trauma Unit, Galilee Medical Center, Nahariya, Israel (Weiss).

Authors' contributions
IJ and IW contributed equally to this work. IJ, YH and BK designed the research. YH, KP and AG performed the research and analyzed the data. ZS and RA collected data and performed statistical analysis. IJ and IW wrote the paper. All authors made important intellectual contributions to the manuscript, and all authors approved the final version before submission.

Competing interests
The authors declare that they have no competing interests.

Author details
[1]Trauma Unit, Assaf Harofeh Medical Center, Zerifin 7030000, Israel, affiliated with the Sackler Faculty of Medicine, Tel Aviv University, Tel Aviv, Israel. [2]National Center for Trauma and Emergency Medicine Research, Gertner Institute for Epidemiology and Health Policy Research, Sheba Medical Center, 52621 Tel Hashomer, Israel. [3]Surgical Division, Hillel Yaffe Medical Center, 38100 Hadera, Israel. [4]Trauma Unit, Hillel Yaffe Medical Center, 38100 Hadera, Israel.

References

1. Pallett JR, Sutherland E, Glucksman E, Tunnicliff M, Keep JW. A cross-sectional study of knife injuries at a London major trauma Centre. Ann R Coll Surg Engl. 2014;96:23–6.
2. Biffl WL, Kaups KL, Pham TN, et al. Validating the western trauma association algorithm for managing patients with anterior abdominal stab wounds: a western trauma association multicenter trial. J Trauma. 2011;71:1494.
3. Benjamin E, Demetriades D. Nonoperative Management of Penetrating Injuries to the abdomen. Curr Trauma Rep. 2015;1(2):102–6.
4. Biffl WL, Leppaniemi A. Management guidelines for penetrating abdominal trauma. World J Surg. 2015;39(6):1373–80.
5. Como JJ, Bokhari F, Chiu WC, Duane TM, Holevar MR, Tandoh MA, et al. Practice management guidelines for selective nonoperative management of penetrating abdominal trauma. J Trauma. 2010;68:721–33.
6. Nance FC, Cohn I. Surgical judgment in the management of stab wounds of the abdomen. Ann Surg. 1969;170:569–80.
7. Navsaria PH, Berli JU, Edu S, Nicol AJ. Non-operative management of abdominal stab wounds-an analysis of 186 patients. S Afr J Surg. 2007;45:128–30. 32
8. Friedmann P. Selective management of stab wounds of the abdomen. Arch Sur. 1968;96:292–5.
9. Renz BM, Feliciano DV. The length of hospital stay after an unnecessary laparotomy for trauma: a prospective study. J Trauma. 1996;40:187–90.
10. Ocampo H, Yamaguchi M, Mackabee J, Ordog G, Fleming A. Selective management of posterior stab wounds. J Natl Med Assoc. 1987;79:283–8.
11. Salim A, Sangthong B, Martin M, Brown C, Plurad D, Inaba K, et al. Use of computed tomography in anterior abdominal stab wounds. Arch Surg. 2006;141:745–50. discussion 750–2
12. Fletcher TB, Setiawan H, Harrell RS, Redman HC. Posterior abdominal stab wounds: role of CT evaluation. Radiology. 1989;173:621–5.
13. Holmes JF, McGahan JP, Wisner DH. Rate of intra-abdominal injury after a normal computed tomographic scan in adults with blunt trauma. Am J Emerg Med. 2012;3:574–9.
14. Inaba K, Okoye OT, Rosenheck R, Melo N, Branco BC, Talving P, et al. Prospective evaluation of the role of computed tomography in the assessment of abdominal stab wounds. JAMA Surg. 2013;148:810–6.
15. Kessel B, Peleg K, Hershekovitz Y, Khashan T, Givon A, Ashkenazi I, et al. Abdominal stab wounds in Israel, 1997–2004: significant increase in overall incidence and prevalence of severe injury. Isr Med Assoc J. 2008;10:135–7.
16. Casali M, Di Saverio S, Tugnoli G, Biscardi A, Villani S, Cancellieri F, et al. [Penetrating abdominal trauma: 20 years experience in a western European trauma center]. [article in Italian]. Ann Ital Chir. 2008;79:399–407.
17. Rozen WM, Ma EH, Jones IT, Judson RT. Emerging epidemic in Australia: abdominal stab wounds. Twenty-four months at a major trauma Centre. Emerg Med Australas. 2007;19:262–8.
18. Cothren CC, Moore EE, Warren FA, Kashuk JL, Biffl WL, Johnson JL. Local wound exploration remains a valuable triage tool for the evaluation of anterior abdominal stab wounds. Am J Surg. 2009;198:223–6.
19. Omari A, Bani-Yaseen M, Khammash M, Qasaimeh G, Eqab F, Jaddou H. Patterns of anterior abdominal stab wounds and their management at Princess Basma teaching hospital, north of Jordan. World J Surg. 2013;37:1162–8.
20. Chestovich PJ, Browder TD, Morrissey SL, Fraser DR, Ingalls NK, Fildes JJ. Minimally invasive is maximally effective: diagnostic and therapeutic laparoscopy for penetrating abdominal injuries. J Trauma Acute Care Surg. 2015;78:1076–83. discussion 1083-5

3

Outcome of elderly emergency department patients hospitalised on weekends

Steffie H. A. Brouns[1,2*†], Joyce J. Wachelder[1,2†], Femke S. Jonkers[1], Suze L. Lambooij[1], Jeanne P. Dieleman[3] and Harm R. Haak[1,2,4]

Abstract

Background: Studies investigating different medical conditions and settings have demonstrated mixed results regarding the weekend effect. However, data on the outcome of elderly patients hospitalised on weekends is scarce. The objective was to compare in-hospital and two-day mortality rates between elderly emergency department (ED) patients (≥65 years) admitted on weekends versus weekdays.

Methods: A retrospective cohort study of emergency department visits of internal medicine patients ≥65 years presenting to the emergency department between 01 and 09-2010 and 31–08-2012 was conducted. The weekend was defined as the period from midnight on Friday to midnight on Sunday.

Results: Data on 3697 emergency department visits by elderly internal medicine patients (mean age 78.6 years old) were included. In total, 2743 emergency department visits (74.2%) resulted in hospitalisation, of which 22.9% occurred on weekends. Comorbidity and urgency levels were higher in patients admitted on weekends. In-hospital mortality was 11.4% for patients admitted on weekends compared with 8.9% on weekdays (OR 1.3, 95%CI 0.99–1.8). Two-day mortality was 3.2% in patients hospitalised on weekends versus 1.9% on weekdays (OR 1.7, 95%CI 0.99–2.9). Multivariable adjustment for age, comorbidity and triage level demonstrated comparable in-hospital and two-day mortality for weekend and week admission (ORadj 1.2, 95%CI 0.9–1.7 and ORadj 1.5, 95%CI 0.8–2.6, resp.).

Conclusion: A small weekend effect was observed in elderly internal medicine patients, which was not statistically significant. This effect was partly explained by a higher comorbidity and urgency level in elderly patients hospitalised on weekends than during weekdays. Emergency care for the elderly is not compromised by adjusted logistics during the weekend.

Keywords: Emergency service, hospital, Aged, Outcome and process assessment (health care)

Background

Emergency departments (EDs) offer acute care for critically ill patients 24 h a day. However, numerous studies have identified a shortfall in the quality of care at EDs during the weekend and demonstrated an association between weekend admission and adverse outcomes, such as increased in-hospital mortality, which has been labelled as "the weekend effect" [1–5].

Several explanations for the weekend effect have been proposed, such as the different organisation of the health care system at the weekend, including a decreased staffing level, less experienced personnel and reduced availability of diagnostic resources [3, 6, 7]. In addition, the higher weekend mortality may reflect differences in the patient characteristics, such as disease severity [8]. However, previous studies in various settings and different medical conditions have demonstrated mixed results regarding the existence of the weekend effect [1–3, 9, 10].

* Correspondence: S.Brouns@mmc.nl
[†]Equal contributors
[1]Department of Internal Medicine, Máxima Medical Centre, 5600 BM Eindhoven/Veldhoven, the Netherlands
[2]Maastricht University, Department of Health Services Research, and CAPHRI School for Public Health and Primary Care, 6229 ER Maastricht, the Netherlands
Full list of author information is available at the end of the article

It is well-established that ED visits and hospitalisation of elderly patients are associated with poor outcome, such as morbidity, institutionalisation and mortality [11, 12]. To date, it is unknown as to whether the weekend effect adds to the risk of adverse events in the elderly population and if additional control measures tailored to the elderly population are needed. We designed a study to examine the effect of weekend admission following an ED visit on patient outcome in the frail elderly population. The primary objective of the study was to estimate the differences in mortality (in-hospital mortality, 2-day mortality and 30-day mortality) for elderly internal medicine patients (≥ 65 years old) admitted from the ED during the weekend as compared with weekdays.

Methods

Study design, setting and population

A retrospective cohort study was performed in a 550-bed teaching hospital, the Máxima Medical Centre, in the Netherlands [13]. Around 28,000 patients visit the ED annually, of which approximately 15% require assessment by an internist. The internist assesses patients within the field of endocrinology, immunology, vascular disease, infectious disease, geriatrics, nephrology, haematology, and oncology. The primary mode of referral in the Dutch emergency care system is by the general practitioner (GP) [14]. Self-initiated visits, ambulance arrivals and referral by a medical specialist are other modes of referral. The staffing level during the week at the ED for the internal medicine consists of 2 residents during daytime (8:00–21:00) and 1 resident during the evening and night (21:00–8:00). In the weekend, there is only 1 resident available during daytime, 1 in the evening and 1 at night. This resident also covers the occupied beds on the wards for the internal medicine during the evening and night as well as the pulmonology and cardiology wards during the night.

All elderly patients, aged ≥65 years old, visiting the ED for internal medicine, and being admitted between 1st September 2010 and 31st August 2012 were included. The unit of analysis was hospital admission following an ED visit, allowing multiple admissions per patient. One abstractor extracted the administrative data of all patients. This person was blinded to the study hypothesis, and information bias was minimised by using standard data collection forms. No informed consent of the patients deemed to be necessary because of the retrospective design, and therefor exemption of ethical approval was acquired by the Ethics Committee of MMC.

Data collection

For each ED visit, the following data were obtained from electronic patient and hospital records: age, gender, medical history (past diagnoses), and current medication use. Organisational factors pertaining to the ED visits were: day and time of ED visit, mode of referral, seniority of the first treating physician on the ED, and number of diagnostic procedures (laboratory tests, a culture test, magnetic resonance imaging, computed tomography, ultrasound, and ultrasonography or electrocardiogram). Information on the triage level, vital parameters (i.e. blood pressure, and heart rate), laboratory assessments (C-reactive protein (CRP) and leukocyte count), and ED diagnosis was retrieved to estimate the severity of the illness at the ED. The date of admission and discharge were gathered. Follow-up lasted from the date of the ED visit until 1 year of follow-up was reached, the date of death or the date of last available information whichever was earliest.

Definitions

Visits were categorised into weekend and weekday visit based on the date and time of admission from the ED visit. In accordance with previous studies investigating the weekend effect, the weekend was defined as the period from midnight on Friday until midnight on Sunday [1]. Daytime was defined as 8 am – 5 pm, evening was defined as 5 pm – 23 pm and night was defined as 23 pm – 8 am, corresponding to the different shifts at our hospital. Dutch national holidays were considered as weekend, because the organisation is the same as in weekends (N = 53). Mode of referral was categorised into referral by a GP, ambulance or medical specialist, and self-referral. The triage level was based on the five-level Manchester Triage System (MTS) [15], and was categorised into the following groups: urgent (red and orange), moderate (yellow) and low (green). Triage category blue is not used at our ED. The seniority of the first physician on ED was categorised into a medical student in last year of medical education, a non-trainee resident, a trainee resident or a medical specialist (internist or emergency physician). Medical history, and ED diagnosis, as documented in the ED records, were categorised according to the International Classification of Disease-10 (ICD-10) [16]. The diagnosis group "miscellaneous" consisted of the following categories: diseases of the musculoskeletal system, eye and adnexa, ear and mastoid process, skin and subcutaneous tissue and external injury or trauma and poisoning. The ICD-10 category "Symptoms, signs and abnormal clinical and laboratory findings, not elsewhere classified" was renamed into "aspecific complaints". The Charlson comorbidity index (CCI) was calculated to assess the comorbidity levels of the patients. ED length of stay (ED-LOS) was defined as the time (in minutes) between ED arrival and ED discharge or admission.

Outcome measures

The primary outcome of this study was the mortality rate of elderly ED patients admitted during the weekend as compared with admissions on weekdays. The in-hospital mortality rate, the two-day mortality rate, and the 30-day mortality rate were calculated from the day of admission.

Statistical analysis

All statistical analyses were performed using SPSS (IBM SPSS Statistics for Windows, version 22.0, Armonk, New York). Differences in characteristics between patients admitted on weekends or on weekdays were compared using the Chi-square test for categorical variables. Numerical variables were tested using the Mann-Whitney U test, and unpaired T-test, depending on the number of groups and the distribution pattern of the variable. Missing data were categorised as "unknown" and included in the analysis of categorical parameters in order to explore the influence of missing values. Logistic regression analysis was performed to test differences in mortality rates and to estimate the effect of covariates on patient outcomes. The odds ratios (OR) and the corresponding 95% confidence interval (CI) were calculated as indicated. Admission on weekdays served as the reference category for weekends. Multivariable analysis was performed in order to estimate the effect of age, CCI and severity of illness (triage level) on mortality and to calculate adjusted OR (ORadj). To evaluate the effect of readmissions on the results, we performed a sensitivity analysis including only the first admission following an ED visit in the analysis. In addition, a second sensitivity analysis was performed in order to evaluate the effect of daytime admission on weekdays versus on weekends on mortality rate. A two-sided p-value < 0.05 was considered significant.

Results

Population

A total of 3697 ED visits for internal medicine by 2798 elderly patients were registered, of which 2743 (74.2%) ED visits resulted in a hospital admission. The mean age at admission was 78.2 years old (SD 7.7). A total of 2114 (77.1%) admissions were during weekdays, and 629 (22.9%) were during the weekend (Fig. 1). A recurrent ED visit was recorded for 675 (24.6%) of the hospitalised elderly patients during the study period.

Patient characteristics

Patient characteristics, such as mean age, gender, and medication use of elderly patients admitted from the ED on weekdays and weekends were comparable (Table 1). Week admissions were associated with a lower CCI than weekend admissions (2.4 versus 2.6 respectively, $p = 0.041$). The seniority of the first physician on the ED differed significantly between weekends and weekdays, mainly due to the absence of medical students and more trainee residents during the weekend (Table 1). Elderly patients admitted on weekends had undergone more diagnostic testing in the ED than those admitted on weekdays (mean 3.6 versus 3.4, $p = 0.009$). The ED-LOS was comparable between weekend and weekday presentation to the ED (162 min and 165 min, respectively, $p = 0.176$). Hospital length of stay (LOS) among patients admitted during weekends (median 5 days, IQR 2-11) was shorter than on weekdays (median 6 days, IQR 2-12, $p = 0.031$).

Severity of illness

Elderly patients admitted during weekends more often had a high urgency level (20.0%) in the ED compared with patients admitted on weekdays (15.8%, $p < 0.001$) (Table 2). The laboratory parameters and vital parameters were comparable among patients admitted on weekends and weekdays (Table 2). The majority of elderly patients

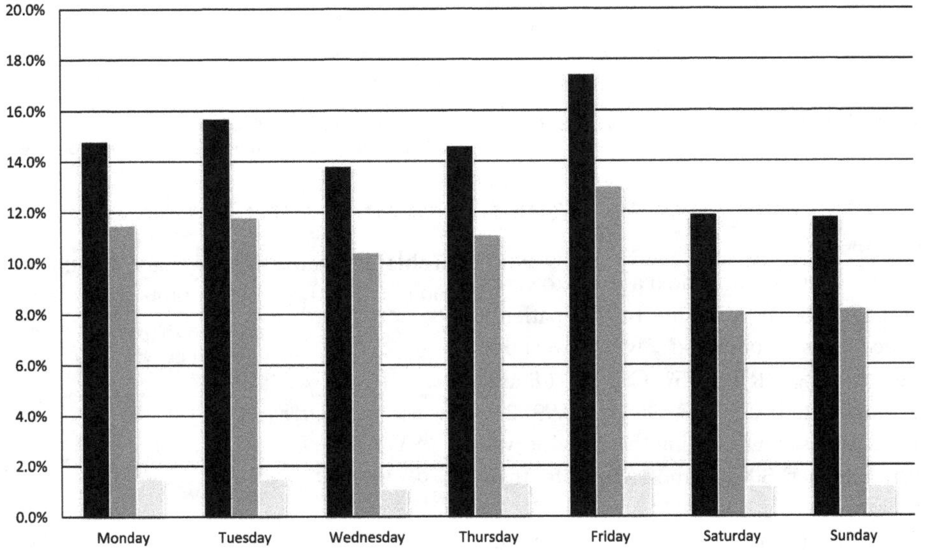

Fig. 1 Percentages of elderly patients presenting to the ED, hospitalized, and the in-hospital mortality. Black square: Percentage of patients presenting to the ED categorised by day of the week. Dark gray square: Percentage of patients admitted following the ED visit categorised by day of the week. Light gray square: In-hospital mortality rate (% of total no. of patients admitted) categorised by day of ED presentation

Table 1 Characteristics of emergency department (ED) visits by elderly patients

	Week admission (*N* = 2114)	Weekend admission (*N* = 629)
Mean age (SD)	78.2 (7.8)	78.0 (7.5)
No. of male participants (%)	943 (44.6)	291 (46.3)
CCI, mean (SD)*	2.4 (2.1)	2.6 (2.3)
Unknown CCI (%)	6 (0.3)	5 (0.8)
Number of drugs, mean (SD)	7.0 (4.1)	6.8 (4.0)
Unknown medication use (%)	348 (16.4)	82 (13.0)
Time of presentation **		
Daytime (8 am – 5 pm) (%)	1356 (64.1)	341 (54.2)
Evening (5 pm – 23 pm) (%)	602 (28.5)	211 (33.5)
Night (23 pm – 8 am) (%)	156 (7.4)	77 (12.2)
Mode of presentation **		
General practitioner (%)	1628 (77.0)	437 (69.5)
Ambulance (%)	181 (8.6)	87 (13.8)
Specialist (%)	170 (8.0)	40 (6.3)
Self-referral (%)	135 (6.4)	65 (10.3)
Seniority of first physician on ED**		
Medical student (%)	177 (6.3)	12 (1.4)
Non-trainee resident (%)	883 (31.2)	271 (30.8)
Trainee resident (%)	1561 (55.2)	538 (61.1)
Medical specialist (%)	160 (5.7)	43 (4.9)
Unknown (%)	45 (1.6)	17 (1.9)
Number of diagnostic tests, mean (SD)*	3.4 (1.9)	3.6 (2.0)
ED-LOS in minutes (IQR)	165 (130–204)	162 (129–201)
Hospital LOS in days (IQR) *	6 (2–12)	5 (2–11)

SD standard deviation, *CCI* Charlson comorbidity index, *ED* emergency department, *ED-LOS* emergency department length of stay, *LOS* length of stay, *IQR* interquartile range
P-values for week versus weekend admission: using the Chi-square test, unpaired t-test (normally distributed) or Mann-Whitney U test (not normally distributed).
* = $0.001 < p < 0.05$; ** = $p < 0.001$

Table 2 Clinical characteristics of elderly patients admitted following an ED visit

	Week admissions N = 2114	Weekend admissions N = 629
No. of admissions per triage level **		
Urgent (%)	333 (15.8)	126 (20.0)
Moderate (%)	1165 (55.1)	372 (59.1)
Low (%)	603 (28.5)	126 (20.0)
No triage (%)	13 (0.6)	5 (0.8)
ED diagnosis		
Aspecific complaints (%)	631 (29.8)	189 (30.0)
Circulatory/respiratory (%)	247 (11.7)	66 (10.5)
Infectious (%)	189 (8.9)	65 (10.3)
Digestive (%)	187 (8.8)	67 (10.7)
Miscellaneous (%)	187 (8.8)	68 (10.8)
Neoplasm/haematological (%)	186 (8.8)	42 (6.7)
Endocrine/metabolic (%)	174 (8.2)	36 (5.7)
Genitourinary (%)	146 (6.9)	47 (7.5)
Unknown (%)	167 (7.9)	49 (7.8)
Initial vital signs, median (range)		
Systolic pressure (mmHg)	138 (64–270)	137 (50–270)
Not measured (%)	82 (3.9)	16 (2.5)
Heart rate (min^{-1})	84.0 (35–180)	84.0 (46–200)
Not measured (%)	404 (19.1)	145 (23.1)
Laboratory, median (range)		
No laboratory test (%)	96 (4.5)	25 (4.0)
CRP (mg/L)	36.0 (0.1–674)	39.0 (0.1–674)
CRP not measured (%)	20 (0.9)	3 (0.5)
Leucocytes (× $10^3/mm^3$)	9.4 (0.2–239)	9.2 (0.2–198)
Leucocytes not measured (%)	11 (0.5)	1 (0.2)

P-values for week versus weekend admission, using the Chi-square test, unpaired t-test (normally distributed) or Mann-Whitney U test (not normally distributed).
* = $0.001 < p < 0.05$. ** = $p < 0.001$
SD standard deviation, *CCI* Charlson comorbidity index, *ED* emergency department, *ED-LOS* emergency department length of stay, *LOS* length of stay

presented with aspecific complaints (29.8% weekend and 30.0% weekday).

Weekend mortality rates

Analysis of the mortality rates demonstrated a trend towards a higher in-hospital and two-day mortality rate of patients hospitalised on weekends compared with weekday admission (11.4% versus 8.9%; OR 1.3, 95% CI 0.99–1.8 and 3.2% versus 1.9%; unadjusted OR 1.7, 95%CI 0.99–2.9, respectively). Weekend admission following the ED visit was not associated with a higher 30-day mortality rate than weekday admission (Table 3).

After multivariable adjustment for age, CCI, urgency level and number of diagnostic tests in-hospital mortality rates for weekend and week admission was comparable (ORadj 1.2, 95%CI 0.9–1.7). Additionally, the adjusted

Table 3 Mortality rates of elderly patients hospitalised following an ED visit on weekends compared with weekdays

	Weekend admission N = 629	Weekday admission N = 2114	OR (95%CI)	ORadj (95%CI)
In-hospital mortality rate (%)	72 (11.4)	189 (8.9)	1.3 (0.99–1.8)	1.2 (0.9–1.7)
2-day mortality rate (%)	20 (3.2)	40 (1.9)	1.7 (0.99–2.9)	1.5 (0.8–2.6)
30-day mortality rate (%)	96 (15.3)	286 (13.5)	1.2 (0.9–1.5)	1.1 (0.8–1.4)

Multivariable analyses included weekend/weekday admission, age, Charlson comorbidity index, triage level, and number of diagnostic tests on ED.
OR odds Ratio, *CI* confidence Interval, *ORadj* adjusted odds ratio

two-day mortality was similar for weekend and weekday admission (ORadj 1.5, 95%CI 0.8–2.6).

The sensitivity analysis, performed to evaluate the effect of readmissions on in-hospital mortality outcome, revealed similar results (OR 1.2, 95%CI 0.8–1.7) for the in-hospital mortality rate. Moreover, the outcome was not different for 2-day and 30-day mortality after sensitivity analysis. The second sensitivity analysis demonstrated a higher in-hospital mortality rate among elderly patients hospitalised during daytime on weekdays compared with on weekends (13.2% versus 9.3%; OR 1.5, 95%CI 1.03–2.1). After multivariable adjustment for age, CCI, urgency level and the number of diagnostic tests, the in-hospital mortality for daytime admission on weekdays and on weekends was similar (ORadj 1.3, 95%CI 0.95–1.99). The 2-day and 30-day mortality was comparable among elderly patients hospitalised during daytime on weekdays and weekends.

Discussion

In this study, we observed a small weekend effect in elderly internal medicine patients (≥ 65 years old), which was not statistically significant. This effect was partly explained by a generally higher comorbidity level and a higher urgency level in elderly patients hospitalised on weekends than during weekdays. Additionally, the 2-day and 30-day mortality demonstrated no difference between weekend admissions and week admissions.

Our results offer insight into the outcome of elderly internal medicine patients admitted from the ED on the weekends, for which existing literature is scarce. The in-hospital mortality rate of elderly patients hospitalised during weekends was 11.4%, which is higher than the 4.2–5.2% found in other studies examining a general population [2, 4]. As our study population consisted solely of elderly patients, a higher mortality rate is to be expected. The weekend effect might be overestimated in this complex population with multi-morbidity [11, 12], because of the reduced access of home care and difficulty of discharge to a hospice during weekends, which might contribute to a higher in-hospital mortality rate [17].

Our study is one of the first studies to examine the weekend effect among elderly patients. Only one earlier study demonstrated the existence of a weekend effect in an elderly population, focusing on patients with substantial head trauma, and found a mortality rate of 9.3% [18]. In contrast to the presumed increased risk of poor health outcomes of elderly internal medicine patients admitted from the ED during the weekend, we found no evidence supporting the existence of a weekend effect in this population after adjustment for important confounders.

Other studies reported conflicting results on the existence of a weekend effect [4–6, 10]. We focused on elderly internal medicine patients admitted following an ED visit, whereas the presence of the weekend effect is potentially related to specific acute diagnoses, such as ruptured abdominal aortic aneurysm, acute epiglottitis, stroke and myocardial infarction [1, 2]. These are all diseases requiring immediate and accurate assessment, intervention and adequate coordination, which could be compromised during the weekend. In our analyses, these acute complex diagnoses were not included, because these are not managed by the internist at the ED in the Netherlands. However, we provide useful insight into the potential added risk of other domains or diseases within the ED.

The discrepancy with other studies might be due to the difference in health care organisation of various countries. It is plausible that certain health care systems, or even individual health centres, create a weekend effect [5, 19, 20]. The majority of studies on the weekend effect have been conducted in the United States, Canada and the United Kingdom [1–6]. The health care system in the Netherlands differs from these countries, as emergency departments cooperate intensely with the ambulance services and GPs. Moreover, the acute care system depends on the gatekeeping role of GPs, whom are obligated to offer emergency care 24 h a day and provide an important safety net [14]. Consequently, our findings suggest that, despite the possible reduction in staffing and services provided on the ED, the Dutch acute care system seems effective in the management of acutely ill elderly patients during the weekend.

Since the main supposed causes of the weekend effect are of an organisational nature, such as decreased availability of diagnostic resources, and less experienced ED personnel [3, 5, 7], we analysed these factors to gain more insight into the potential determinants of the weekend effect. Remarkably, comparison of in-hospital mortality following daytime admission on weekdays versus weekends, which represents the main contrast in availability of resources, reveals no differences after adjustment for severity of illness. Elderly patients admitted on weekends used even more diagnostic resources and had shorter hospital length of stay compared with patients admitted on weekdays, contradicting previous studies of reduced access to the necessary resources and treatment [1].

A strength of our study was the assessment of confounders, such as the severity of illness of elderly ED patients hospitalised on weekends or weekdays, which contributes important information to existing evidence [2, 3, 8]. We found a higher comorbidity and urgency level among elderly patients hospitalised during weekends than on weekdays, which could be explained by a delay in presentation to the ED [8]. However, the difference in the severity of illness of elderly patients presenting to our ED on weekdays versus weekends did not appear to influence their health outcomes, as mortality (in-hospital mortality, 2-day and 30-day mortality) was comparable between both groups. This might be caused by a more thorough assessment and timely treatment on the ED in these patients with a higher triage level. Another possible explanation is appropriate referral by primary care during weekends, with subsequent early intervention. This could clarify the absence of a weekend effect in our study and may verify the adequate acute health care organisation and referral by primary care.

Our results may have several limitations being retrospective and observational by nature. Firstly, there is a potential for bias, because of the use of administrative data with the possibility of coding errors. Due to missing values, we were unable to apply a standardised tool, such as the Acute Physiology and Chronic Health Evaluation Score, to assess the severity of illness. Instead, we analysed surrogate markers for the severity of illness, such as triage level, vital parameters, and laboratory measurements. The effect of incomplete data was assessed by including this information in the analyses. A second limitation is the single centre setting, which may compromise the generalisability of the results. However, to the best of our knowledge, so far no similar study has been done yet regarding the weekend effect in the Netherlands. Furthermore, the organisation of acute care system in other centres and countries should be considered in interpreting our results, although we can also learn from the differences in this respect. Third, the relatively small number of patients may have led to reduced reliability of our results. It is possible that the sample size of the study was too small to exclude the presence of a weekend effect with sufficient statistical power. Fourth, although we corrected for confounders, such as severity of illness, residual confounding may still be present.

Conclusion

Our results demonstrate a slightly higher in-hospital mortality rate in elderly internal medicine patients hospitalised on weekends compared with weekdays. However, adjustment for a higher comorbidity and higher urgency level showed there is no independent causal association between weekend effect and in-hospital mortality. This suggests that emergency care in the Netherlands is not compromised by different logistics during the weekend, and appears to provide adequate emergency care to elderly patients.

Acknowledgements
Not applicable.

Funding
No funding was received.

Authors' contributions
SB conceived the study, and designed the protocol, SB and JW collected and analysed the data. HH supervised the conduct of the study and data collection. SB and JW drafted the manuscript, and all authors contributed substantially to its revision. SB and JW take responsibility for the paper as a whole. All authors read and approved the final manuscript.

Competing interests
The authors declare that they have no competing interests.

Author details
Department of Internal Medicine, Máxima Medical Centre, 5600 BM Eindhoven/Veldhoven, the Netherlands. [2]Maastricht University, Department of Health Services Research, and CAPHRI School for Public Health and Primary Care, 6229 ER Maastricht, the Netherlands. [3]Máxima Medical Centre Academy, Máxima Medical Centre, Eindhoven/Veldhoven, the Netherlands. [4]Department of Internal Medicine, division of general medicine, section acute medicine, Maastricht University Medical Centre, 6229 HX Maastricht, the Netherlands.

References

1. Bell CM, Redelmeier DA. Mortality among patients admitted to hospitals on weekends as compared with weekdays. N Engl J Med. 2001;345(9):663–8.
2. Aylin P, Yunus A, Bottle A, Majeed A, Bell D. Weekend mortality for emergency admissions. A large, multicentre study. Qual Saf Health Care. 2010;19(3):213–7.
3. Cram P, Hillis SL, Barnett M, Rosenthal GE. Effects of weekend admission and hospital teaching status on in-hospital mortality. Am J Med. 2004;117(3):151–7.
4. Sharp AL, Choi H, Hayward RA. Don't get sick on the weekend: an evaluation of the weekend effect on mortality for patients visiting US EDs. Am J Emerg Med. 2013;31(5):835–7.
5. Powell ES, Khare RK, Courtney DM, Feinglass J. The weekend effect for patients with sepsis presenting to the emergency department. J Emerg Med. 2013;45(5):641–8.
6. Carr BG, Reilly PM, Schwab CW, Branas CC, Geiger J, Wiebe DJ. Weekend and night outcomes in a statewide trauma system. Arch Surg. 2011;146(7):810–7.
7. Becker DJ. Weekend hospitalization and mortality: a critical review. Expert Rev Pharmacoecon Outcomes Res. 2008;8(1):23–6.
8. Jairath V, Kahan BC, Logan RFA, Hearnshaw SA, Travis SPL, Murphy MF, Palmer KR. Mortality from acute upper gastrointestinal bleeding in the United Kingdom: does it display a "weekend effect". Am J Gastroenterol. 2011;106:1621–8.
9. Concha P, Gallego B, Hillman K, Delaney GP, Coiera E. Do variations in hospital mortality patterns after weekend admission reflect reduced quality of care or different patients cohort? A population-based study. BMJ Qual Saf. 2013;0:1–8.
10. Metcalfe D, Perry DC, Bouamra O, Salim A, Lecky FE, Woodford M, Edwards A, Costa ML. Is there a 'weekend effect' in major trauma? Emerg Med J. 2016;33(12):836–42.
11. Samaras N, Chevalley T, Samaras D, Gold G. Older patients in the emergency department: a review. Ann Emerg Med. 2010;56(3):261–9.
12. Aminzadeh F, Dalziel WB. Older adults in the emergency department: a systematic review of patterns of use, adverse outcomes, and effectiveness of interventions. Ann Emerg Med. 2002;39(3):238–47.
13. Brouns SH, Stassen PM, Lambooij SL, Dieleman J, Vanderfeesten IT, Haak HR. Organisational factors induce prolonged emergency department length of stay in elderly patients - a retrospective cohort study. PLoS One. 2015;10(8):e0135066.

14. Holmes JL. Emergency medicine in the Netherlands. Emerg Med Australas. 2010;22(1):75–81.
15. Mackway-Jones K. Manchester triage group: emergency triage: 2nd ed. Oxford: Bmj Publishing Group; 2005.
16. Needham DM, Scales DC, Laupacis A, Pronovost PJ. A systematic review of the Charlson comorbidity index using Canadian administrative databases: a perspective on risk adjustment in critical care research. J Crit Care. 2005; 20(1):12–9.
17. Lapointe-Shaw L, Bell CM. It's not you, it's me: time to narrow the gap in the weekend care. BMJ Qual Saf. 2013;0:1–3.
18. Schneider EB, Hirani SA, Hambridge HL, Haut ER, Carlini AR, Castillo RC, Efron DT, Haider AH. Beating the weekend trend: increased mortality in the older adult traumatic brain injury (TBI) patients admitted on weekends. J Surg Res. 2012;177(2):295–300.
19. James MT, Wald R, Bell CM, Tonelli M, Hemmelgarn BR, Waikar SS, Chertow GM. Weekend hospital admission, acute kidney injury, and mortality. J Am Soc Nephrol. 2010;21(5):845–51.
20. Ruiz M, Bottle A, Aylin PP. The global comparators project: international comparison of 30-day in-hospital mortality by day of the week. BMJ Qual Saf. 2015;24(8):492–504.

4

HEMS inter-facility transfer: a case-mix analysis

Damien Di Rocco[1], Mathieu Pasquier[2], Eric Albrecht[3], Pierre-Nicolas Carron[2] and Fabrice Dami[2*]

Abstract

Background: Helicopter emergency medical services (HEMS) are popular rescue systems despite inconsistent evidence in the scientific literature to support their use for primary interventions, as well as for inter-facility transfer (IFT). There is little research about IFT by HEMS, hence questions remain about the appropriateness of this method of transport. The aim of this study was to describe a case-mix of operational and medical characteristics for IFT activity of a sole HEMS base, and identify indicators of over-triage.

Methods: This is a retrospective study on HEMS IFT over 36 months, from January 1st 2013 to December 31st 2015. Medical and operational data from the database of the Emergency Department of Lausanne University Hospital, which provides the emergency physicians for this helicopter base, were reviewed. It included distance and time of flight transport, type of care during flight, and estimated distance of transport if conducted by ground.

Results: There were 2194 HEMS missions including 979 IFT (44.6%). Most transfers involved adults (> 17 years old; 799 patients, 81.6%). Forty patients (4.1%) were classified as having benefitted from resuscitation or life-saving measures performed in flight, 615 (62.8%) from emergency treatment and 324 (33.1%) from simple clinical examination. The median distance by air between hospitals was 35.4 km. The estimated median distance by road was 47.7 km. The median duration time from origin to destination by air was 12 min.

Conclusions: This case-mix of IFTs by HEMS presents a high severity. There are many signs in favour of over-triage. We propose indicators to help choosing whether HEMS is the most appropriate mean of transport to perform the transfer regarding patient condition, geography, and medical competences available aboard ground ambulances; this may reduce over-triage.

Keywords: Inter-facility transfer (IFT), Helicopter emergency medical services (HEMS), Case-mix, Over-triage

Background

Helicopter emergency medical services (HEMS) are popular rescue systems despite inconsistent evidence in the scientific literature to support their use for primary interventions, as well as for inter-facility transfer (IFT) [1–5]. For IFT, the main added values of the helicopter are speed of patient transport, and sometimes medical competences if not available in ground ambulances (GA). IFT can either upgrade the level of care (to a trauma centre or university hospital) or downgrade it (to make room in those trauma centres or university hospitals) [6].

In contrast to direct transport from the scene of injury, there has been much less research about IFT by HEMS; hence, questions remain about the appropriateness of this method of transport. Furthermore, research on this topic has been mainly limited to specific types of disease (STEMI, stroke, spinal injury) and not on whole HEMS case-mixes [7, 8]. To the best of our knowledge, there is no generally accepted guideline that would help choose the most appropriate transport method for IFT, nor definition of over-triage when using the helicopter to perform those IFTs.

The aim of this study is to describe a single HEMS IFT case-mix and its severity, and identify over-triage through operational and medical indicators.

* Correspondence: Fabrice.Dami@chuv.ch
[2]Emergency Department, Lausanne University Hospital (CHUV), Bugnon 46, 1011 Lausanne, Switzerland
Full list of author information is available at the end of the article

Methods

Setting.

The State of Vaud (western Switzerland) has one trauma centre (Lausanne University Hospital), seven regional hospitals and many private clinics that are distributed equally over its territory. Most hospitals have a GA which they can use for transfers. All GAs are staffed with at least one paramedic. They use State protocols for autonomous intravenous access, cardiopulmonary resuscitation procedures, defibrillation and emergency medication administration. They are not allowed to manage upper airway disposals (intubation, laryngeal mask or tube) or continuous drug infusions (vasopressors, anaesthesia and sedation); these procedures require the presence of an emergency physician (EP). EPs are scarcely available to conduct IFT by GA as hospitals want to keep these scare resources within their emergency department. Therefore, HEMS which are staffed with their own EP and paramedic are regularly used to perform those transfers. Switzerland is very well covered for its area of 41,300 km^2 (16,000 mile^2), with 20 medically equipped helicopters from private companies during the daytime, and 8 during the night. In this State, requests for IFT by the helicopter are made by the hospital medical team in charge of the patient; there is no triage either from the HEMS companies or from dispatch centres regarding secondary transport.

Study design.

This was a retrospective study, carried out on data from January 1st 2013 to December 31st 2015 (36 months). All data were extracted from the database of the Emergency Department of the Lausanne University Hospital which staffs the EPs for this HEMS. Pre-hospital medical charts are completed by EPs and then checked by medical supervisors.

Measurements and outcomes.

Demographics (age and sex), diagnosis and operational data (distances, origin and destination, date, time of day and duration of flight) were collected. Patients who were 17 years of age and under were included in a paediatric subgroup. Outcome at 48 h (mortality, ICU or ward stay, discharge) was obtained from hospital charts. Diagnosis was grouped into nine clinical categories (*heart and vessel disease, traumatology, neurology, pneumology, obstetrics, paediatrics, toxicology, psychiatry* and *miscellaneous*). Patient care provided during transfer was classified into three care categories by EPs: *simple clinical examination, emergency treatment* and *resuscitation or life-saving manoeuvres.* Simple clinical examination consisted of simple monitoring of the patient during the flight. Emergency treatment consisted of administering any medication (continuously or not) including fluid resuscitation, even if it was started in the hospital, or to pursue ongoing ventilation. Resuscitation consisted of gestures and manoeuvres necessary to maintain the patient's life, such as cardiac massage, defibrillation or intubation. Specific treatments requiring the presence of an EP in this system (continuous drug infusion or airway management) were collected. Distances of journeys by road were calculated using Google Maps®; major differences between flight and ground distances for the same IFT may reveal geographical constraints (e.g. mountains, water).

Data were integrated into an Excel® spreadsheet, and processed and analysed using Stata© (Stata, Statistical Software 14.2, Stata Corporation, College Station, TX, USA).

Results

During the study period, there were 2194 HEMS missions including 982 IFT (44.8%). Three patients were excluded as they died before take-off; the final group included 979 patients (Fig. 1) (Table 1). Most missions involved adults (> 17 years old) (799; 81.6%). There were 772 (78.8%) transfers from regional hospitals to a university hospital, 139 (14.2%) from a university hospital to a regional hospital, 36 (3.7%) from a regional hospital to another regional hospital and 32 (3.3%) from a university hospital to another university hospital. Trauma patients represent 15.5% of the case-mix. Forty patients (4.1% of total) were classified as having benefitted from *resuscitation or life-saving measures* performed in flight, 615 (62.8%) from an *emergency treatment* and 324 (33.1%) from a *simple clinical examination.* Table 2 lists the fate of all patients at 48 h, regarding the type of care performed *en route.*

Operational characteristics (Table 3).

The median distance by air between hospitals was 35.4 km. The median distance by road calculated using Google Maps® was 47.7 km. The overall duration from origin to destination by air was 12 min.

There were 270 (27.6%) transfers during weekends, and 361 (36.9%) night transfers (7 pm–7 am).

Discussion

The decision to use HEMS is a sensitive topic, and there is no unambiguous evidence in favour or against its use for IFT in the literature; studies are carried out in different health policy settings and in different geographical environments; their results cannot be directly transposed to other EMS. Some studies have described factors (e.g. distance, geography) that influence the use of HEMS for IFT [9–11]; some demonstrated either a survival advantage [1, 12, 13] or disadvantage [2, 11] for injured patients. Moreover, most of these studies take into account only one category of pathology and not the whole case-mix, as this study proposes [8, 9].

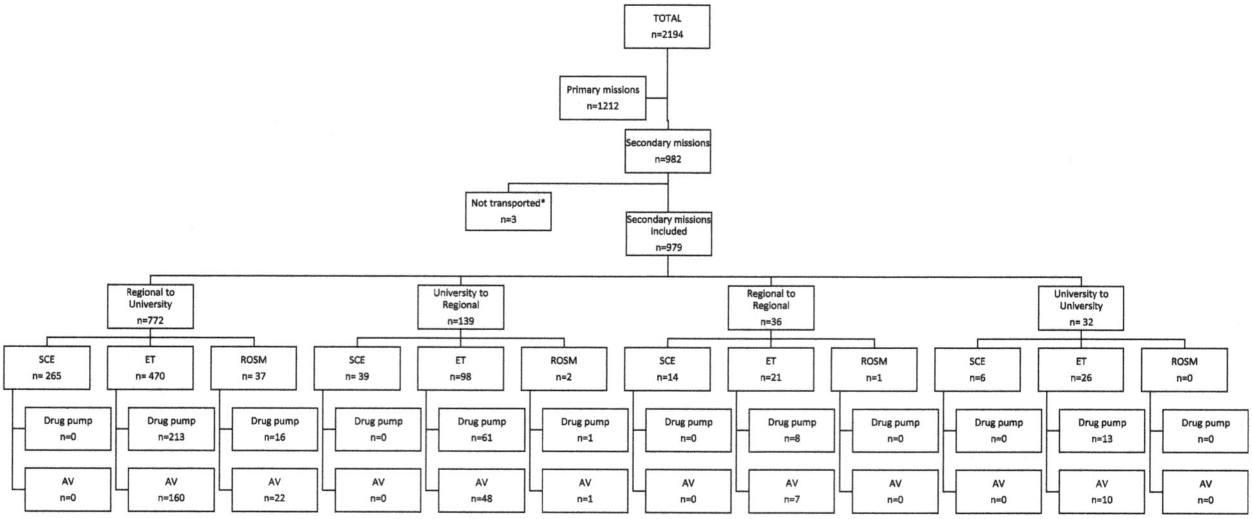

Fig. 1 Inter-facility transfer flowchart. SCE: simple clinical examination, ROSM: resuscitation or life-saving manoeuvres, ET: emergency treatment, AV: assisted ventilation (intubated/tracheotomised). *not transported: died before take-off

The analysis of the case-mix, the first aim of the study, shows that 425 (43.4%) patients were hospitalised in an ICU at 48 h, which demonstrates the severity of this case-mix. There were few trauma cases in this case-mix, which could be explained by efficient sorting performed during on-scene missions, and a consequently low re-transfer rate, as previously published in this HEMS [14]. Out of the 974 IFT, 772 (79%) patients were transported from a regional hospital to a university hospital (upgrading the level of care).

The measure of over-triage, the second aim of the study, is complex and must take into account many different indicators. For example, upgrading the level of care or the severity conditions at 48 h mentioned above are not indicators that can justify the use of HEMS by themselves.

If speed is needed by the referral team, then distance by air and ground have to be taken into account. If they are very different (e.g. affected by mountains, water), the probability that HEMS may be faster is high. Regarding this issue, some have proposed using distances between hospitals or the expected duration of transfer to justify the use of HEMS [15, 16], but there is no consensus on a cut-off distance or time for which the helicopter should be used [5]. Kristiansen et al. showed an increase in the use of HEMS proportional to the distance to be covered, and a decrease in mortality for transfers by HEMS ≥100 km [15]. Another study recommends considering HEMS for distances ≥30 km by road for IFT [16]. If we transpose these values to our study, we note that 738 (75%) missions were above the 30 km proposed limit, and 70 (7%) above the 100 km limit. It should however be highlighted that although a helicopter can cover a greater distance than a GA in a given time, it is not always the fastest method of transfer [5]. Indeed, it takes longer to install a patient in a helicopter than in a GA. Take-off and landing procedures also take longer than starting an ambulance engine [17]. In this area, although hospital landing zones are open 24/24, they are often located on roof tops or at some distance from emergency departments. Finally, it should be mentioned that most hospitals have a GA service nearby, which may be at the patient's bedside somewhat quicker than HEMS. When looking for speed, the estimated global time of transfer from the call to the arrival at destination should be estimated by air versus ground.

In some EMS, GA medical competences are sometimes estimated to be insufficient to handle the patient and therefore HEMS is requested. This is the case in this study, as paramedics cannot handle intubation, mechanical ventilation or continuous drugs. When looking at the *simple clinical examination* group, the main possible added value of HEMS was speed of transport to exclude and/or treat a time-sensitive condition (i.e. STEMI, stroke, angiography, or neurosurgery) after having received all necessary treatment in the local hospital. When analysing in detail the diagnosis declared by EPs for this category, we can retrospectively hypothesise that some of them may not have needed HEMS as advanced medical competences were not required (head trauma with GCS 14, spine trauma without neurological deficit, pneumonia, intoxication, alcohol abuse). When looking ate the *emergency treatment* group, the vast majority did not benefit from ventilation or continuous drug treatment. The medical files were not retrospectively checked to determine whether continuous treatment could have

Table 1 Patients' clinical characteristics including demographics, medical equipment according to the type of care provided, and clinical category (*n* = 979)

Demographic	
All	
n (%)	979 (100)
Gender male, n (%)	594 (60.7)
Age (mean ± SD) (range)	50.7 ± 26.9 (1–95)
Adults	
n (%)	799 (81.6)
Gender male, n (%)	487 (49.7)
Age (mean ± SD) (range)	60.8 ± 18.1 (18–95)
Paediatric patients	
n (%)	180 (18.4)
Gender male, n (%)	107 (10.9)
Age (mean ± SD) (range)	6.1 ± 5.1 (1–17)
Care category (= n) (%)	
Simple clinical examination	324 (33.1)
Intubated before transfer	0 (0)
Tracheotomized before transfer	0 (0)
Infusion pumps	0 (0)
Emergency treatment	615 (62.8)
Intubated before transfer	205 (20.9)
Tracheotomized before transfer	20 (2.0)
Infusion pumps	295 (30.1)
Resuscitation or life-saving measures	40 (4.1)
Intubated before transfer	23 (2.3)
Tracheotomized before transfer	0 (0)
Infusion pumps	17 (1.7)
Clinical category (= n) (%)	
Heart/vessel disease	252 (25.7)
Myocardial infarct	103 (10.5)
Chest pain	38 (3.9)
Cardiac arrest	28 (2.9)
Cardiac insufficiency	17 (1.7)
Aortic abdominal aneurysm ruptured	14 (1.4)
Other	52 (5.3)
Traumatology	152 (15.5)
Mild TBI (GCS 14–15)	29 (3)
Blunt abdominal trauma	24 (2.5)
Moderate TBI (GCS 9–13)	13 (1.3)
Severe TBI (GCS 3–8)	13 (1.3)
Other trauma	73 (7.5%)
Neurology	123 (12.6)
Stroke	85 (8.7)
Status epilepticus	16 (1.6)
Epilepsy	14 (1.4)
Other	8 (0.8)
Pneumology	85 (8.7)
Obstetrics	58 (5.9)
Paediatrics	46 (4.7)
Toxicology	25 (2.6)
Psychiatry	3 (0.3)
Miscellaneous	235 (24)

SD standard deviation, *GCS* Glasgow Coma Scale, *TBI* traumatic brain injury
*Continuous drugs used: norepinephrine, dopamine, dobutamine, propofol, clonidine, sodium nitroprusside, labetalol, alteplase, heparin, isosorbide dinitrate, nitroglycerin, atosiban

been interrupted for the duration of transfer, allowing paramedics to take care of the patient from this category without EP.

HEMS should be used for IFT if medical competences that exceed GA competences are needed or may be needed during transfer, or if speed is needed and the estimated time from call to arrival at the destination is faster with a helicopter. In the setting described, the hospital physician in charge of the patient performs this triage, but they are often not aware of paramedic competences and do not have the information on GA availability. Ideally, a dispatch centre should decide whether to allow HEMS transfers or not based on the need of HEMS for primary missions, the patient's condition, the suspected pathology and time gained by using HEMS for IFT. This would require advanced medical competences within the dispatch centre; it may also allow the treatment to be simplified wherever possible, to enable the GA to take care of the patient.

In the future, to better understand the use of HEMS for IFT and thus be able to propose new guidelines, it should be mandatory to prospectively document the reason why physicians choose HEMS instead of GA, in particular if it is a matter of speed or level of care. It should also be mandatory to evaluate whether ongoing continuous treatment can be stopped briefly or not. The dispatch centre should be capable of deciding whether to use HEMS for IFT rather than in-hospital physicians; all of those measures may contribute to a reduction in the over-use of HEMS for IFT.

The results point out that there are numerous signs of over-triage in this case-mix, regarding either the flight distances, clinical categories, medical procedures performed during flight, and diagnosis of patients. However, we lack two critical pieces of information to fully circumscribe the issue: the reason why HEMS is requested (speed? Medical competences?) and the estimate time

Table 2 Patients' 48 h outcome according to the type of care provided

Outcome at 48 h (= n)	Total (n = 979)	Type of care		
		Simple clinical examination (*n* = 324) (33.1%)	Emergency treatment (*n* = 615) (62.8%)	Resuscitation or life-saving measures (*n* = 40) (4.1%)
Hospitalized in intensive care unit	425 (43.4)	75 (7.7)	325 (33.2)	25 (2.6)
Hospitalized in intermediate care unit	196 (20)	96 (9.8)	96 (9.8)	4 (0.4)
Hospitalized in ward division	181 (18.5)	70 (7.2)	108 (11.0)	3 (0.3)
Transfer to another institution	88 (9)	42 (4.3)	45 (4.6)	1 (0.1)
Hospitalized and returned home	44 (4.5)	34 (3.5)	10 (1.0)	–
Not hospitalized, discharged	9 (0.9)	4 (0.4)	5 (0.5)	–
Died: 0–1 h (after admission)	3 (0.3)	1 (0.1)	–	2 (0.2)
Died: 1–6 h	3 (0.3)	–	3 (0.3)	–
Died: 6–24 h	19 (1.9)	–	14 (1.4)	5 (0.5)
Died: 24–48 h	11 (1.1)	2 (0.2)	9 (0.9)	–

Table 3 Operational characteristics

	HEMS	Road (estimated)
Total missions, n	979	979
Median distance (km) (IQR)	35.4 (22.5-–40.2)	47.7 (30.5–71.1)
< 30 km, n (%)[a]	342 (34.9)	241 (24.6)
≥ 100 km, n (%)[¶]	37 (3.8)	70 (7.1)
Median duration (min) (IQR)	12 (10–15)	
Flow of transfers & clinical classification		
University to university	32 (3.3%)	
Simple clinical examination	6 (0.6)	
Emergency treatment	26 (2.7)	
Resuscitation or life-saving measures	0 (0)	
Regional to regional	36 (3.7%)	
Simple clinical examination	14 (1.4)	
Emergency treatment	21 (2.1)	
Resuscitation or life-saving measures	1 (0.1)	
University to regional	139 (14.2%)	
Simple clinical examination	39 (4.0)	
Emergency treatment	98 (10.0)	
Resuscitation or life-saving measures	2 (0.2)	
Regional to university	772 (78.8%)	
Simple clinical examination	265 (27.1)	
Emergency treatment	470 (48.0)	
Resuscitation or life-saving measures	37 (3.8)	
Night mission 7 pm–7 am	361 (36.9%)	

IQR: interquartile range
[a]Expert recommendation by Kim et al. study, [¶]expert recommendation by Kristiansen et al. study

saved using HEMS versus GA for each IFT, taking into account the time from the alarm and the fact that an ambulance may already be at the hospital.

There will always be a certain amount of over-triage in the use of HEMS for transfer and we should accept it. The question, as always, is how much is too much?

Limitations.

This is a monocentric and retrospective study. The data available could not define whether primary missions needing HEMS had to go by ground because of transfer activity with the helicopter. The reason why physicians required HEMS instead of a GA for transfer is not known, as it is not documented in hospital or pre-hospital charts. The category used to describe the treatment received during flight is not a validated standard. Air and ground distances were estimated using Google Maps®. The elapsed time between HEMS activation and arrival at the patient's bedside was not described, as some transfers were 'scheduled', meaning that the crew was asked to take off within a specific delay (30–90 min). Only the duration of transport by HEMS was measured, rather than the entire process from the alarm to the arrival of HEMS at the receiving facility. No direct comparison was made with a GA; therefore, we cannot assess whether using HEMS for those transfers was quicker than if they had been performed by GA. This study did not intend to measure under-triage, as this would have required the operational characteristics of ground IFTs.

This study took place in a specific setting (geography, paramedics' autonomy, absence of EPs in GAs), and may not be applicable elsewhere.

Conclusions

The case-mix of IFTs by HEMS analysed presents a high severity. There are many signs in favour of over-triage. We propose indicators to help to determine whether HEMS is the most appropriate to perform the transfer regarding patient condition, geography, and medical competences available on-board GA; this may reduce over-triage.

Abbreviations

EMS: Emergency medical service; EP: emergency physician; GA: Ground ambulance; HEMS: Helicopter emergency medical service; ICU: Intensive care unit; IFT: Inter-facility transfer; ISS: Injury severity score; STEMI: ST-elevation myocardial infarction

Competing interests.

The authors declare that they have no competing interests.

Authors' contributions.

DDR generated, analysed and interpreted the data, and was a major contributor in writing the manuscript. FD analysed and interpreted the transfer data, and was a major contributor in writing the manuscript. PNC, EA and MP critically revised the manuscript for important intellectual content, and approved the final version to be published. All authors read and approved the final manuscript.

Author details

Medical Student, Faculty of Medicine, University of Lausanne, Lausanne, Switzerland. [2]Emergency Department, Lausanne University Hospital (CHUV), Bugnon 46, 1011 Lausanne, Switzerland. [3]Department of Anaesthesia, Lausanne University Hospital, Lausanne, Switzerland.

References

1. Boyd CR, Corse KM, Campbell RC. Emergency inter-hospital transport of the major trauma patient: air versus ground. J Trauma. 1989 Jun;29(6):789–94.
2. Arfken CL, Shapiro MJ, Bessey PQ, Littenberg B. Effectiveness of helicopter versus ground ambulance services for inter-facility transport. J Trauma. 1998 Oct;45(4):785–90.
3. Hill AD, Fowler RA, Nathens AB. Impact of inter-hospital transfer on outcomes for trauma patients: a systematic review. J Trauma Inj Infect Crit Care. 2011 Dec;71(6):1885–901.
4. Ryb GE, Dischinger P, Cooper C, Kufera JA. Does helicopter transport improve outcomes independently of emergency medical system time? J Trauma Acute Care Surg. 2013 Jan;74(1):149–56.
5. Karanicolas PJ, Bhatia P, Williamson J, Malthaner RA, Parry NG, Girotti MJ, et al. The fastest route between two points is not always a straight line: an analysis of air and land transfer of non-penetrating trauma patients. J Trauma Inj Infect Crit Care. 2006 Aug;61(2):396–403.
6. Koval KJ. Are patients being transferred to level-I trauma centres for reasons other than medical necessity? J Bone Jt Surg Am. 2006 Oct 1;88(10):2124.
7. Galvagno Jr SM, Sikorski R, Hirshon JM, Floccare D, Stephens C, Beecher D, et al. Helicopter emergency medical services for adults with major trauma. In: Cochrane Database of Systematic Reviews [Internet]. John Wiley & Sons, Ltd; 2015 [cited 2016 Mar 1]. Available from: http://onlinelibrary.wiley.com/doi/10.1002/14651858.CD009228.pub3/full
8. Foster NA, Elfenbein DM, Kelley W Jr, Brown CR, Foley C, Scarborough JE, et al. Comparison of helicopter versus ground transport for the inter-facility transport of isolated spinal injury. Spine J. 2014 Jul 1;14(7):1147–54.
9. Stewart K, Garwe T, Bhandari N, Danford B, Albrecht R. Factors associated with the use of helicopter inter-facility transport of trauma patients to tertiary trauma centres within an organised rural trauma system. Prehospital Emerg Care Off J Natl Assoc EMS Physicians Natl Assoc State EMS Dir. 2016; 20(5):601–8.
10. Stewart KE, Cowan LD, Thompson DM, Sacra JC. Factors at the scene of injury associated with air versus ground transport to definitive care in a state with a large rural population. Prehosp Emerg Care. 2011 Mar 9; 15(2):193–202.
11. Brown JB, Stassen NA, Bankey PE, Sangosanya AT, Cheng JD, Gestring ML. Helicopters improve survival in seriously injured patients requiring inter-facility transfer for definitive care. J Trauma Inj Infect Crit Care. 2011 Feb; 70(2):310–4.
12. Moylan JA, Fitzpatrick KT, Beyer AJ, Georgiade GS. Factors improving survival in multisystem trauma patients. Ann Surg. 1988 Jun;207(6):679–85.
13. Campbell R, Corse K, Boyd C. Impact of inter-hospital air transport on mortality in a rural trauma system. Ann Emerg Med. 1989 Apr;18(4):474.
14. Carron P-N, Taffe P, Ribordy V, Schoettker P, Fishman D, Yersin B. Accuracy of pre-hospital triage of trauma patients by emergency physicians: a retrospective study in western Switzerland. Eur J Emerg Med. 2011 Apr; 18(2):86_93.
15. Kristiansen T, Lossius HM, Søreide K, Steen PA, Gaarder C, Næss PA. Patients Referred to a Norwegian Trauma Centre: effect of transfer distance on injury patterns, use of resources and outcomes. J Trauma Manag Outcomes [Internet]. 2011 Dec [cited 2017 Sep 3];5(1). Available from: https://doi.org/10.1186/1752-2897-5-9.

5

Prevalence and outcome of injury in patients visiting the emergency Department of Yirgalem General Hospital, Southern Ethiopia

Abel Negussie[1*], Andarge Getie[2], Elias Manaye[3] and Tamrat Tekle[4]

Abstract

Background: Traumatic injuries continue to be an important cause of morbidity and mortality in the developing world. Despite the high burden of injury in Ethiopia, the occurrence and health impact have not received due attention. The aim of the study was to assess the prevalence and outcome of injury among patients visiting the Emergency Department (ED) of Yirgalem General Hospital, southern Ethiopia.

Methods: A facility-based prospective cross sectional study was conducted from March, 27 – April, 30/2017. The final calculated sample size was 353 and all eligible trauma patients who visited the ED of Yirgalem General Hospital during the study period were included in the study. Data was collected using a checklist which was adapted from the WHO injury surveillance guideline. The data were entered and analyzed using SPSS version 19.

Results: A total of 346 patients, who visited the ED during the study period, participated in the study and of them, 171 (49.4%) were injury cases. Unintentional injuries accounted 123 (71.9%) of the total injuries and the age group ≤24 years (48.2%) was the most commonly affected age group. More than half (51.4%) of unintentional injury cases were due to Road Traffic Injuries (RTIs) and 48 (28%) of the cases were attributed to interpersonal violence (assault). The majority of patients, 97 (56.7%), had a minor or superficial injury (like bruises and minor cuts), 44 (25.7%) had a moderate injury and 16 (9.3%) had severe type of injury requiring intensive medical/surgical management; and RTIs accounted for 11 (68%) of all severe injuries.

Conclusion: The prevalence of injury was considerably high in Yirgalem General Hospital. Road Traffic Injuries (RTIs) accounted for the majority of severe injury cases; therefore, appropriate prevention strategies should be strengthened and implemented against RTIs. We also suggest that children and young adults should be educated in schools and work environments to prevent injuries/accidents.

Keywords: Injury, Prevalence, Outcome, Facility-based, Southern Ethiopia

Background

Injuries continue to be an important cause of morbidity and mortality in the developed and developing world. According to WHO Global Burden of Disease (GBD) estimates, in 2008, 5.1 million people died worldwide every year as a result of injuries and violence. This account for around 9% of the world's deaths and the majority of injury related deaths are unintentional or "accidental" with road traffic crashes, falls and drowning ranking among the main causes [1]. In the past few decades, due to urbanization, industrialization, rapid motorization, and unsafe driving, the risk of accidents have increased, contributing a large burden of mortality and morbidity, especially in developing countries [2]. Road Traffic Injuries (RTIs) are among the leading causes of death and lifelong disability globally and according to the 2015 WHO global status report on road safety, about 1.25

* Correspondence: abelnegussie@ymail.com
[1]Department of Social and Population Health, Yirgalem Hospital Medical College, Yirgalem, Ethiopia
Full list of author information is available at the end of the article

million people die annually on the world's roads, with 20–50 million sustaining non-fatal injuries [3].

Traumatic injuries represent a significant and growing disease burden in the developing world, and now it is one of the leading causes of death in economically active adults in many low and middle income countries (LMICs) [4]. LMICs represent more than 90% of global road traffic deaths and RTI death rates are highest in the African region. In developing countries, injury ranks third as a major cause of death and permanent disability among the adult population next to tuberculosis and HIV/AIDS [5]. The main reason of this burden of injuries is due to lack of organized efforts to reduce its occurrence; and the cost-effectiveness of injury prevention and emergency treatment in these resource limited settings is not yet well understood as the development of emergency care systems is in its nascence [6].

In Ethiopia, like that of other developing countries, injuries are common and the 2008 national report on road safety indicated that nearly 19,000 road traffic accidents occurred per year, claiming over 2500 lives and property worth of US$ 56 million [7]. Even though some previous studies done in other regions of the country indicated high burden of injury, the occurrence and increasing public health importance haven't received due attention and a comprehensive injury data still remains limited [8–10]. It is also important to provide local data on the rate of injuries which might serve as a baseline data for local authorities and health care planners to implement appropriate injury prevention strategies. The aim of this study was to describe the magnitude and outcome of injuries requiring ED visit in Yirgalem General Hospital, southern Ethiopia.

Methods

Study design and setting

A hospital-based prospective cross sectional study was conducted from March, 27 – April, 30/2017 at ED of Yirgalem General Hospital. Yirgalem General Hospital is found in Yirgalem town and it is one of the General Hospitals in the South, Nations, Nationalities and Peoples Region (SNNPR). The hospital was established in January 1966 and it serves about 4.2 million people. The hospital had four main departments (Medical, Surgical, Pediatrics and Gynecology/Obstetric wards), three special care units (Medical Intensive Care Unit, Neonatal Intensive Care Unit and Surgical recovery Room) and five clinics (Eye, Anti-retro viral Treatment, Dental, TB and MDR-TB clinics).

In the Ethiopian health care system, hospitals are structured as Primary, General and Specialized hospitals. Primary hospital (to cover 60,000–100,000 people) is established at district or primary care level; and the coverage of General and Specialized hospitals extends to larger portions of the population providing services to 1–1.5 million and 3.5–5 million people, respectively. Though the study was done in Yirgalem General Hospital, it may give the overall picture of the burden of injury at EDs of similar hospitals found in the country.

Study participants

All eligible patients who visited the ED of Yirgalem General Hospital during the study period (March, 27 – April, 30/2017) were included in the study. Patients who died before arrival with unknown cause were excluded from the study. The required sample size to estimate the prevalence of injury was calculated using $P = 0.32$ [8], confidence interval = 95% and margin of error (d) = 5%. As a result of adding non-response rate of 5% to the initially estimated sample size, the final sample size became 353.

Data collection procedure

Data was collected using a checklist which was adapted from the WHO injury surveillance guideline and comprised of items regarding the socio-demographic characteristics; and the mechanism, severity and outcome/type of injury cases. Data was collected by three clinical nurses who took a 2 days training on detail contents of the checklist. The filled checklists were checked for completeness and proper filling by the investigators to assure data quality.

Data processing and analysis

The data were entered and analyzed using SPSS version 19. Frequency distribution and percentage calculations were made to describe the socio-demographic characteristics of study participants; and also the mechanism, severity and outcome of injury cases were examined using measures of descriptive statistics.

Operational and standard definitions

- ***Injury:*** *Any instance of physical damage to the body or body part.*
- ***Intentional injury:*** *Categorized as interpersonal violence (including violence against intimate partner), collective violence (including war) and self-directed violence (suicide).*
- ***Psychoactive substance:*** *Is defined as psychoactive ingredients that alter mood, cognition and behaviour.*
- ***Outcome of the injury:*** *the intent of the injury that results on the victim like fracture, dislocation, laceration and abrasion.*
- ***Severity of injury***
  No injury: *Patient who had no accessible injury and no need of any intervention.*

Minor injury: *Patient who had minor injury or superficial injury (*e.g. *Bruises, minor cut) requiring cleaning of the area.*
Moderate injury: *Patient who had moderate injuries requiring some sort of skilled treatment such as fracture stabilization and suturing of wounds.*
Severe injury: *Patient who had severe injuries requiring intensive medical/surgical management (*e.g. *internal haemorrhage, moderate/severe head injuries).*

- ***Unintentional injury:*** *Comprises road traffic injuries, fires, falls and drowning.*

Results

Out of the total 353 patients who visited the ED during the study period, 346 of them agreed to participate in the study with a response rate of 98%; and of them, 171 (49.4%) were injury cases. Most study participants were males (67.3%), under the age group of 25 (48.2%), Sidama (77.2%) by ethnicity and Protestant (59.5%) by religion. Regarding the educational status of the participants, almost half 166 (48%) of them had attended primary education. Furthermore, students and farmers accounted 97 (28%) and 81 (23.4%) of the total ED cases, respectively (Table 1).

The prevalence of injury was found to be 49.4% and unintentional injuries accounted 123 (71.9%) of the total injuries. More than half of the cases, 88 (51.4%), were due to RTIs followed by interpersonal violence (assault), 48 (28%), and falling accident, 24 (14%). Other less common causes of injury were burning, choking and injuries during use of industrial machineries (Fig. 1). Most assaults, 9 (18.3%), had used club/stick followed by hit/attack by a person, 7 (14.2%).

Of the total injury cases, 57 (33.3%), 42 (24.6%), 16 (9.3%) and 15 (8.7%) of the injured patients had a bruise/superficial injury, cuts/bites/open wound, fracture and concussion, respectively (Table 2). The majority of patients, 97 (56.7%), had a minor or superficial injury (like bruises and minor cuts), 44 (25.7%) had a moderate injury and 16 (9.3%) had severe type of injury requiring intensive medical/surgical management. Most importantly, RTIs alone accounted for 11 (68%) of all severe injuries. Our study found that 53 (31%) of the injured patients had a history of alcohol consumption before 6 Hrs. of the trauma. Of them, 26 (49%) had encountered assault and 10 (5.8%) had used psychoactive substance in addition to alcohol.

Most frequent affected body parts were head, neck and face – 45 (26.3%). Upper extremity, 39 (22.8%), and trunk injuries, 25 (14.6%), were also common (Fig. 2). The majority of the cases, 135 (78.9%), were treated as outpatients, 27 (15.7%) were admitted and 9 (5.2%) were referred to other hospitals for further investigation and management. All outpatient and inpatient cases, 162 (100%), were discharged with improvement and follow-up.

Discussion

The study found that half of all emergency visits were due to traumatic injuries. This result is higher when compared to other similar study findings [8, 11], but is relatively comparable to the report of a study done in Amhara Regional State Referral Hospitals, Ethiopia (55.6%) [9]. This

Table 1 Socio-demographic characteristics of study participants visiting the Emergency Department of Yirgalem General Hospital, southern Ethiopia, from March 27 – April 30/ 2017; (*n* = 346)

Variable	Categories	Frequency	Percent
Age	≤24	167	48.2
	25–59	158	45.6
	≥60	21	6.1
Sex	Male	233	67.3
	Female	113	32.7
Ethnicity	Sidama	267	77.2
	Amhara	42	12.1
	Oromo	30	8.7
	Others	7	2
Religion	Protestant	206	59.5
	Orthodox	112	32.4
	Muslim	28	8.1
Marital Status	Married	187	54
	Single	156	54.1
	Others	3	0.9
Residence	Urban	159	46
	Rural	187	54
Monthly Income (In Ethiopian Birr per month)	< 660	138	39.9
	660–1600	106	30.6
	> 1600	102	29.5
Educational level	Illiterate	87	25.1
	Primary education	166	48
	Secondary education	64	18.5
	Higher education	29	8.4
Occupational status	Student	97	28
	Farmer	81	23.4
	Unemployed	62	17.9
	Civil servant	34	9.8
	Trader of any kind	25	7.2
	Daily laborer	19	5.4
	Driver	18	5.2
	Construction worker	10	2.9

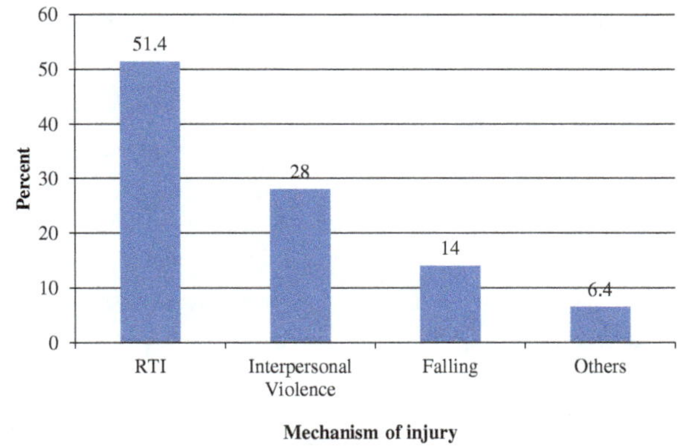

Fig. 1 Mechanism of injury in patients visiting the Emergency Department of Yirgalem General Hospital, southern Ethiopia, from March 27 - April 30/2017; N = 171; blue square Mechanism of injury

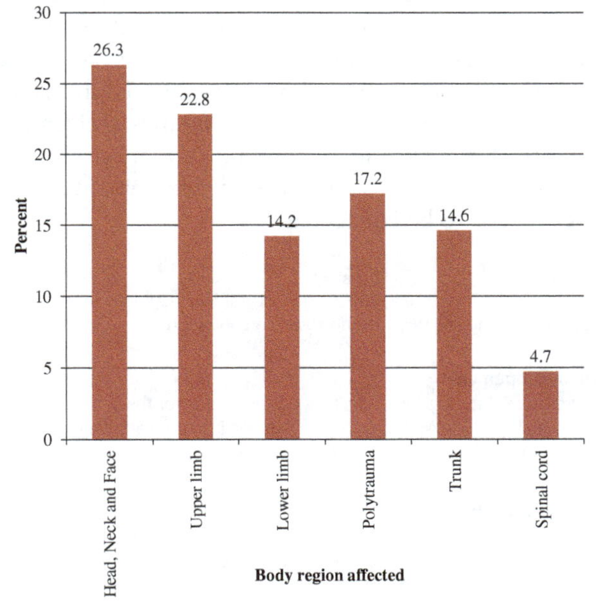

Fig. 2 Body part affected by the injury in patients visiting the Emergency Department of Yirgalem General Hospital, southern Ethiopia, from March 27–April 30/2017; $N = 171$; red square Body region affected

difference in the magnitude of injury cases may be due to differences in study time and setting; or differences in the level and number of facilities studied. The most common cause of injury was found to be RTIs which is similar to the findings of other researches [4, 9, 11]. Furthermore, a greater number of injury victims were under the age of 25 compared to those aged 25–59 or to those aged 60 years and older, which signifies the possible economic impact of the problem as the productive age group of the society is being affected. The possible explanation for this may be is that, this age group is in active working years of life and it is time of practicing independent life out of parental supervision. This finding is also in line with other previous studies [5, 10].

Our study also indicated that RTI was the most common cause of injury contributing to more than half of the total unintentional injuries. This result is higher than the finding of a study done at Regional referral hospitals in Amhara region, Ethiopia. This may be due to lack of well-established road for pedestrians, as the primary victims of RTIs were the pedestrians, and no separate pathways for domestic animals in the study area, or due to the difference in study time and setting [9].

Table 2 Type of injury in patients visiting the Emergency Department of Yirgalem General Hospital, southern Ethiopia, from March 27 - April 30/2017, ($n = 171$)

Type of injury	Frequency	Percent (%)
Bruise	57	33.3
Cut/open wound	42	24.6
Strain	18	10.5
Fracture	16	9.3
Concussion	15	8.7
Dislocation	8	4.6
Organ system	5	2.9
Concussion and open wound	6	3.5
Concussion and organ system	3	1.7
Others	10	5.8

We found that minor or superficial injuries were the leading injury outcomes and unlike our finding, a study done in Jimma, Ethiopia, showed that most of the cases were with moderate injury [9]. Moreover, a study done at Tikur Anbessa Specialized Referral Hospital, Addis Ababa, reported that fractures were the primary outcome of injuries [8]. This discrepancy may be attributed to a difference in status of the hospitals in the health care delivery system. Most importantly, RTIs alone accounted more than half of the severe injuries, in our study. In addition, the majority of injury patients were treated and discharged as outpatients, which is comparable to other studies done elsewhere [10, 11].

Limitations of the study

Even though the study indicated the prevalence and outcome of injury among emergency department patients, it is a descriptive facility based study and lacks generalizability to the total target population. Additionally, patients who had visited the emergency department during a specific period were considered and a possible selection bias may present.

Conclusions

Our study found that the prevalence of injury was considerably high in Yirgalem General Hospital, and the age group of ≤24 years was the most affected age group.

RTIs accounted half of all severe injury cases; therefore, appropriate prevention strategies should be strengthened and implemented against RTIs. We also suggest that children and young adults should be educated in schools and work environments to prevent injuries/accidents as they are the most affected group. Furthermore, future studies which focus on identifying determinant factors of RTIs need to be conducted.

Abbreviations
ED: Emergency Department; LMICs: Low and middle income countries; RTI: Road traffic injury; WHO: World Health organization

Acknowledgements
We are grateful to Yirgalem Hospital Medical College for the facilitation of this research project. We thank Yirgalem General Hospital and Emergency Department staffs for their unlimited assistance.

Authors' contributions
Conceived and designed the study: AN AG EM TT. Performed the data collection: AG EM TT. Analysed the data and interpreted the results: AN AG EM TT. Supervised the conduct of the study: AN. Wrote the manuscript: AN. Critically reviewed the manuscript: AG EM TT. All authors read and approved the final submitted manuscript.

Competing interests
The authors declare that they have no competing interests.

Author details
[1]Department of Social and Population Health, Yirgalem Hospital Medical College, Yirgalem, Ethiopia. [2]Administration for Refugee and Returnee Affairs (ARRA), Addis Ababa, Ethiopia. [3]Department of Internal Medicine, Wollo University, Dessie, Ethiopia. [4]Dawro General Hospital, SNNPR, Dawro, Ethiopia.

References
1. Bartolomeos K, Kipsaina C, Grills N, Ozanne-Smith J, Peden M, editors. Fatal injury surveillance in mortuaries and hospitals: a manual for practitioners. Geneva: World Health Organization; 2012.
2. Mohammad Fararoei, Seyed Javad Sadat, Mohammad Zoladl: Epidemiology of Trauma in Patients Admitted to an Emergency Ward in Yasuj *inpress:* 2016 e30572 .
3. World Health Organization. Global status report on road safety 2015. Geneva: World Health Organization; 2015.
4. Haagsma JA, Graetz N, Bolliger I, et al. The global burden of injury: incidence, mortality, disability-adjusted life years and time trends from the global burden of disease study 2013. Inj Prev. 2015; 0:1–16
5. World Health Organization: Road Traffic Injuries: Fact sheet. 2015. http://www.who.int/mediacentre/factsheets/fs358/en/index.html
6. GBD. 2013 Mortality and Causes of Death Collaborators: Global, regional, and national age-sex specific all-cause and cause-specific mortality for 240 causes of death, 1990-2013: a systematic analysis for the global burden of disease study 2013. Lancet. 2015;385(9963):117–71. https://doi.org/10.1016/S0140-6736(14)61682-2.
7. National Road Safety Coordinating Office Ethiopia: Overview of the Road Safety in Ethiopia. 2008.
8. Tadesse B, Tekilu S, Nega B, Seyoum N. Pattern of injury and associated variables as seen in the emergency Department at Tikur Anbessa Specialized Referral Hospital, Addis Ababa, Ethiopia. East Central Afr J Surg. 2014;19(1):73–82.
9. Bashah DT, Dachew BA, Tiruneh BT. Prevalence of injury and associated factors among patients visiting the Emergency Departments of Amhara Regional State Referral Hospitals, Ethiopia: a cross-sectional study. BMC Emerg Med. 2015;15(20):3.
10. Woldemichael K, Berhanu N. Magnitude and pattern of injury in Jimma University specialized hospital, south West Ethiopia. Ethiop J Health Sci. 2011;21(3):155–65.
11. Ogendi JOK, Ayisi JG. Causes of injuries resulting in a visit to the emergency department of a Provincial General Hospital, Nyanza, western Kenya. Afr Health Sci. 2011;11(2):255–61.

6

Management and outcomes of patients presenting with sepsis and septic shock to the emergency department during nursing handover

Sami Alsolamy[1], Atheer Al-Sabhan[2], Najla Alassim[2], Musharaf Sadat[3], Eman Al Qasim[4], Hani Tamim[4,5] and Yaseen M Arabi[3,4,6,7*]

Abstract

Background: Clinical handover is an important process for the transition of patient-care responsibility to the next healthcare provider, but it may divert the attention of the team away from active patients. This is challenging in the Emergency Department (ED) because of highly dynamic patient conditions and is likely relevant in conditions that requires time-sensitive therapies, such as sepsis. We aimed to examine the management and outcomes of patients presenting with sepsis and septic shock to the ED during nursing handover.

Methods: This retrospective cohort study was conducted at a 115-bed ED and more than 200,000 annual ED visits, within a 900-bed academic tertiary care center. Data on Surviving Sepsis Campaign (SSC) bundle elements and hospital mortality were collected for all ≥14-year-old patients who presented to the ED with a diagnosis of sepsis and septic shock between January 1, 2011 and October 30, 2013. Our primary outcome was time to antibiotics, were other SSC bundle elements and mortality counted as secondary outcomes. Patients were divided into two groups: 1) handover time group, comprising patients who presented an hour before or after the start of handover time (6–8 AM/PM), and 2) non-handover time group, comprising patients who presented over the remaining 20 h.

Results: During the study period, 1330 patients presented with sepsis or septic shock (228, handover time group; 1102, non-handover time group). No significant differences were found between the handover time and non-handover time groups, respectively, in median time to antibiotic administration (100 [interquartile range (IQR) 57–172] vs. 95 [IQR 50–190] minutes; $P = 0.07$), median time to serum lactate result (162 [IQR 108–246] vs. 156 [IQR 180–246] minutes; $P = 0.33$) and median time to obtain blood culture (54 [IQR 36–119] vs. 52 [IQR 28–103] minutes; $P = 0.52$), and hospital mortality rate (29.4% vs. 28.9%; $P = 0.89$).

Conclusion: No significant differences were found in median time of SSC bundle elements or hospital mortality between patients who presented during the handover and non-handover times.

Keywords: Sepsis, Handover, Nursing

* Correspondence: arabi@ngha.med.sa
[3]Intensive Care Department, King Abdulaziz Medical City, Riyadh, Kingdom of Saudi Arabia
[4]King Saud Bin Abdulaziz University for Health Sciences, King Abdullah International Medical Research Center, Riyadh, Kingdom of Saudi Arabia
Full list of author information is available at the end of the article

Background

Handover is an essential process in the Emergency Department (ED), as patient care is provided in a continuum around the clock manner; it follows, staff must work in shifts [1]. Handover is defined as a transition of care, responsibility, and future management or disposition plans to the next healthcare provider [2]. This definition applies to all health care workers, including physicians, nurses, and care assistants.

Nursing handover is a complex process that requires effective transfer of all required patient information in the most time-efficient manner. This process needs good communication skills and time management. Trivial miscommunication may lead to delivery of inaccurate or incomplete data, resulting in delayed care or other adverse effects [3, 4]. Nursing handover time has been recognized as a time where adverse events are more likely to occur [4]. In addition, the quality of handover has a direct effect on the quality of patient care over the following shift [5]. In the ED, this complexity is further increased because new patients, in stable or unstable condition, can arrive at any time, regardless of the handover time. A prospective observational study addressing ED handover problems revealed deficiencies in the handover processes [4]. These deficiencies were mainly noted in communication and disposition of information [4]. In another study that assessed the differences in information retention between various handover styles, the authors concluded that purely verbal handover processes are even more prone to serious data loss [6]. The lack of transfer of some information during the handover process may significantly reduce the overall quality of patient care [4, 7]. Therefore, it is crucial to investigate delays in treating patients arriving at the ED during handover time.

Reviewing the literature, we found ED handover studies that focused on evaluating the quality of care transfer, the need to initiate a standardized tool to aid the process, and on reporting handover-related errors and adverse events. Interestingly, we did not find any studies that investigated the effect of handover time on the patients with time-sensitive disorders who visited the ED during the nursing handover time. Sepsis is an important time-sensitive condition in which delays in providing care, such as delays in antibiotic administration, are associated with adverse outcomes. In particular, delays in antibiotic administration have been shown to be associated with a 7.6% decrease in survival for each hour of delay in antimicrobial administration during the 6 h after the first hour of documented hypotension [8]. In this study, we aimed to evaluate the direct impact of handover time on the management of sepsis. We compared different processes measurements to reflect the quality of sepsis care, including the time to intravenous antibiotic administration, time to serum lactate result and time to obtain blood culture among patients who arrived at the ED during the nursing handover time in comparison to those who arrived at other times. We hypothesized that arrival at the ED during the nursing handover period is associated with delay in management of septic patients, and with worse outcomes.

Methods

Study design and setting

The study was performed in a large, urban, tertiary-care ED with an Emergency Medicine Residency Program. The ED is staffed with board-certified emergency medicine physicians, and has 115 beds. The number of annual ED visits range from approximately 200,000 to 214,000 per year at this 900-bed academic tertiary care center. In this study, we used data from the Sepsis Database, collected as part of a quality improvement project conducted by the Intensive Care and Emergency Medicine Departments. The Sepsis Database used the 2008 and 2012 Surviving Sepsis Campaign (SSC) tools.

Selection of participants

We included all patients aged ≥14 years who were admitted to the ED with a diagnosis of sepsis and septic shock between January 1, 2011 and October 30, 2013. In our institution, nursing shifts are 12-h based in all departments. Nursing handover process is done at the bedside using both verbal and written forms. The form used in our institution is SBAR (Situation, Background, Assessment, Recommendation) [9], which must be filled by the endorsing nurse to the receiving nurse. For operative purposes, sepsis was defined as systemic inflammatory response syndrome with acute organ dysfunction secondary to documented or suspected infection. Septic shock was defined as sepsis with persistent hypotension after fluid resuscitation with at least 20 mL/kg of crystalloid (or equivalent) [10]. Patients were identified as having sepsis or septic shock based on clinical assessments performed by the ED physicians. We divided these patients into two groups: 1) a handover time group that included patients who visited the ED an hour before or an hour after the handover time (6–8 AM and PM), and 2) a non-handover time group that included patients who arrived at the ED over the remaining 20 h. We chose the 2-h duration to study the effect of the handover because nurses typically start to prepare for the handover one hour prior to the handover time, and handover sessions can last almost an hour after their initiation.

Methods and measurements

We extracted the following data from the Sepsis Database: ED arrival time, source of infection, physical examination findings, laboratory findings, time-to-antibiotic administration (from arrival to ED), time-to-lactate results and time-to-obtaining blood culture, mechanical ventilation requirement, and hospital mortality [10]. The primary study outcome was the time-to-antibiotic administration, time-to-lactate results and time-to-obtaining blood culture. The study was approved by the Institutional Review Board of Ministry of National Guard-Health affairs, and the informed consent requirement was waived.

Data analysis

Because of the skewed data distribution, we have presented data as median and inter-quartile range for continuous variables, and frequency and proportion for categorical variables. Continuous variables were compared between two groups using the *t*-test, and categorical values were compared using the chi-square test. All data management and analysis was performed with SAS (version 9.1; SAS Institute, Inc., Cary, NC).

Results

Baseline characteristics

Over the study period, 1330 patients fulfilled the diagnostic criteria for sepsis and septic shock, and were included in the final analysis: 228 patients in the handover time group and 1102 patients in the non-handover time group.

The presenting characteristics of patients who arrived during the handover time and those who arrived during the non-handover time are presented in Table 1. The predominant sources of infection in both groups were pneumonia and urinary tract infection. Patients presenting with septic shock made up 38.6% of patients in the handover time group and 40.9% of patients in the non-handover time group. The proportion of patients requiring mechanical ventilation was similar in both groups (29%). Lastly, non-handover group did not differ from handover group patients in terms of initial signs and symptoms nor lab results (Table 1).

Processes of care and outcomes

All patients received antibiotics, and median time-to-antibiotic administration showed a tendency of being longer in the handover time group (100 [IQR 57–172] minutes) as compared to the non-handover time group (95 [IQR 50–190] minutes; $P = 0.07$). The distribution of median time-to-antibiotic administration by hour of day is presented in Fig. 1. The median time-to-lactate results in the handover time group (162 [IQR 108–246] minutes) was not significantly different from that in the non-handover time group (156 [IQR 180–246] minutes; $P = 0.33$). The median time-to-obtaining blood cultures in the handover time group (54 [IQR 36–119] minutes) was not significantly different from that in the non-handover time group (52 [IQR 28–103] minutes; $P = 0.52$). The hospital mortality rate in the handover time group (29.4%) was not significantly different from that in the non-handover time group (28.9%; $P = 0.89$).

Table 1 The presenting characteristics of patients who arrived during the handover time and those who arrived during the non-handover time

	Handover time	Non-Handover time	*P*-value
All patients	*N* = 228	*N* = 1102	
Source of sepsis, no. (%)			
Pneumonia	103 (45.2)	499 (45.3)	0.98
Urinary tract infection	32 (14)	173 (15.7)	0.53
Acute abdominal infection	15 (6.6)	80 (7.3)	0.72
Soft tissue infection	6 (2.6)	42 (3.8)	0.38
Other infections	84 (36.8)	376 (34.1)	0.43
Signs and Symptoms, no. (%)			
Temperature > 38 °C	57 (25)	281 (25.5)	0.87
Temperature < 36 °C	6 (2.6)	41 (3.7)	0.42
Acutely altered mental status	47 (20.6)	217 (19.7)	0.75
Chills and rigors	2 (0.9)	18 (1.6)	0.39
Heart Rate > 90/min	201 (88.2)	945 (85.8)	0.34
Respiratory Rate > 20/min	197 (86.4)	928 (84.2)	0.40
Hypotension*	75 (32.9)	332 (30.1)	0.41
Hypoxia*	75 (32.9)	332 (30.1)	0.41
Laboratory Findings, no. (%)			
Leukocytosis*	99 (43.4)	452 (41)	0.50
Leukopenia*	14 (6.1)	49 (4.5)	0.27
Increased creatinine*	13 (5.7)	99 (9)	0.10
Thrombocytopenia*	8 (3.5)	33 (3)	0.68
Hyperbilirubinemia*	5 (2.2)	41 (3.7)	0.25
Hyperlactatemia*	100 (43.9)	458 (41.6)	0.52
Coagulopathy*	13 (5.7)	57 (5.2)	0.74

*Hypotension: systolic blood pressure < 90, mean arterial pressure < 65 or systolic blood pressure decrease > 40 mmHg from baseline, *Hypoxia: oxygen requirement to maintain oxygen saturation > 90%, *Leukocytosis: WBC count > 12 Å~ 109/L, *Leucopenia: white blood cell count < 4 Å~ 109/L, *Increased creatinine: creatinine increase > 176.8 mmol/L, *Thrombocytopenia: platelet count < 100 Å~ 109/L, *Hyperbilirubinemia: bilirubin > 34.2 mmol/L, *Hyperlactatemia: lactate > 2 mmol/L, *Coagulopathy: international normalized ratio (INR) > 1

Discussion

Handovers are pivotal junctures and integral process in the continuity of care in every patient's clinical course. To the best of our knowledge, the idea of handover time as a possible distractor that might delay urgent patient care is not addressed in current literature. We aim to shed light on the duration of handover process as a possible time where patient care is affected. In this study, we evaluated the direct effect of nursing handover process on patient care. We used a sepsis database to compare ED processes and outcomes between patients who arrived at the ED during nursing handover time and those who arrived during non-handover time.

Our results showed a trend of longer time-to-antibiotic administration in handover group, however this was not

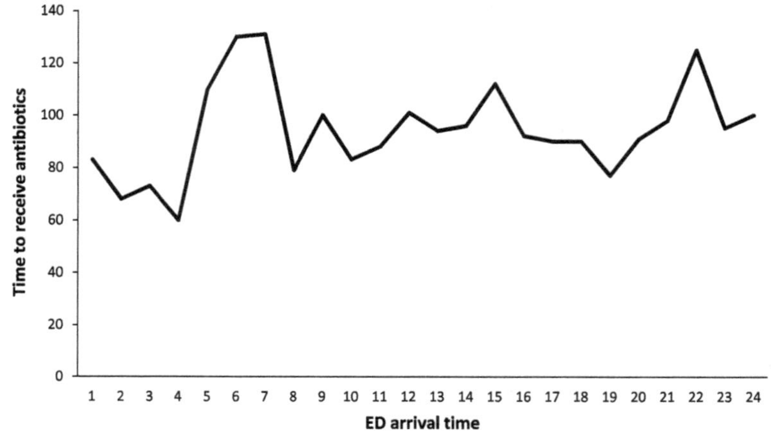

Fig. 1 The distribution of median time-to-antibiotic administration by hour of day with the arrival in ED

clinically nor statistically significant. Nonetheless, the clinical value is unconvincing; as 5 min' difference, might be minor when it comes to antibiotic delivery. It follows, additional studies with another time sensitive assessment tools are needed to address the clinical outcome of this delay, and how to prevent it. We found no significant association between ED nursing handover and time-to- lactate results or time-to-obtaining blood culture, or hospital mortality in patients admitted with a diagnosis of sepsis and septic shock. This could be explained by our ED nurses are vigilant with alerts and our institution was conducting SSC with constant reminders of early management and septic alerts [11]. Consequently, our results may not reflect the situation in institutions with different methods of handover.

A prospective observational study addressing ED handover problems revealed deficiencies in the handover processes [4]. These deficiencies were mainly noted in communication and disposition of information [4]. In another study that assessed the differences in information retention between various handover styles, the authors concluded that purely verbal handover processes are even more prone to serious data loss [6]. In light of that, researchers have been developing new tools to ease the process and grant adequate transfer of information [9]. These tools have been shown to improve nursing handover [12–19].

The main strengths of our study include the numbers of patients included, detailed data collection, the tertiary academic setting with numerous complex and critically ill patients, and standardized data collection using the SSC tools. As a retrospective cohort study, the present study has some important limitations. Foremost, the study aimed to evaluate the direct impact of handover time on time to time-to-antibiotic administration, time-to-lactate results, and time-to-obtaining blood culture, as surrogate indicators of the quality of sepsis and septic shock management. Nonetheless, other important measures in sepsis management were not investigated such as time to effective fluid resuscitation. Additionally, there is inherent variation and subjectivity in the handover process among ED nursing staff might have underpowered our results. Lastly, because of the retrospective nature of this study and the fact that it was conducted in a busy ED, others factors, such as ED overcrowding and boarding patients in ED, could have affected the study results.

Conclusion

This is one of the first reports of the impact of ED nursing handover on time-sensitive interventions that involve multiple tasks performed by ED nurses. Due to the retrospective nature, patient population with single pathology, and our structured handover process that might have reflected on the results of this study. Future studies are still needed to explore ED functionality during the handover time.

Abbreviations

ED: Emergency department; IQR: Interquartile range; SAS: Statistical analysis software; SSC: Surviving sepsis campaign

Acknowledgements

None

Funding

None

Authors' contributions

SS: conception, acquisition of data, design, analytical plan, drafting of the manuscript and critical revision of the manuscript for important intellectual content, approval of the final version to be published. AA, MS and YA: Drafting of the manuscript and critical revision of the manuscript for important intellectual content, approval of the final version to be published. NA and EQ: Drafting of the manuscript, data acquisition and critical revision of the manuscript for important intellectual content, approval of the final version to be published. HT: Statistical analysis and critical revision of the manuscript for important intellectual content, approval of the final version to be published.

Competing interests
The authors declare that they have no competing interests.

Author details
[1]Emergency Medicine and Intensive Care Department, College of Medicine, King Saud Bin Abdulaziz University for Health Sciences, King Abdulaziz Medical City, Riyadh, Kingdom of Saudi Arabia. [2]Emergency Medicine Department, King Abdulaziz Medical City, Riyadh, Kingdom of Saudi Arabia. [3]Intensive Care Department, King Abdulaziz Medical City, Riyadh, Kingdom of Saudi Arabia. [4]King Saud Bin Abdulaziz University for Health Sciences, King Abdullah International Medical Research Center, Riyadh, Kingdom of Saudi Arabia. [5]Department of Internal Medicine, American University of Beirut-Medical Center, Beirut, Lebanon. [6]College of Medicine, King Saud Bin Abdulaziz University for Health Sciences, Riyadh, Kingdom of Saudi Arabia. [7]Respiratory Services, King Abdulaziz Medical City, Riyadh, Kingdom of Saudi Arabia.

References
1. Krogstad U, Hofoss D, Hjortdahl P. Continuity Of hospital care: beyond the question of personal contact. BMJ. 2002;324:36–8. https://doi.org/10.1136/bmj.324.7328.0a.
2. Odell A. Communication theory and the shift handover report. Br J Nurs. 1996;5:1323–6. https://doi.org/10.12968/bjon.1996.5.21.1323.
3. Thomas EJ, Studdert DM, Burstin HR, et al. Incidence and types of adverse events and negligent care in Utah and Colorado. Med Care. 2000;38:261–71. https://doi.org/10.1097/00005650-200003000-00003.
4. Ye K, McD Taylor D, Knott JC, Dent A, MacBean CE. Handover in the emergency department: deficiencies and adverse effects. Emerg Med Australas. 2007;19:433–41. https://doi.org/10.1111/j.1742-6723.2007.00984.x.
5. Gage W. Evaluating handover practice in an acute NHS trust. Nurs Stand. 2013;27:43–50. https://doi.org/10.7748/ns2013.07.27.48.43.e7753.
6. McFetridge B, Gillespie M, Goode D, Melby V. An exploration of the handover process of critically ill patients between nursing staff from the emergency department and the intensive care unit. Nurs Crit Care. 2007;12:261–9. https://doi.org/10.1111/j.1478-5153.2007.00244.x.
7. Spoelstra-de Man AME, Girbes ARJ. Comment on "surviving sepsis campaign: international guidelines for management of severe sepsis and septic shock: 2008" by Dellinger et al. Intensive Care Med 2008;34:1160–1162; author reply 1163-1164. doi:https://doi.org/10.1007/s00134-008-1089-5.
8. Kumar A, Roberts D, Wood KE, et al. Duration of hypotension before initiation of effective antimicrobial therapy is the critical determinant of survival in human septic shock*. Crit Care Med. 2006;34:1589–96. https://doi.org/10.1097/01.CCM.0000217961.75225.E9.
9. Thomas CM, Bertram E, Johnson D. The SBAR communication technique: teaching nursing students professional communication skills. Nurse Educ. 2009;34(4):176–80.
10. Rhodes A, Evans LE, Alhazzani W, et al. Surviving sepsis campaign: international guidelines for Management of Sepsis and Septic Shock: 2016. Crit Care Med. 2017;45:486–552. https://doi.org/10.1097/CCM.0000000000002255.
11. Alsolamy S, Al Salamah M, Al Thagafi M, Al-Dorzi HM, Marini AM, Aljerian N, et al. Diagnostic accuracy of a screening electronic alert tool for severe sepsis and septic shock in the emergency department. BMC medical informatics and decision making. 2014;14(105)
12. Bergs J, Lambrechts F, Mulleneers I, Lenaerts K, Hauquier C, Proesmans G, et al. A tailored intervention to improving the quality of intrahospital nursing handover. International emergency nursing. 2017;
13. Breuer RK, Taicher B, Turner DA, Cheifetz IM, Rehder KJ. Standardizing postoperative PICU handovers improves handover metrics and patient outcomes. Pediatric critical care medicine : a journal of the Society of Critical Care Medicine and the World Federation of Pediatric Intensive and Critical Care Societies. 2015;16(3):256–63.
14. Agarwal HS, Saville BR, Slayton JM, Donahue BS, Daves S, Christian KG, et al. Standardized postoperative handover process improves outcomes in the intensive care unit: a model for operational sustainability and improved team performance*. Crit Care Med. 2012;40(7):2109–15.
15. Ting WH, Peng FS, Lin HH, Hsiao SM. The impact of situation-background-assessment-recommendation (SBAR) on safety attitudes in the obstetrics department. Taiwanese journal of obstetrics & gynecology. 2017;56(2):171–4.
16. Martin HA, Ciurzynski SM. Situation, Background, Assessment, and Recommendation-Guided Huddles Improve Communication and Teamwork in the emergency department. Journal of emergency nursing: JEN : official publication of the Emergency Department Nurses Association. 2015;41(6):484–8.
17. Graan SM, Botti M, Wood B, Redley B. Nursing Handover from ICU to cardiac ward: standardised tools to reduce safety risks. Australian critical care : official journal of the Confederation of Australian Critical Care Nurses. 2016;29(3):165–71.
18. Achrekar MS, Murthy V, Kanan S, Shetty R, Nair M, Khattry N. Introduction of situation, background, assessment, recommendation into nursing practice: a prospective study. Asia-Pacific journal of oncology nursing. 2016;3(1):45–50.
19. Marmor GO, Li MY. Improving Emergency department medical clinical handover: barriers at the bedside. Emergency medicine Australasia : EMA. 2017;29(3):297–302.

7

The feasibility, acceptability and preliminary testing of a novel, low-tech intervention to improve pre-hospital data recording for pre-alert and handover to the Emergency Department

David Fitzpatrick[1*], Douglas Maxwell[2] and Alan Craigie[3]

Abstract

Background: Poor communication during patient handover is recognised internationally as a root cause of a significant proportion of preventable deaths. Data used in handover is not always easily recorded using ambulance based tablets, particularly in time-critical cases. Paramedics have therefore developed pragmatic workarounds (writing on gloves or scrap paper) to record these data. However, such practices can conflict with policy, data recorded can be variable, easily lost and negatively impact on handover quality.

Methods: This study aimed to measure the feasibility and acceptability of a novel, low tech intervention, designed to support clinical information recording and delivery during pre-alert and handover within the pre-hospital and ED setting. A simple pre and post-test design was used with a historical control. Eligible participants included all ambulance clinicians based at one large city Ambulance Station ($n = 69$) and all nursing and physician staff ($n = 99$) based in a city Emergency Department.

Results: Twenty five (36%) ambulance clinicians responded to the follow-up survey. Most felt both the pre-alert and handover components of the card were either 'useful-very useful' ($n = 23$ (92%); and $n = 18$ (72%) respectively. Nineteen (76%) used the card to record clinical information and almost all (n = 23 (92%) felt it *'useful'* to *'very useful'* in supporting pre-alert. Similarly, 65% ($n = 16$) stated they *'often'* or *'always'* used the card to support handover. For pre-alert information there were improvements in the provision of 8/11 (72.7%) clinical variables. Results from the post-test survey measuring ED staff ($n = 37$) perceptions of handover demonstrated small ($p < 0.05$) improvements in handover in 3/5 domains measured.

Conclusion: This novel low-tech intervention was highly acceptable to ambulance clinician participants, improving their data recording and information exchange processes. However, further well conducted studies are required to test the impact of this intervention on information exchange during pre-alert and handover.

Keywords: Paramedic, Ambulance, Emergency department, Handover, Pre-alert, Intervention, Feasibility

* Correspondence: david.fitzpatrick@stir.ac.uk
[1]Faculty of Health Sciences and Sport, University of Stirling, Stirling FK9 4LA, Scotland
Full list of author information is available at the end of the article

Background

Poor communication during patient handover is recognised internationally as a root cause of a significant proportion of preventable deaths [1] and as such is named as one the of the top five World Health Organisation improvement priorities [2]. Despite the introduction of a number of recommended strategies to reduce this harm, the handover phase of care continues to impact negatively on patient outcome [3–6]. It is widely accepted that handover of patients in any clinical setting carries significant risk [7]. However, handover of critically ill or injured patients from the pre-hospital to Emergency Department (ED) team carries additional risk due to the time critical nature of the process and multiple human factors involved in dealing with stressful clinical events [5, 8]. Such knowledge has led to calls for further, more rigorous research into handover, and to develop solutions to support handover in diverse environments [5, 9, 10].

Despite the limited evidence on pre-hospital to ED handover practice, a number of pragmatic options, informed by theory, have been recommended. These include for example, the development of shared mental models, standardisation of approach (an agreed handover system and format/mnemonic) applied at the interface between professional domains, and the introduction of technology to support and enhance the process [5, 7, 11]. But unfortunately, cultivating a movement towards a shared mental model has remained a challenge with evidence of considerable inconsistencies in mnemonic usage and preference both nationally and internationally [12–15]. Beyond these higher level, theoretically informed systems and processes, there are other more fundamental and pragmatic challenges to consider and address.

Recording clinical data used during handover accurately and with ease is incredibly challenging during the delivery of prehospital care. These data are the cornerstone of clinical handover, independently or aggregated, they provide an immediate clinical impression of the patient's condition [16, 17]. Excluding some of these essential variables during pre-alert or handover may delay subsequent life-saving interventions [18, 19]. The importance of developing tools to support the recording and handover of these data is established in the study by Bhabra et al. [20] who identified only 33% of data is retained on first handover when relying on memory alone, but where a standardized, printed form was used, 99% of information was retained. Rightly, therefore, attention has recently been directed towards the use of technology in supporting both data capture and handover with the development of natural language generation software [21, 22] and in exploring ambulance clinicians use of electronic patient report forms [23]. Hardware placed in ambulances to support the recording of clinical data used during handover is often in tablet form. However, this technology is not always carried by ambulance clinicians to the patient's side, particularly in those incidents that are time-critical. Consequently, data is often retrospectively entered, post-handover. And whilst technology continues to advance in this area, more rapid and accessible methods are required now to support the recording of essential clinical data in the high acuity patient.

Pragmatic workarounds have been developed by ambulance clinicians and currently it is not uncommon for clinical data to be recorded on the back of a gloved hand or on scrap paper [21, 24, 25]. However, there are potential infection control risks with the former and neither practice necessarily comply with data protection legislation. Additionally, data recorded will be variable and with heavy contamination of gloves being a particular problem in these environments, glove changes can be frequent [26]. As such, both gloves or paper will be easily discarded or lost.

There currently exists a paucity of evidence, and therefore understanding and knowledge, on how ambulance clinicians can best record and deliver information essential for handover. There is therefore an immediate need to investigate and develop more pragmatic and low-tech solutions to record information that supports information exchange between ambulance clinicians and ED staff.

Methods

This project aimed to measure the feasibility and acceptability of a novel intervention designed to support clinical information recording and delivery during pre-alert and handover within the pre-hospital and ED setting.

Design and setting

A simple pre and post-test design was used with a historical control. The Scottish Ambulance Service (SAS) is a national service covering 30,420 sqm, serving a population of 5.4 million [27] and responding to around 650,000 emergency calls per annum [28]. The service is primarily set within an Anglo-American model of care [29] whereby road based Paramedics and Emergency Medical Technicians (EMT) deliver the majority of care. At the time of study the service operated within 5 geographical Divisions (North, East, South, West and West Central). The study was undertaken in West Central Division, which covers the most densely populated areas in the West of Scotland. Our intervention hospital and ambulance station were therefore located in a busy urban setting in the centre of Glasgow; population 606,000. During the 3 month study period (February to April 2017) the ED received 22,913 patients [30], with Ambulance Clinicians at the intervention station responding to circa 5339 emergency calls during the same time period [31].

Participants

Eligible participants included all ambulance clinicians ($n = 69$) based at one city centre Ambulance Station and all nursing and physician staff ($n = 99$) based in the ED of a large city hospital in Glasgow. The ambulance station selected was the largest in Glasgow and, as such, provided a broad demographic pool of clinicians; clinical grade EMT's 45% [$n = 31$] vs. Paramedic 55% [$n = 38$]) and clinical experience (service in years range from 1 to 40). Due to organisational time pressures we intentionally kept to a minimum the data requested from ED staff and so only demographic data on job title was sought (Nurse/Physician). All ED participants were invited to complete the respective pre and post-test questionnaires.

Intervention design

The intervention design was informed by the collective results of two unpublished studies i) a survey investigating handover in the pre-hospital domain and ii) a pre-test survey of handover practices of local ambulance clinicians ($n = 23/69$; 33%). A study stakeholder group was formed to synthesize the results of both along with published evidence and particularly within the context of existing challenges affecting key points in the handover process: pre-handover, arrival, handover and post-handover [7]. A specific focus was retained on the technical aspects of information recording in both the prehospital and in-hospital settings. The stakeholder group consisted of front line ambulance clinicians ($n = 6$), an Emergency Medicine physician and ED registrar, senior paramedic managers ($n = 4$), an applied health service researcher and a Union representative. Infection Control and Data Protection Leads from the SAS ensured compliance with existing legislation and authorised the final prototype used in testing.

A graphic design expert designed the card based on the stakeholder group's requirements. The prototype intervention consisted of a double-sided A6 card in high contrast colour with pre-alert and handover clinical information requirements on opposing sides. Corresponding boxes for clinical variables were available for writing in with a marker pen. Included variables and final mnemonic choice were based on the synthesized data and a compromise on both the needs of the ambulance clinicians and ED staff. The variables included were known prognostic indicators (individually or collectively) for degrees of severity in injury and illness [32, 33].

The intervention was piloted in a simulated setting with prehospital critical care practitioners and physicians prior to being finalised. The simulation led to a change in physical format from a card encased in a sealable plastic cover to a stand-alone, high density plastic card (Additional file 1). A number of pens were tested and a type selected that ensured rapid dry and non-smudge properties. To support the concept of a shared mental model, an A4 'ambulance form' (AF) was developed for use within the ED (Additional file 2). This consisted of a pre-printed A4 sheet placed next to the ambulance radio located within the ED; this is the radio system that receives pre-alert calls from ambulance clinicians who are bringing in critically ill patients. The AF content duplicated the information provided on the ambulance pre-alert and handover card.

Intervention procedure

Ambulance clinicians ($n = 69$) at the participating station were each issued a personal issue pre - alert and handover card (PAHC) with pens. An instruction notice was placed at various strategic locations around the ambulance station. Cards were to be used in time-critical cases with both the pre-alert and handover sections to be completed contemporaneously with assessment at appropriate times during care. During pre-alert and handover clinical information would be delivered in the sequence provided on the PAHC. For data protection purposes recording of date of birth and surname was not permitted. Post incident, these data were transferred onto the electronic patient report form in the ambulance as per usual practice. In accordance with infection control procedures the cards were cleaned using Tuffie© wipes and dried with a paper towel.

Within the ED, those receiving the ambulance pre-alert were instructed to record all clinical information provided via the radio call in the respective boxes on the AF. On arrival within the ED ambulance clinicians then verbally delivered the clinical information in the sequence provided on PAHC. Receiving staff would record this handover information in the respective sections on their AF.

Data collection tools

Pre-test measures

Subjective During February 2016 opinions of ED staff on ambulance clinician handover were measured via a short online survey (Additional file 3). In the absence of rigorously validated and accepted measures of perceptions of pre-alert and handover quality in the ED, the survey development was informed through key elements of handover identified in the study by Ledema et al. [3] along with the clinical experiences of study investigators. Due to the significant pressures of the ED environment, the survey was deliberately designed to be short and succinct and thus reduce time required for completion. Five domains of handover were measured using a five point Likert scale (1- Always to 5 – Never). The domains measured were: i) Structure ii) standardised iii) Focus iv) repetition avoidance and v) interruption avoidance. Potential participants ($n = 99$) received an e-mail containing a link to the online survey along with information on the project. Consent was presumed by completion of the questionnaire. These data formed the historic control.

Objective Base-line data on pre-alert and handover were extracted from the month preceding the intervention introduction (January 2017) using the paper-based AF which had already been introduced for use by ED staff. Key clinical data were recorded on these sheets during the pre-alert and handover. Ambulance Clinicians in the intervention station were not made aware of the study prior to its commencement.

Post-test measures

Subjective Following the 3 month intervention test period (February – April 2017) questionnaires were sent to both ED and Ambulance Clinicians during May 2017. Ambulance clinicians were sent a paper-based questionnaire (Additional file 4), while ED staff were invited again, via e-mail, to complete the online questionnaire (Additional file 3). The different questionnaire formats reflected the operational environments for each clinical group and were designed to improve response rates. Ambulance Clinicians are established as hard to reach populations in questionnaire based research and traditionally deliver low response rates [34–36]. The decision to use paper-based surveys for ambulance clinicians was informed by the predictable difficulties experienced with a highly mobile workforce, their inability to access computers and past studies undertaken in similar settings [37, 38] that used evidence informed methods [39, 40] which had previously provided improved response rates. The questionnaire for ambulance clinicians focused on measuring the feasibility and acceptability of the prompt card. Questions consisted of Likert scales and dichotomised yes/no responses. ED staff repeated the same questions used in the pre-test questionnaire. This permitted comparisons between the pre-test (historical control) and post-test measures.

Prior to distribution, questionnaires were assessed for ease of completion and comprehension. This led to a small number of changes in wording to aid comprehension. Again participants were provided with a cover letter and information sheet with consent presumed by completion of the questionnaire. For ambulance clinician participants pens were provided in the invitation envelops and a cardboard 'post box' located in the ambulance station mess room to facilitate ease of completion and submission.

Objective Ambulance Forms were routinely completed by ED Nurses during handover and collected by receptionists thereafter. These forms were divided into i) a pre-alert information section and ii) a handover information section and included the same variables as were presented in the ambulance clinician's pre-alert and handover cards. Frequency counts were used to measure clinical variables recorded during both the pre-alert and handovers provided by ambulance clinicians. These data permitted pre and post-test data comparisons to be made on the interventions impact.

Analysis

Data were recorded on Microsoft Excel 2010 prior to conversion to Statistical Package for the Social Sciences (SPSS) (v.21). Descriptive statistics were used to present the results of the questionnaire. Chi Square tests were used to compare the frequency counts between the hospital pre-alert pre and post-test objective data. Mann Whitney U analysis was used to compare the median ratings of the pre and post-test measures on opinions of handover quality.

Results

Ambulance participants

A four week intervention run-in period from 1st to 28th February was permitted to enable ambulance clinicians and ED staff to familiarise with the intervention. During the 3 month study period ambulance clinicians at the intervention station responded to 5339 call and conveyed 1938 (30%) of these patients to the participating ED. There were approximately 160 (20/week) pre-alerts made to the ED during this time period. Thirty six percent of ambulance clinicians ($n = 25$) completed the post-test questionnaire; paramedics 70.8% ($n = 18$) vs Technicians 29.2% ($n = 7$). The median length of service in years was 16 (IQR 8–30).

Acceptability and perceived utility of intervention

Ninety six percent ($n = 24$) of participants reported receiving the intervention. Most felt both the pre-alert and handover components of the card were 'useful' to 'very useful' (92%; $n = 23$ for pre-alert and 72%; $n = 18$) for handover). In measuring the utility of the intervention, questions focused on the use of the card, its legibility, format and pen performance. Over three quarters of responders (76%; $n = 19$) reported using the card to record clinical information and almost all (92%; $n = 23$) felt it *'useful'* to *'very useful'* in supporting pre-alert. A small proportion 16% ($n = 4$) reported recording information on back of gloved hand and 8% ($n = 2$) still relying on memory. Almost two thirds of participants (65%; $n = 16$) stated they 'often' or 'always' used the card for handover.

The pen was perceived to perform well with 60% rating it either 'good' (12%; $n = 3$) or 'very good' (48%; $n = 12$). However, a small proportion (12%; $n = 3$) rated the pen as either 'poor' or 'very poor'. Perceptions on the cards legibility in both bright or poor lighting were also sought. Sixty four percent ($n = 16$) rated it as 'easy' (24%; $n = 6$) or 'very easy' (40%; $n = 10$) to read in bright lighting and 56% (n = 16) 'easy' (24%; n = 6) or 'very easy' (32%; $n = 8$) to read in poor lighting. Forty percent (n = 10) were neutral in their response.

Emergency department participants

Thirty seven percent ($n = 37/99$) of ED Staff responded to the pre-test questionnaire; Doctors 63.2% ($n = 24$) and Nurses 36.8% ($n = 13$). Slightly less responded to the post-test questionnaire; 29% ($n = 29/99$); Doctors 48% ($n = 14$) and Nurses 52% ($n = 15$).

Perceptions of handover quality

ED staff (Nurses and Physicians) were asked to rate their experiences of different aspects of Ambulance Clinician handover (as per 'domains' outlined in methods section previously). The overall responses in the pre-test survey were relatively neutral but clearly demonstrated a requirement for improvement in each of the handover domains measured. Results from the post-test survey demonstrated small but statistically significant improvements in perceptions of handover in 3/5 domains measured (Table 1).

Objective measure of pre-alert information

Ambulance pre-alert forms were routinely used within the ED throughout both the pre-and post-test stages of the study. To provide an indication of any change in handover clinical information provision data were taken from three time points i) the month leading up to the intervention introduction, ii) the end of week 5 (after the 4 week bedding in period) and iii) at week 8. Figure 1 demonstrates the trend in variables provided during pre-alert starting at beginning of week 5 of intervention period. Frequency counts and proportions of the variables recorded during pre-alert are presented in Table 2. There was a statistically significant improvement in the delivery of 2/7 (29%) clinical variables during pre-alert. However, non-significant improvements were apparent in the remaining five other clinical variables. Small, non-significant reductions, were also noted in three other variables. Overall demonstrable improvements were identified in 8/12 (67%) variables.

Analysis of the handover section of the ambulance forms within the ED proved problematic. Of the forms that were collected only 32/57 (56%) had at least one of the data fields completed. Only 10.5% ($n = 6$) were fully completed and as a result comparisons with pre-test data were not undertaken. And so, whilst the results suggest a perceived improvement in the quality of handover this could not be measured more objectively as had originally been planned.

Discussion

We aimed to test the feasibility and acceptability of a novel low tech intervention to support the prehospital recording and delivery of clinical information for use by ambulance clinicians during pre-alert and handover. Our measures focused on ambulance clinician's perceptions of the intervention and both subjective and objective elements of the pre-alert and handover process from the ED clinician's perspectives. We also sought to determine whether the data collection tools developed for this study would be sufficient in providing useful measures of improvement in a larger trial.

Acceptability of the intervention

Our study has determined that, overall, Ambulance Clinician participants felt the intervention was useful to very useful, using it to both record and support the delivery of clinical information in the majority of pre-alert and handovers. The perceptions of participating ED staff on handover quality were also positive with significant improvements in 3 out of 5 handover domains measured and small, non-significant improvements in the remaining 2 domains. During pre-alert, despite statistically significant improvements in the provision/recording of only $n = 2$ (29%) clinical variables, overall, positive trends were identified in $n = 8$ (67%) variables. Had we extended final measures beyond the 12 weeks, permitting more familiarity with the intervention and embedding in clinical practice, these figures may have continued to improve.

Table 1 Comparing ED clinicians pre-test and post-test perceptions of handover (Likert scale – 1 = always to 5 = never). Mann-Whitney *U* test comparing median responses

Aspect of handover measured	Pre-test survey results Median (IQR[a])	Post-test survey results Median (IQR[a])	*p*-value (U)
Is structured	3 (2–3)	2 (2–3)	0.126
Is standardised	4 (2–4)	2 (2–3)	<.001
Is focussed	2 (2–3)	2 (2–2.75)	0.223
Avoids repetition	3 (2–3)	2 (2–2.75)	0.014
Avoids interruptions	3 (2.25–4)	2 (2–3)	0.003

[a]*IQR* Inter-quartile range

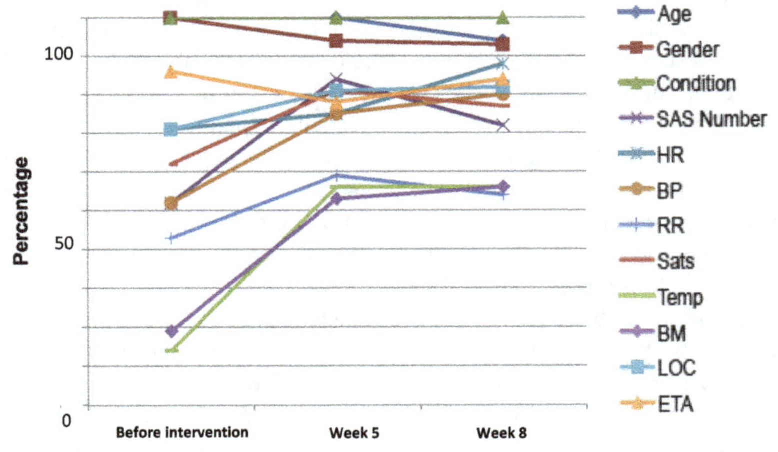

Fig. 1 Trends in clinical variables provided during pre-alert

Feasibility of the introduction of the low-tech intervention

Our intervention was designed to be intuitive, practical and one that, with minor modification, would seamlessly replace existing clinical data recording practices when managing high acuity patients. As such we decided that no formal education would be provided to ambulance clinicians to support the interventions introduction (with the exception of station notices). There were possible risks associated with this approach however. Educational practices within the host ambulance service frequently consist of clinical bulletins posted in station boards or distributed via e-mail and intranet. The efficacy of this educational format has not been formally measured in this setting, however some research has established that similar 'online' forms of education for ambulance clinicians does not necessarily improve adherence to guidance [24]. Additionally, other studies strongly advocate education and training in handover ([25, 41]. The finding that this deliberately pragmatic and considered approach was well accepted by participating clinicians, and that so many ambulance clinicians reported using the intervention for its intended purpose were therefore welcome. This also may suggest that this intuitive intervention could be introduced on a larger scale in future trials with little requirements for formal education.

Initial assessment of the interventions ability to share clinical data

Although this study was not designed or powered to address the question of intervention efficacy, we accessed the data recorded on the AF's within the ED to identify trends. Previous work using similar measures [42] determined that an average 50% of clinical variables were received from ambulance clinicians during handover, but that only 72.9% of the information received was documented by ED staff. Although

Table 2 Recorded frequencies of pre-alert variables provided to ED pre and post-test

Pre-alert variable	Pre-test forms % ($n = 21$)	Post-test forms % ($n = 32$)	% change	p-value chi square
Call sign	52.4% ($n = 11$)	71.9% ($n = 41$)	+19.5	.379
Age	100% ($n = 21$)	100.0% ($n = 32$)	n/a	n/a
Gender	100% ($n = 21$)	93.8% ($n = 30$)	- 6.2	.243
Injury/Illness	100% ($n = 21$)	100% ($n = 32$)	n/a	n/a
LOC[a]	71.4% ($n = 15$)	83.9% ($n = 26$)	+12.5	.281
Resps[a]	42.9% ($n = 9$)	59.3% ($n = 19$)	+16.4	.239
Sats[a]	61.9% ($n = 13$)	81.3% ($n = 26$)	+19.4	.118
Heart rate[a]	71.4% ($n = 15$)	75% ($n = 24$)	+3.6	.773
Blood pressure[a]	52.4% ($n = 11$)	75% ($n = 24$)	+22.6	.089
Blood Glucose[a]	19% ($n = 4$)	53.1% ($n = 17$)	+34.1	.013*
Temp[a]	14.3% ($n = 3$)	56.3% ($n = 18$)	+42	.002*
ETA	85.7% ($n = 18$)	78.1% ($n = 25$)	-7.6	.490

[a]Clinical variables only

*Chi square analysis with an alpha level of 0.05 (exact Sig. [2-sided])

we only report on pre-alert rather than handover data, our pre-intervention average for vital signs provided/recorded was 47.6%, slightly lower than those reported by Carter et al. [42]. However, post intervention, our proportion of clinical variables provided/recorded improved to an average of 69.4%; a 46% increase and proportionately higher than in the study by Carter et al. [42]. Although we were unable to objectively determine if these improvements were as a direct result of the intervention, no other changes in pre-alert or handover were introduced during the study period. And so these identified difference are likely to be a result of the intervention and provide an indication that it may have positively impacted on data provision during pre-alert.

It should be noted too that we are also comparing different stages and forms of communication to those presented in the study by Carter et al. [42] i.e. pre-alert via radio call v's face-to-face handover. There are distractions and pressures likely to present during a face-to-face handover in the ED that do not exist during radio communication; the patient for one. These are likely to impact on the amount and quality of data provided and recorded during handover and may therefore negatively impact on the proportions of variables recorded [25, 41]. Our study does however highlight the importance of this pre-alert phase of information exchange prior to the physical handover. The ability to provide timely and accurate clinical information prior to arrival, and handover, at the ED has been shown to improve care in specific time critical conditions [43, 44]. It is advisable therefore that such pre-arrival information is considered as an essential and central component of the broader handover process and system.

Our measured indications of improvements may also have been influenced by the introduction of a common system for use by both ambulance and ED clinicians. We fostered the shared mental model concept [7] by ensuring both professional groups used the same mnemonic and as such a common understanding of clinical variables required and provided was developed within the system. Ensuring a common expectation on the provision of specific clinical variables has also been shown to improve efficacy of handover [45]. The ability to manually and accurately record pre-alert information contemporaneously [20] negates the requirement for information retention during periods of high cognitive demand and also appears to have supported this process. Either these individual components, or their cumulative parts, may have contributed to the improvement in perceptions of ED participants and the proportion of clinical data provided or recorded during pre-alert.

Notably there were no statistically significant improvements in two of the subjective handover domains measured; *'structured'* and *'focused'*. On reviewing the AF format it was clear that the sequence of clinical data boxes, particularly in the pre-alert section, did not match the sequence provided on the ambulance PAHC. It is highly probable that this had an impact on the flow of pre-alert and handover recording by ED staff and may partially explain why there were no perceived improvements in these variables measured. This was valuable learning and as such changes will be incorporated into future interventions to ensure continuity of clinical variable sequence in both the PAHC and AF.

Challenges and considerations for recording tools aimed at measuring pre-alert and handover data

ED staff consistently used the ambulance pre-alert section of the form to record the pre-alert information thus suggesting this section of the form was a useful and feasible measurement tool. It should be noted that there are likely to be occasions whereby ambulance clinicians, working alone in the rear cab of an ambulance, will be required to prioritise vital signs measured. For example, during management of an unconscious patient the absolute need to provide airway management will take priority over a temperature recording. Similarly the check and identified presence of a radial pulse in a time critical patient serves as a proxy measure of blood pressure and may replace, at least in the short term, the need to record a blood pressure. It is likely therefore that these practical elements may partly explain the variability in frequency counts and inability to consistently reach 100% of clinical variables provided during pre-alert. It also highlights the difficulties in ensuring that all clinical variables are 'always' provided during pre-alert and handover. Occasionally, this is not feasible and should be considered as a limitation to any objective measure.

However, problems were encountered with the completion of the handover section. There were two elements that may have influenced this. Firstly, in our ED site handover data from ambulance clinicians were not always recorded on the AF contemporaneously. This is not unusual in the ED setting. Well known pressures on ED's i.e. crowding and capacity issues lead to distractions known to impact on the accuracy of information recording [41], and perhaps on a reliance on recall of verbal information, previously identified as a contributor to information loss [20, 41, 46]. Secondly, and perhaps a more significant contributor to data loss, were our data collection methods. To ensure data capture, clerical staff were instructed to photocopy the AF's at (or very near to) the time of handover. Ironically this may have led to forms being removed too early and before full completion. Thus, the investigators enthusiasm to capture data early is likely to have had a significant impact on the recording of handover data. These combined factors, therefore, are probable contributors to the loss of information on AF's. Essentially, future studies must ensure rigorous and timely methods of data recording to support the objective measure of the handover component of new interventions. Consideration of an observational component via video recording [47] or an external, supernumerary, observer for contemporaneous note taking would also be helpful and advisable in future studies.

These identified issues also highlight the complex nature of the handover process and the need for investigation beyond just the technical aspects [7]. Low tech or high tech interventions may provide solutions to support the recording and delivery of known essential clinical information during handover, however, more research is clearly required to investigate the non-technical and system elements of ambulance clinician to ED handover. Such systems will undoubtedly require multi-modal interventions to ensure the accurate transfer of clinical information during high acuity situations. As such, our novel low-tech intervention tested in this small-scale study may perhaps be viewed upon as one small component of a larger system of handover. A system that needs further development of multiple components in order to address both the technical and non-technical aspects of handover. Only when these multiple elements of handover are addressed will any true improvements in handover quality and safety be realised.

Strengths and limitation

This was a small-scale study to measure utility and acceptability of a novel intervention. It was conducted in one large city centre ambulance station in Scotland. However, the results were positive and demonstrated the ease at which a simple, pragmatic intervention could be introduced within the prehospital domain. The ambulance clinician response rate was low (36%, $n = 25$) and, as such, is prone to response bias. However, in terms of demographics we found no difference in median length of service between study participants ($Mdn = 16$; IQR 8–30) and overall station population ($Mdn = 15$; IQR 3.5–23.75); $U = 715$; $p = 0.247$. Similarly, there were no difference between proportions of grade; paramedics 55% ($n = 38$) vs 70.8% ($n = 18$) and Technicians 45% ($n = 31$) vs 29.2% ($n = 7$); χ^2 $(1, N = 94) = 1.83$, $p = 0.176$. Despite these similarities in demographics, low response rates and small sample size limit the results generalisability to the wider ambulance population and as such these results should be interpreted with caution. However, the study was not designed to be generalisable or provide a definitive answer to the interventions effectiveness on improving handover. The 'Hawthorne effect' may also have been present during this study with a positive impact on ambulance clinicians pre-alert and handover behaviours [48]. Further research is planned on a larger scale across one Division in Scotland.

The key learning that has taken place during the undertaking of this study will support improvements to methods used to further test both the subjective and objective efficacy of the intervention. Specifically these will include the introduction of additional evidence based methods to improve response rates to questionnaires with consideration also to the addition of online access (via our cab-based computer systems), the need for qualitative components by way of interviews and the use of video footage or observers to objectively record elements of handover.

Conclusion

These results suggest that the introduction of a low tech, novel intervention is very acceptable to ambulance clinicians, intuitive to use, requires little education on use and positively supports their contemporaneous data recording and information exchange processes. Although there are some data to suggest the effectiveness of the intervention in its ability to improve information sharing during pre- alert and handover, this study was neither designed nor powered to do this. However, the overall positive results suggest that further well conducted studies to test an updated intervention, based on feedback provided, are worthwhile. Importantly, future studies should carefully consider, in the absence of advanced data sharing technology, how information required for pre-alert and handover can be recorded contemporaneously to minimise data loss. This will be essential from both a patient safety perspective and to more objectively measure the impact of any future handover intervention.

Abbreviations

AF: Ambulance Form; ED: Emergency Department; EMT: Emergency Medical Technician; PAHC: Pre-alert and Handover Card; SAS: Scottish Ambulance Service

Acknowledgements

Stakeholder Group: Mr. Ian Middlemiss, Mrs. Mary Mulligan, Mr. Keith Colver, Mr. Colin Crookston. Intervention design: Dr. Mary Steele. For feedback on questionnaire design and intervention Ms. Nicola Lawrie, Ms. Laura Adam. Mrs. Susan Wilson for advice on infection control. We also wish to thank Emergency Medical Retrieval Service (EMRS) clinicians for trialling the prototype during simulation. Mr. Derek Milligan for providing data on participating ambulance station call numbers. Significant thanks to all Scottish Ambulance Service Ambulance Clinicians and ED staff who participated in this study.

Additional thanks to the reviewers who provided incredibly constructive feedback that supported the improvement of our manuscript.

Funding

The Scottish Ambulance Service kindly funded the printing of pre-alert/ handover cards.

Authors' contributions
DM came up with the original concept. All three authors DF, DM and AC contributed to the study design and write-up. DF and DM undertook the analysis of data. All authors have read and approved the manuscript.

Competing interests
The authors declare that they have no competing interests.

Author details
[1]Faculty of Health Sciences and Sport, University of Stirling, Stirling FK9 4LA, Scotland. [2]Royal Alexandra Hospital Paisley, NHS Greater Glasgow and Clyde, Corsebar Rd, Paisley, Glasgow PA2 9PN, Scotland. [3]Scottish Ambulance Service , 28 Laverockhall St, G21 4AB, Glasgow, Scotland.

References
1. Abdellatif A, Bagian JP, Barajas ER, Cohen M, Cousins D, Denham CR, Horvath D. Communication during patient hand-overs. Joint Commission Journal on Quality and Patient Safety. 2007;33(7):439–42.
2. Jensen SM, Lippert A, Ostergaard D. Handover of patients: a topical review of ambulance crew to emergency department handover. Acta Anasthesial Scand. 2013;57:964–70.
3. Iedema R, Ball C, Daly B, et al. Design and trial of a new ambulance-to-emergency department handover protocol: 'IMIST-AMBO'. BMJ Qual Saf. 2012;21(8):627–33.
4. Bost N, Crilly J, Wallis M, Patterson E, Chaboyer W. Clinical handover of patients arriving by ambulance to the emergency department – a literature review. International Emergency Nursing. 2010;18(4):210–20.
5. Wood K, Crouch R, Rowland E, Pope C. Clinical handovers between prehospital and hospital staff: literature review. Emerg Med J. 2015;32:577–81.
6. Abraham J, Kannampallil T, Patel VL. A systematic review of the literature on the evaluation of handoff tools: implications for research and practice. Journal of the American Medical Informatics Association: JAMIA. 2014;21(1):154–62.
7. Manser T, Foster S. Effective handover communication: an overview of research and improvement efforts. Best Pract Res Clin Anaesthesiol. 2011; 25(2):181–91.
8. Thakore S, Morrison W. A survey of the perceived quality of patient handover by ambulance staff in the resuscitation room. Emerg Med J. 2001; 18:293–6.
9. Manser T. Fragmentation of patient safety research: a critical reflection of current human factors approaches to patient handover. J Public Health Res. 2013;2(3):e33. https://www.jphres.org/index.php/jphres/article/view/jphr.2013.e33/186. Accessed 31 May 2018
10. Riesenberg LA, Davis R, O'Hagan E. Handoff Research: The Good, the Bad, and the Ugly: Proceedings of the International Symposium on Human Factors and Ergonomics in Health Care. 2016;5(1):106–11. https://doi.org/10.1177/2327857916051026. Accessed 31 May 2018
11. Dawson S, King L, Grantham H. Review article: improving the hospital clinical handover between paramedics and emergency department staff in the deteriorating patient. Emerg Med Australas. 2013;25:393–405.
12. Joint Royal College Ambulance Liaison Committee. UK Ambulance Service Clinical Practice Guidelines. Bridgewater: Association of Ambulance Chief Executives, Calls Publishing Ltd; 2016. p. 224.
13. Clinical Quality & Patient Safety Unit, Queensland Ambulance Service, 2016. Clinical practice procedures: other/clinical handover: Queensland Government; 2016. https://www.ambulance.qld.gov.au/docs/clinical/cpp/CPP_Clinical%20handover.pdf. Accessed 1 June 2018
14. Healthcare Improvement Scotland. Scottish Patient Safety Programme Safe in our Hands: SBAR Guide. NHS Scotland. 2017. https://ihub.scot/media/1841/spsp_sbar_guider2.pdf. Accessed 1 June 2018.
15. Department of Health [Ireland]. Communication (Clinical Handover) in Acute and Children's Hospital Services. National Clinical Guideline No. 11 November 2015. ISSN 2009-6259. https://health.gov.ie/wp-content/uploads/2015/12/NCG-No-11-Clinical-Handover-Acute-and-Childrens-Hospital-Services-Full-Report.pdf. Accessed 1 June 2018.
16. Sbiti-Rohr D, Kutz A. Christ-Crain M for the ProHOSP study group, et al. the National Early Warning Score (NEWS) for outcome prediction in emergency department patients with community-acquired pneumonia: results from a 6-year prospective cohort study. BMJ Open. 2016; https://doi.org/10.1136/bmjopen-2015-011021
17. Mochizuki K, Shintani R, Mori K, Sato T, Sakaguchi O, Takeshige K, Nitta K, Imamura H. Importance of respiratory rate for the prediction of clinical deterioration after emergency department discharge: a single-center, case-control study. Acute Medicine & Surgery. 2017;4(2):172–8. http://doi.org/10.1002/ams2.252
18. Brown R, Warwick J. Blue calls—time for a change? Emerg Med J. 2001; 18:289–92.
19. Sheppard JP, Mellor RM, Greenfield S on behalf of the CLAHRC BBC investigators, et al. The association between prehospital care and in-hospital treatment decisions in acute stroke: a cohort study. Emerg Med J. 2015;32:93–9.
20. Bhabra G, Mackeith S, Monteiro P, Pothier DD. An experimental comparison of handover methods. Ann R Coll Surg Engl. 2007;89(3):298–300.
21. Mort A, Fitzpatrick D, Schneider A, et al. Pre-hospital technology research: reflecting on a collaborative project between ambulance service and academia. J Paramed Pract. 2015;7(4):184–91.
22. Schneider AH, Mort A, Kindness P, Mellish C, Reiter E, Wilson P. Using technology to enhance rural resilience in pre-hospital emergencies. Scott Geogr J. 2015;131:194–200. https://doi.org/10.1080/14702541.2014.978810.
23. Porter et al. ERA Electronic Records in Ambulances to support the shift to out of hospital care: challenges, opportunities and workforce implications. National Institute for Health Service Research. 2017. Online at: https://www.journalslibrary.nihr.ac.uk/programmes/hsdr/144722/#/. [Accessed 12/09/2017].
24. Ebben RH, van Grunsven PM, Moors ML, et al. A tailored e-learning program to improve handover in the chain of emergency care: a pre-test post-test study. Scandinavian Journal of Trauma, Resuscitation and Emergency Medicine. 2015;23:33. https://doi.org/10.1186/s13049-015-0113-3.
25. Evans SM, Murray A, Patrick I, et al. Clinical handover in the trauma setting: a qualitative study of paramedics and trauma team members. Qual Saf Health Care. 2010;19:e57.
26. Infection Control Team, 2016. Health Protection Scotland:National Infection Control Manual. Version 2.5.1 NHS National Services Scotland, 2016. http://www.nhslothian.scot.nhs.uk/Services/A-Z/InfectionControl/InfectionControlManual/CP001.pdf. Accessed 1 June 2018.
27. National Records of Scotland. Scotland Population – Key statistics. 2018. https://www.nrscotland.gov.uk/statistics-and-data/statistics/scotlands-facts/population-of-scotland . Accessed 1 June 2018.
28. Scottish Ambulance Service. Annual Report 2015/16. 2016. http://www.scottishambulance.com/userfiles/file/TheService/Annual%20report/201606_SAS%20AnnualReport%20201601_13full.pdf. Accessed 1 June 2018.
29. Dick WF. Anglo-American vs. Franco-German emergency medical services system. Prehospital and Disaster Medicine. 2003;18(01):29–37.
30. ISD Scotland. NHS performs: Glasgow Royal Infirmary – emergency department activity (main sites): number of attendances. Scotland: Information Services Division; 2017. http://www.nhsperforms.scot/hospital-data/indicator-hospital?hospitalid=20&indicatorid=1. Accessed 5 Oct 2017
31. Scottish Ambulance Service. Audit of Emergency Ambulance Calls. Edinburgh: Scottish Ambulance Service; 2017.
32. Royal College of Physicians. National Early Warning Score (NEWS): Standardising the assessment of acute illness severity in the NHS. Report of a working party London: RCP; 2012.
33. O'Driscoll BR, Howard LS, Earis J on behalf of the British Thoracic Society Emergency Oxygen Guideline Group, et al. BTS guideline for oxygen use in adults in healthcare and emergency settings. Thorax. 2017;72:ii1–ii90.
34. Schneider A., Vaudry P., Mort A., Mellish C., Reiter E., and Wilson P. 2013. MIME - NLG in Pre-hospital Care. In Proceedings of 14th European Natural Language Generation Workshop (ENLG).
35. McLelland G, Flynn D, Rodgers H, Price C. A survey of UK paramedics' views about their stroke training, current practice and the identification of stroke mimics. British Paramedic J. 2016;1(2):4–15.
36. Colver K, Fitzpatrick D, Cooper M, Ward J. Paramedic practitioner: a survey of scope of practice and development requirements. Emerg Med J. 2016;33:e10.
37. Duncan EAS, Fitzpatrick D. Improving self-referral for diabetes care following hypoglycaemic emergencies: a feasibility study with linked patient data analysis. BMC Emerg Med. 2016;16(13) https://doi.org/10.1186/s12873-016-0078-1.
38. Fitzpatrick D, McKenna M, Rooney K, Beckett D, Pringle N. Improving the management and care of people with sepsis. Emergency Nurse. 2014;22(1):18–24.
39. Dillman DA. Mail and Internet surveys: The tailored design method–2007 Update with new Internet, visual, and mixed-mode guide. Hoboken: Wiley; 2011.
40. McColl E, Jacoby A, Thomas L, Soutter J, Bamford C. Design and use of questionnaires: a review of best practice applicable to surveys of health service staff and patients. Health Technol Assess. 2002;5(31):1–256.

41. Talbot R, Bleetman A. Retention of information by emergency department staff at ambulance handover: do standardised approaches work? Emerg Med J. 2007;24(8):539–42.
42. Carter AJE, Davis KA, Evans LV, Cone DC. Information loss in emergency medical services handover of trauma patients. Prehospital Emergency Care. 2009;13(3):280–5.
43. McLean S, Egan G, Connor P, et al. Collaborative decision-making between paramedics and CCU nurses based on 12-lead ECG telemetry expedites the delivery of thrombolysis in ST elevation myocardial infarction. Emerg Med J. 2008;25:370–4.
44. Carberry M, Harden J. A collaborative improvement project by an NHS emergency department and Scottish ambulance paramedics to improve the identification and delivery of sepsis 6. BMJ Open Quality. 2016;5 https://doi.org/10.1136/bmjquality.u212670.w5049.
45. Pezzolesi C, Manser T, Schifano F, Kostrzewski A, Pickles J, Harriet N, Warren I, Dhillon S. Human factors in clinical handover: development and testing of a 'handover performance tool' for doctors' shift handovers. Int J Qual Health Care. 2013;25(1):58–65.
46. Nagpal K, Vats A, Ahmed K, et al. An evaluation of information transfer through the continuum of surgical care: a feasibility study. Ann Surg. 2010; 252(2):402–7.
47. Lyon R, Crawfor A, Crookston C, Short S, Clegg G. The combined use of mechanical CPR and a carry sheet to maintain quality resuscitation in out-of-hospital cardiac arrest patients during extrication and transport. Resuscitation. 2015;93:102–6.
48. Landsberger HA. Hawthorne revisited, Ithaca, the new york state school of industrial and labor relations; 1958. p. 132.
49. NHS Health Research Authority decision tool. Medical Research Council: Is my study research? 2017. Available online: http://www.hra-decisiontools.org.uk/research/. Accessed 20 Dec 2017.

8

Methicillin resistant *Staphylococcus Aureus* in emergency department patients

Muna Al Jalaf[1†], Hanan Fadali[1†], Rasha Alanee[1], Firas Najjar[1], Zulfa Al Deesi[2], Rania M. Seliem[2] and Eric J. Nilles[3,4*]

Abstract

Background: Since the 1990s, community-associated methicillin resistant *staphylococcus aureus* (CA-MRSA) has emerged as an important global cause of skin and soft tissue infections. Little is known about the epidemiology of this pathogen in the Middle East.

Methods: We conducted a prospective observational study in a single large teaching hospital in Dubai to identify the incidence of community-acquired methicillin resistant *staphylococcus aureus* (MRSA) among ambulatory patients presenting with purulent skin and soft tissue infections. We performed wound cultures and administered standard questionnaires to 100 cases presenting to the emergency department. Bivariate and multivariate analyses were performed to identify risk factors for MSRA versus other pathogens.

Results: The prevalence of MRSA was 23% (18/78) among 78 culture-positive isolates and 29% (18/62) among Staphylococcus-positive isolates. 74% received antibiotics of which 4/74 (5%) received antibiotics appropriate for CA-MRSA infections. Multivariate adjusted analysis identified playing contact sports (OR 5.9 [95% CI 1.3–27.1]) and female sex (OR 6.3 [95% CI 1.6–24.8]) as independent risks for MRSA infection.

Conclusions: This is the first study to describe the epidemiology of CA-MRSA in the ambulatory setting in the Middle East and demonstrates a substantial proportion of cases presenting with skin and soft tissue infections were CA-MRSA. Although most skin and soft tissue infections are abscesses for which the cornerstone of treatment is high quality incision and drainage, if adjunct antibiotics are prescribed in this setting, CA-MRSA-active antibiotics should be considered.

Keywords: Community-associated methicillin resistant *staphylococcus aureus*, MRSA, United Arab Emirates, Middle East, Emergency, SSTI, Abscess, Skin infection, Antibiotic resistance

Background

During the 1990s community-acquired MRSA (CA-MRSA) emerged in populations without exposure to health facilities and without traditional risk factors for MRSA [1, 2]. CA-MRSA infections exhibit different epidemiological characteristics, are resistant to fewer antibiotics, and express different toxin producing genes including, notably, the Panton-Valentine leucocidin a bicomponent toxin associated with recurrent skin and soft tissues infections (SSTIs) and necrotizing pneumonia [3].

CA-MRSA has emerged as a major global cause of purulent skin and soft tissues infections but little is known about the epidemiology of CA-MRSA in the Middle East [3–5] and no studies in the region have examined the prevalence of CA-MRSA in ambulatory settings. Given the absence of epidemiological data on this emerging pathogen we performed a cross-sectional observational study examining the prevalence of MRSA in purulent SSTI in ED patients in the United Arab Emirates (UAE). A secondary objective was to identify risk factors and clinical features of MRSA.

* Correspondence: enilles@bwh.harvard.edu
†Equal contributors
[3]Department of Emergency Medicine, Brigham & Women's Hospital, Boston, USA
[4]Harvard Medical School, Boston, USA
Full list of author information is available at the end of the article

Methods

From January 2011, we prospective enrolled a convenience sample of 100 adult patients presenting with purulent SSTIs to the emergency department (ED) of Rashid Hospital and Trauma Centre, a 599-bed public, tertiary-care, urban teaching hospital in Dubai that serves a largely poor migrant worker population. The annual ED census is ~ 140,000. Approximately 85–90% of the Dubai population are expatriates with the majority originating from the Indian subcontinent.

Prior to study enrollment, standardized study protocol training was conducted for ED physicians and nurses including enrollment criteria, questionnaire administration, and culture swab collection. After obtaining consent, enrolling clinicians collected standardized information on epidemiological and clinical features, potential risk factors, treatment and disposition (Table 1). Exclusion criteria included patients below the age of 18 years, hospitalization within the previous week, Bartholin, odontogenic or perianal abscesses, and infected post-operative incisional sites. We defined community-acquired MRSA according to United States Centers for Disease Control and Prevention criteria: (1) Positive culture for MRSA as an outpatient or within 48 h of hospital admission; (2) No medical devices or indwelling catheters that are permanently placed though the skin; (3) No history of MRSA infections; and (4) No recent history of hospitalization or residence in nursing home or long-term care facility. [6] Antibiotic sensitivity testing was performed using standard MIC and disk diffusion RH sensitivity methods.

Crude and adjusted analyses using logistical regression to identify variables associated with MRSA versus other bacterial isolates were performed using IBM SPSS (V 19). A multivariate model using backward stepwise elimination was performed using all risk variables. Significance assumes $p < 0.05$ or an Odds Ratio (OR) that does not cross one.

Ethics approval and consent to participate

All study participants provided written informed consent to participate in this study. The Medical Research Committee of the Dubai Health Authority, UAE, approved this study (October 2010).

Results

Between January 2011 and June 2012, 99 patients with purulent SSTI infections were enrolled in the study and provided 100 culture samples (one patient with recurrent SSTI provided two specimen cultures 6 weeks apart); 75 (75%) were male with a median age of 30 (range 16–64); 74 (74%) were expatriates and 26% Emirati nationals. A bacterial culture isolate was identified in 78 patients including 44 methicillin-sensitive

Table 1 Univariate risk factors for MRSA infection versus other bacterial pathogens among emergency department patients with purulent skin and soft tissue infections

Variable	Sub-variable	MRSA (n = 18)	%	Other bacteria (n = 60)	%	Odds Ratio (95% CI)
Sex	Female	8	44%	12	20%	3.2 (1.0–9.9)
Nationality	Emirati national[a]	5	28%	14	23%	1.3 (0.4–4.2)
Accommodation	Shared	6	33%	19	32%	REF
	Home	9	50%	29	48%	1.0 (0.3–3.3)
	Camp	2	11%	9	15%	1.4 (0.2–8.5)
Past Medical History[b]	Yes	1	6%	9	15%	0.3 (0.0–3.8)
Risk factors	Incarcerated in past year	1	6%	0	0%	
	Play contact sports	5	28%	8	13%	2.5 (0.7–8.9)
	HH member with skin infection	1	6%	2	3%	0.6 (0.2–2.3)
	Recent hospitalization[c]	1	6%	3	5%	0.4 (0.1–5.9)
	ICU stay in past year	0	0%	0	0%	
Recent skin infection	Abscess/cellulitis	3	17%	15	25%	0.6 (0.2–2.4)
Antibiotic use last 3 months	Yes	5	28%	19	32%	1.3 (0.5–4.0)
MRSA suspected by clinician	Yes (vs no or not sure)	2	11%	2	3%	3.6 (0.5–27.3)
Current infection	Multiple abscesses/lesions	4	22%	4	7%	3.9 (0.9–17.7)
	Associated cellulitis	15	83%	48	80%	1.5 (0.4–6.0)

[a]Versus expatriates
[b]Included diabetes, hypertension, asthma, thalassemia, coronary artery disease, osteosarcoma. Some with multiple medical problems
[c]Past 3 months
HH Household

Staphylococcus aureus (SSSA) isolates and 18 MRSA isolates; other organisms were isolated from 16 patients. No organism was identified in 22 patients. When considering all patients enrolled, MRSA was isolated in 18 of 100 cases (18%); when considering only positive isolates, 18 of 78 (23%) were MRSA-positive. Of 62 total *S. aureus* isolates, 18 (29%) were MRSA positive. Seventeen of 18 MRSA cases (94%) met the criteria for CA-MRSA (one case had been hospitalized < 3-months prior to enrollment). Potential risk factors stratified by MRSA versus other bacteria isolates are listed in Table 1.

Multivariate adjusted analysis identified female sex (OR 6.3 [95% CI 1.6–24.8]) and playing contact sports (OR 5.9 [95% CI 1.3–27.1]) as independent risks for MRSA infection. A total of 74 patients (74%) received antibiotics of which 4/74 (5%) were antibiotics routinely recommended for CA-MRSA infections including clindamycin (3) and doxycycline (1). All of the 18 MRSA isolates were susceptible to trimethoprim-sulfamethoxazole in addition to vancomycin and linezolid. Isolates were not routinely tested for clindamycin or erythromycin susceptibility. There was no difference in the proportion of MRSA-positive cases versus non-MRSA positive cases requiring hospitalization (11/18, 61% versus 36/60, 60%, $p = 0.33$).

Discussion

We present the first study in the Middle East to describe the epidemiological features of CA-MRSA among ambulatory patients presenting with SSTI. The overall prevalence of MRSA was 18% and the prevalence of MRSA among *S. aureus* isolates was 29%. The CA-MRSA prevalence reported in this study, although not as high as the United States, [7, 8] are similar to those recently reported in a multi-centre European study in which an average of 15% of SSTIs presenting to EDs were CA-MRSA, although substantial geographic variability was reported [9]. A number of studies have examined molecular characteristics of CA-MRSA in the UAE and Middle East or the prevalence of MRSA among laboratory *S. aureus* isolates [10–16] but no regional study has described the prevalence and epidemiology of MRSA among ambulatory patients.

Our study identified female sex and playing contact sports as independent risk factors for MRSA infection. Although playing contact sports is a well described risk factors for CA-MRSA in other settings, the association of female sex with MRSA was unexpected and requires further study. The risk of CA-MRSA versus other bacterial isolate was not different between the local Emirate and expatriate populations. Other risk factors were not identified, perhaps due to the relatively small sample size of this study or due to widespread community transmission of CA-MRSA beyond narrow epidemiological niches, which makes the identification of specific risk factors more challenging. Clinicians were not able to discriminate between MRSA and non-MRSA infections in this study.

Although most SSTI cases were treated with antibiotics, only a small proportion were treated with CA-MRSA-active antibiotics, a finding that is consistent with anecdotal observations that awareness of CA-MRSA as an important cause of purulent SSTI among healthcare providers is low. A substantial and likely increasing proportion of patients in this setting are likely to be infected with MRSA that will not respond to treatment with beta-lactam antibiotics including cephalosporins and combination or newer generation penicillins (for example amoxicillin-clavulanic acid). If antibiotic treatment is being considered as primary or adjunct treatment for purulent SSTI due to CA-MRSA, the Infectious Disease Society of American (IDSA) recommend clindamycin, trimethoprim-sulfamethoxazole, tetracyclines (minocycline, doxycycline) or Linazolid.

Historically, the management of purulent SSTI, particularly abscesses, has been incision and drainage, regardless of whether or not the responsible organism is MRSA. Recent data from the US, however, indicates that treatment with trimethoprim-sulfamethoxazole, which is active against most CA-MRSA strains, in addition to incision and drainage, improves cure rates in ED patients [7]. In that study, however, MRSA prevalence rates were ~45% raising questions about whether trimethoprim-sulfamethoxazole should be prescribed to patients with purulent SSTIs in countries where CA-MRSA prevalence rates may be lower. Regardless, if antibiotics are being considered in addition to standard incision and drainage, clinicians should be aware that in this setting one in four patients presenting to an ED with a purulent SSTI may be infected with CA-MRSA.

Limitations of this study include the small sample size and the longer-than expected enrollment period suggesting cases may have been missed and potentially risking selection bias. No molecular typing of samples was performed which would provide additional insight into the circulating strains and molecular epidemiology of CA-MRSA in the UAE.

Conclusion

Given the global CA-MRSA epidemic will continue to evolve and given the UAE and the Middle East region will likely experience increasing rates of CA-MRSA-related disease in the future, clinicians should be prepared for and comfortable with managing SSTIs and other related conditions.

Abbreviations

CA-MRSA: Community-associated methicillin-resistant *staphylococcus aureus*; ED: Emergency department; IDSA: Infectious Disease Society of American; SSTI: Skin and soft tissue infection

Authors' contributions
MAJ and HF participated in the design of the study, study coordination, data collection, data analysis, and drafting the manuscript. RA participated in data collection and drafting the manuscript. FN participated in the design of the study, study coordination, and drafting the manuscript. ZAD and RS provided laboratory support and participated in study design. EN conceived the study and participated in the design, study coordination, data analysis, and drafting the manuscript. All authors read and approved the final manuscript.

Competing interests
The authors declare that they have no competing interests.

Author details
[1]Department of Emergency Medicine, Rashid Hospital and Trauma Centre, Dubai Health Authority, Dubai, UAE. [2]Laboratory Medicine Department, Rashid Hospital and Trauma Centre, Dubai Health Authority, Dubai, UAE. [3]Department of Emergency Medicine, Brigham & Women's Hospital, Boston, USA. [4]Harvard Medical School, Boston, USA.

References

1. Barrett FF, McGehee RF, Finland M. Methicillin-resistant Staphylococcus aureus at Boston City Hospital. N Engl J Med. 1968;279(9):441–8.
2. Herold BC, Immergluck LC, Maranan MC, Lauderdale DS, Gaskin RE, Boyle-Vavra S, et al. Community-acquired methicillin-resistant Staphylococcus aureus in children with no identified predisposing risk. JAMA. 1998;279(8): 593–8.
3. Zetola N, Francis JS, Nuermberger EL, Bishai WR. Community-acquired meticillin-resistant Staphylococcus aureus: an emerging threat. Lancet Infect Dis. 2005;5(5):275–86.
4. Pallin DJ, Egan DJ, Pelletier AJ, Espinola JA, Hooper DC, Camargo CA. Increased US emergency department visits for skin and soft tissue infections, and changes in antibiotic choices, during the emergence of community-associated methicillin-resistant Staphylococcus aureus. Ann Emerg Med. 2008;51(3):291–8.
5. Qualls ML, Mooney MM, Camargo CA, Zucconi T, Hooper DC, Pallin DJ. Emergency department visit rates for abscess versus other skin infections during the emergence of community-associated methicillin-resistant Staphylococcus aureus, 1997-2007. Clin Infect Dis. 2012;55(1):103–5.
6. Maree CL, Daum RS, Boyle-Vavra S, Matayoshi K, Miller LG. Community-associated methicillin-resistant Staphylococcus aureus isolates and healthcare-associated Infections1. Emerg Infect Dis. 2007;13(2):236–42.
7. Talan DA, Mower WR, Krishnadasan A, Abrahamian FM, Lovecchio F, Karras DJ, et al. Trimethoprim–sulfamethoxazole versus placebo for uncomplicated skin abscess. N Engl J Med. 2016;374(9):823–32.
8. Moran GJ, Krishnadasan A, Gorwitz RJ, Fosheim GE, McDougal LK, Carey RB, et al. Methicillin-resistant Staphylococcus aureus infections among patients in the emergency department. N Engl J Med. 2006;355(7):666–74.
9. Bouchiat C, Curtis S, Spiliopoulou I, Bes M, Cocuzza C, Codita I, et al. MRSA infections among patients in the emergency department: a European multicentre study. J Antimicrob Chemother. 2017;72(2):372–75.
10. Aly M, Balkhy HH. The prevalence of antimicrobial resistance in clinical isolates from gulf corporation council countries. Antimicrob Resist Infect Control. 2012;1:26.
11. Udo EE, Al-Sweih N, Dhar R, Dimitrov TS, Mokaddas EM, Johny M, et al. Surveillance of antibacterial resistance in Staphylococcus aureus isolated in Kuwaiti hospitals. Med Princ Pract. 2008;17:71–5.
12. Dash N, Panigrahi D, Al Zarouni M, Yassin F, Al-Shamsi M. Incidence of community-acquired methicillin-resistant Staphylococcus aureus carrying pantone-valentine leucocidin gene at a referral hospital in United Arab Emirates. APMIS. 2014;122(4):341–6.
13. Sonnevend Á, Blair I, Alkaabi M, Jumaa P, al Haj M, Ghazawi A, et al. Change in methicillin-resistant Staphylococcus aureus clones at a tertiary care hospital in the United Arab Emirates over a 5-year period. J Clin Pathol. 2012;65(2):178–82.
14. Monecke S, Skakni L, Hasan R, Ruppelt A, Ghazal SS, Hakawi A, et al. Characterisation of MRSA strains isolated from patients in a hospital in Riyadh, Kingdom of Saudi Arabia. BMC Microbiol. 2012;12(1):146.
15. Senok A, Somily A, Raji A, Gawlik D, Al-Shahrani F, Baqi S, et al. Diversity of methicillin-resistant Staphylococcus aureus CC22-MRSA-IV from Saudi Arabia and the Gulf region. Int J Infect Dis. 2016;51:31–5.
16. Udo EE, Al-Lawati BA-H, Al-Muharmi Z, Thukral SS. Genotyping of methicillin-resistant Staphylococcus aureus in the Sultan Qaboos University Hospital, Oman reveals the dominance of Panton–valentine leucocidin-negative ST6-IV/t304 clone. New Microbes New Infect. 2014;2(4):100–5.

9

Titration of oxygen therapy in critically ill emergency department patients

Anna S. M. Dobbe[2], Renate Stolmeijer[3], Jan C. ter Maaten[4] and Jack J. M. Ligtenberg[1,4*]

Abstract

Background: Liberal use of oxygen in an emergency situation is common. Today, most health care professionals do not adjust the amount of oxygen given when a saturation of 100% or a PaO2 which exceeds the normal range is reached- which may result in hyperoxia. There is increasing evidence for the toxic effects of hyperoxia. Therefore, it seems justified to aim for normoxia when giving oxygen. This study evaluates whether it is feasible to aim for normoxia when giving oxygen therapy to patients at the emergency department (ED).

Methods: A prospective cohort study was performed at the ED of the University Medical Center Groningen (UMCG). A protocol was developed, aiming for normoxia. During a 14 week period all patients > 18 years arriving at the ED between 8 a.m. and 23 p.m. requiring oxygen therapy registered for cardiology, internal medicine, emergency medicine and pulmonology were included. Statistical analysis was performed using student independent t-test, Mann–Whitney U-test, Fisher's exact test or a Pearson's chi-squared test.

Results: During the study period the study protocol was followed and normoxia was obtained after 1 h at the ED in 86,4% of the patients. Patients with COPD were more at risk for not being titrated to normal oxygen levels.

Conclusions: We showed that it is feasible to titrate oxygen therapy to normoxia at the ED. The study results will be used for further research assessing the potential beneficial effects of normoxia compared to hyper- or hypoxia in ED patients and for the development of guidelines.

Keywords: Emergency medicine, Oxygen inhalation therapy, Hyperoxia, Normoxia, Hypoxia, Titration of oxygen therapy, Emergency department, Critically ill patients, Pulmonary disease, chronic obstructive, Prospective studies, Oxygen

Background

Oxygen is one of the most widely used drugs and is applied in a wide range of medical specialities [1]. Supplemental oxygen is vital in many clinical situations; impaired oxygen delivery in critically ill patients is associated with increased mortality. Therefore, reassuring oxygen delivery has become a cornerstone in resuscitation and liberal use of supplemental oxygen in an emergency situation is common. [2] In acute medical care, toxicity of oxygen therapy is not immediately obvious. Over the past years, several studies have shown the potential harmful effects of hyperoxia, resulting in increased mortality [3–5]. Guidelines for emergency oxygen use have been developed, recommending to aim for normal or near-normal oxygen saturation for all acutely ill patients, such as the British Thoracic Society (BTS) guideline [1]. Despite these studies and guidelines, in real-life the amount of oxygen given is often not decreased if the SaO_2 measured by pulse oximeter is 100%, or if PaO_2 levels are high [5, 6]. Considering that the Emergency Department (ED) is the department where many critically ill patients arrive, it is important to cause no additional harm due to hyperoxia and to treat patients with the right dose of oxygen. The only study outside the ICU (in prehospital setting) aiming for normoxia had to be stopped because it appeared to be not feasible [7]. That is why we investigated if it is feasible to titrate oxygen therapy immediately after arrival at the ED. This prospective

* Correspondence: j.j.m.ligtenberg@umcg.nl
[1]Emergency Department, Internal Medicine, University Medical Center Groningen (UMCG), Hanzeplein 1, 9700, RB, Groningen, The Netherlands
[4]Internist acute medicine, Emergency physician, Emergency Department, University Medical Center Groningen, Groningen, The Netherlands
Full list of author information is available at the end of the article

study evaluates the feasibility of a protocol aiming for normoxia in adult, critically ill patients at the ED.

Methods

Study population & research design

This prospective cohort study was performed at the ED of the University Medical Center Groningen, a tertiary care teaching hospital with 33.000 ED visits/year. During a 14 week period from February until May 2016, consecutive patients > 18 years arriving at the ED, registered for cardiology, internal medicine, pulmonary medicine and emergency medicine, requiring oxygen therapy (according to the judgement of the ambulance nurse, ED nurse or ED physician) were included from 8.00 h a.m. until 23.00 h p.m. The institutional review board of our hospital waived informed consent. Exclusion criteria were: intubated patients or patients requiring immediate intubation, patients with unreliable pulse oximetry recording [8] and patients using bleomycin, because high concentrations of inspired oxygen (FiO2) increases lung toxicity in these patients.

Also, patients with a known specific target saturation due to other causes at presentation were excluded, such as patients with congenital heart disease in whom saturations < 85% were normal.

A protocol was developed aiming for normoxia, defined as PaO_2 9,5–13,5 kPa (70–100 mmHg) or a corresponding oxygen saturation of 94–98%. Hyperoxia was defined - according to normal values used in our hospital - as $PaO_2 >$ 13.5 kPa or $SaO_2 > 98\%$, and hypoxia as $PaO_2 < 9.5$ kPa or $SaO_2 < 94\%$. In consultation with our pulmonologists saturations between 90 and 92% were used to aim for normoxia in patients with known severe COPD (GOLD III or IV), in order to avoid hypercapnia, while further using the same study protocol (Fig. 1). The study protocol is shown in Fig. 1. For example, if a patient was admitted with a non-rebreathing mask (NRM) (15 L O_2/minute, $FiO_2 = \pm$ 0.8) and peripheral oxygen saturation (SaO_2) immediately after arrival was ≥98%, the nurse would apply a Ventimask (VM) 40% with 10 L O_2/minute ($FiO_2 = \pm$ 0.4). If after 5 min, in arterial blood gas analysis PaO_2 was still > 13.5 kPa or (peripheral) SaO_2 was ≥98%, oxygen was titrated towards an oxygen saturation (SaO_2) between 94 and 98%, preferably administered by a nasal oxygen cannula. If the patient was admitted with a nasal oxygen cannula and SaO_2 was ≥94% immediately after arrival, oxygen was titrated towards a SaO_2 between 94 and 98%. If SaO_2 was < 94%, a VM 40% with 10 L O_2/minute (FiO_2 = ± 0.4) would be applied and the same procedure as described above would be followed. Patients with known Chronic Obstructive Pulmonary Disease (COPD) GOLD III of IV dropped out of the study if they became hypercapnic ($PaCO_2 > 6.0$ kPa or > 45 mmHg) in the first hour after arrival. This threshold was chosen in consultation with our pulmonologists to prevent respiratory acidosis caused by relative hyperoxia lowering the respiratory rate. Oxygen saturation values were measured by non-invasive pulse oximetry [Masimo Corporation, CA, USA] and if the treating physician requested an arterial blood gas, PaO_2 as well as oxygen saturation were used [ABL800 flex, Radiometer, Copenhagen, DK].

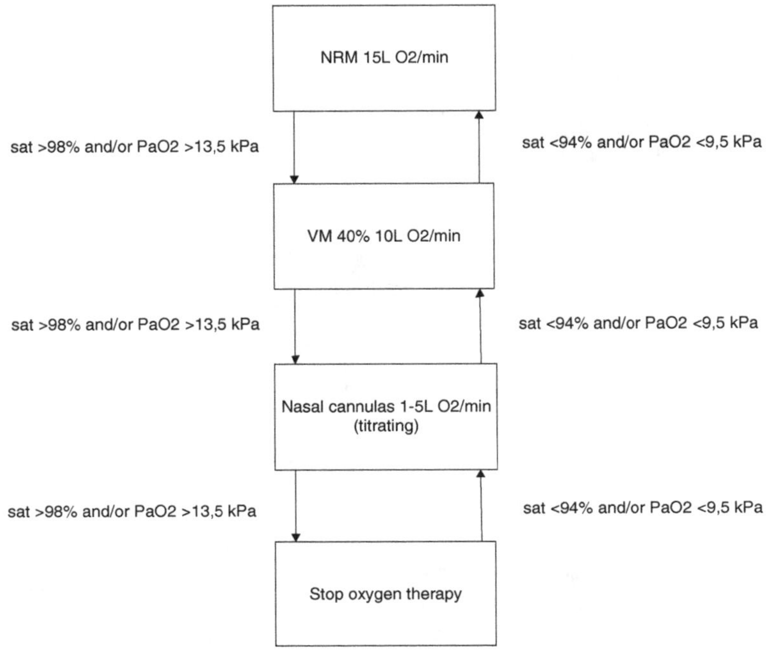

Fig. 1 Study protocol aiming for normoxia. In severe COPD patients the same protocol was used, but saturations were different (92% instead of 98 and 90% instead of 94%)

Data collection

All ED nurses and physicians were educated about the purpose of the study and the protocol. Data was collected using a case report form. The values of SpO_2 and PaO_2 (if available) were measured at ED presentation (T_0), after 5–10 min (T_1), after 1 h (T_2), and after 3 h (T_3) together with the dose of oxygen and the method used to administer oxygen. Vital signs were measured at the same time points. When the patient was admitted to a nursing ward or ICU, the same parameters were also collected 24 h after arrival at the ED (T_4). No advice was given about aiming for normoxia at the nursing ward or ICU. The Modified Early Warning Score (MEWS) was calculated on arrival and after 3 h.

Outcome parameters

The primary outcome parameter was whether the protocol was followed and whether normoxia was obtained. This was based on the measurements made by the pulse oxymeter, to enchance clinical applicability. The protocol was followed when during the time the patient was admitted at the ED (between arrival at the ED and 3 h after arrival at the ED) normoxia was achieved. If only at the final measurement (3 h after arrival at the ED) the SaO_2 was too high or too low, but the first three measurements were in the normal range, it was also concluded that the protocol was followed.

Statistical analysis

Baseline characteristics and results are presented as mean and standard deviation (SD) when normal distribution was assumed by means of a Kolmogorov–Smirnov test. Skewed variables are presented as median and interquartile range. Categorical variables are presented as frequency and percentage. For independent continuous variables with a normal distribution, student independent t-test was used. Other continuous variables were compared using the Mann–Whitney U-test. Categorical variables were compared using Fisher's exact test or a Pearson's chi-squared test. A significance level of $p < 0.05$ was used.

Results

Study population

In the study period 201 patients were screened for inclusion; 162 patients were included. The flowchart of patient inclusion and exclusion is shown in Fig. 2. In 140 patients the protocol was followed and normoxia successfully achieved (86,4%) within 1 h after arrival at the ED. In 7 normoxic patients multiple blood gases were additionally sampled during ED admission, of these 6 were normoxic measuring both SaO2 and PaO2. In 22 patients the protocol was not followed, of which there were 5 known COPD patients who dropped out due the development of hypercapnia in the first hour at the ED. There were different reasons why the

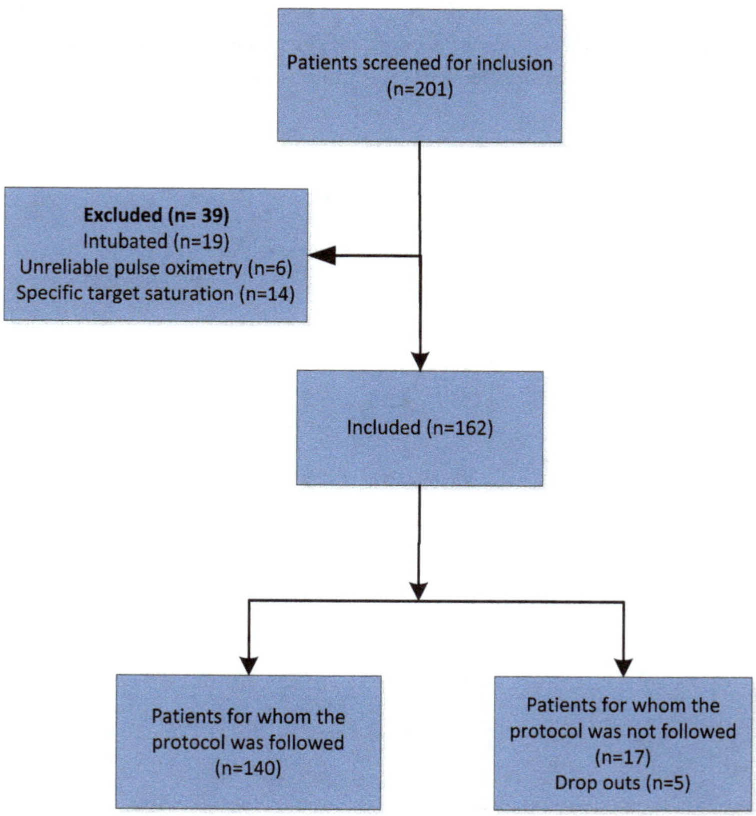

Fig. 2 Flowchart of patient inclusion and exclusion

protocol was not followed in the other 17 patients. The most important observation was that most of these patients suffered from COPD. It appeared that in some COPD patients the threating physician seemed reluctant to follow the protocol, resulting in not reducing oxygen therapy in patients with severe COPD ($n = 11$) or too low oxygen saturations in patients with mild COPD ($n = 3$). For other patients we could not find a specific reason for not following the protocol.

The baseline characteristics of the 162 study patients are shown in Table 1. Significantly more patients had severe COPD (GOLD III or IV) in the group in which the protocol was not followed ($P < 0.001$). This group also received significantly more often oxygen before ED arrival.

Diagnosis at discharge

An overview of the diagnosis at discharge from the ED for the total study population is shown in Table 2. Some patients were discharged with more than one diagnosis. In the group in which the protocol was not followed more patients were discharged with a COPD exacerbation ($P = 0.03$) or with other pulmonary conditions ($P = 0.04$) compared to the group in which the protocol was followed. Other diagnoses at discharge were not significantly different between the patient groups.

Prehospital oxygen

The median PaO_2 of patients arriving with prehospital oxygen was 9.5 (8.1–11.8) kPa. There is an effect of the method of oxygen delivery on causing hyperoxia at T_0. In patients arriving with a NRM, 50% was hyperoxic at T_0 compared to 18% of the patients with oxygen administered via a nasal cannula ($P < 0.001$).

Oxygen saturation at the ED and after 24 h

Figure 3 shows the course of the oxygen saturation at the ED and 24 h after arrival at the ED for all included patients. When patients stopped receiving oxygen therapy and their saturation was > 94% or > 90% in severe COPD patients, they were considered to be normoxic. In some patients their oxygen saturation fluctuated during ED admission, resulting in shifting between hypoxia, normoxia and hyperoxia at the different time points. From the figure it becomes clear that most patients were in the normoxia range after 1 h at the ED. In the first 10 min (T_0-T_1) it was more difficult to attain normoxia, maybe due to the amount of oxygen treatment in the ambulance or due to the number of actions that have to be performed when a patient arrives at the ED. Some patients were normoxic at first but at T_3 they became hypoxic or hyperoxic, probably because they were checked less frequently. When patients were admitted to the ICU or nursing ward, most patients stayed in the normoxia range.

Oxygen saturation of severe COPD patients

In patients with severe COPD the protocol was more often not followed. For this reason, we made a separate graph for this subgroup, shown in Fig. 4.

Table 1 Patient characteristics at ED arrival

Characteristics		Patients in which the protocol was followed ($n = 140$)	Patients in which the protocol was not followed ($n = 22$)	Total (n = 162)	P-value
Male sex [n (%)]		82 (59)	11 (50)	93 (57)	0.45
Age (years)		68 ± 13	68 ± 12	68 ± 13	0.78
Prehospital oxygen	Yes [n (%)]	94 (67)	18 (82)	112 (69)	0.16
Within target at arrival*	Yes [n (%)]	56 (60)	1 (6)	57 (51)	0.00
PaO_2 (kPa)		9 (8–12)	8 (8–11)	9 (8–12)	0.53
Systolic blood pressure (mmHg)		125 (107–141)	137 (119–165)	126 (109–145)	0.04
Diastolic blood pressure (mmHg)		76 (65–89)	76 (65–103)	76 (65–89)	0.49
Heart rate (beats/min)		88 (75–108)	95 (88–120)	91 (78–110)	0.06
Respiratory rate (breaths/min)		21 (18–25)	22 (20–27)	21 (18–25)	0.17
GCS [1–15]**		15 (15–15)	15 (15–15)	15 (15–15)	0.24
MEWS		4 (3–5)	4 (3–6)	4 (3–5)	0.27
Smoking [n (%)]		30 (21)	8 (36)	38 (24)	0.12
Cardiac condition [n (%)]		57 (41)	10 (46)	67 (41)	0.68
COPD GOLD I/II [n (%)]		27 (19)	3 (14)	30 (19)	0.53
COPD GOLD III/IV [n (%)]		14 (10)	11(50)	25 (15)	0.00
Other pulmonary condition [n (%)]		19 (14)	5 (23)	24 (15)	0.26
Neurological condition [n (%)]		1 (1)	1 (5)	2 (1)	0.13

*Within target saturation on arrival at the ED with prehospital oxygen
**GCS, Glasgow Coma Scale

Table 2 Diagnosis at discharge from the ED

Diagnosis at discharge from ED	Protocol was followed [n (%)]	Protocol was not followed [n (%)]	Total [n (%)]	*P*-value
Pneumonia	30 (21)	4 (18)	34 (21)	1.00
Infection	28 (20)	6 (27)	34 (21)	0.41
Heart failure	22 (16)	4 (18)	26 (16)	0.76
Other	23 (16)	1 (5)	24 (15)	0.20
Sepsis	22 (16)	2 (9)	24 (15)	0.54
COPD exacerbation	14 (10)	8 (36)	22 (14)	0.03
Cardiac condition other	17 (12)	0 (0)	17 (11)	0.13
Pulmonary condition other	10 (7)	5 (23)	15 (9)	0.04
Malignancy	11 (8)	1 (5)	12 (7)	1.00
Neurological	6 (4)	1 (5)	7 (4)	1.00

Figure 4 shows that almost half of the severe COPD patients were hyperoxic during the first 3 h after arrival at the ED. Almost none were hypoxic and at T_2 most patients were in the normal range. After being admitted to the nursing ward or ICU, more than half of the severe COPD patients (69%) stayed hyperoxic.

Discussion

To our knowledge, this study is the first to investigate the feasibility of aiming for normoxia in critically ill patients at the ED. A study performed in the prehospital setting was stopped early because it appeared that it was not feasible to titrate prehospital oxygen therapy to normoxia [7]. We found that it is feasible to titrate oxygen therapy aiming for normoxia in critically ill patients at the ED; normoxia was obtained in 86,4% of the patients within 1 h after arrival at the ED. Furthermore, we found that patients for whom the protocol was not followed were mostly severe COPD (GOLD III/IV) patients ($P < 0.001$), patients with an COPD exacerbation ($P = 0.03$) or other pulmonary conditions ($P = 0.04$). The clinical impression the COPD patient made in the ED appeared to influence which saturation was aimed for by the responsible physician, making it difficult to attain the specific target saturations prescribed by our protocol. Future research will need to validate the ideal target saturation for patients with and without risk of hypercapnic respiratory failure. Despite this, in our opinion, COPD patients could also be treated with titrated oxygen therapy. Of the patients who received prehospital oxygen, patients arriving with a NRM were significantly more often hyperoxic ($P < 0.001$) on arrival (T_0) compared to patients arriving with a nasal cannula.

Liberal oxygen use is still common. There is still uncertainty about the ideal target saturation, mostly due to lack of evidence from clinical trials [1]. The majority of studies evaluating aiming for normoxia were performed at the ICU. Most ICU clinicians acknowledge the potential adverse effects of hyperoxia and declare low tolerance for high oxygen levels, but in clinical practice a substantial part of their patients were exposed to high arterial oxygen levels [9]. Another ICU study found that hyperoxia was frequently observed but not resulted in adjustment of the ventilator settings [6]. This study's main strength is that it is a prospective cohort study with inclusion of ED patients with different

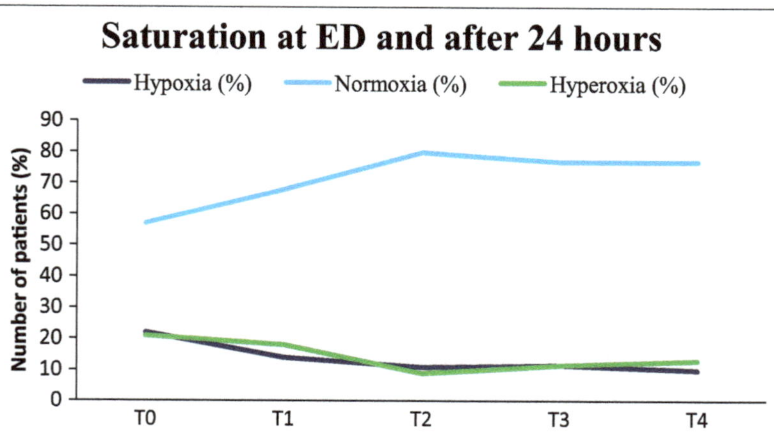

Fig. 3 Course of oxygen saturation for all study patients ($n = 162$). On arrival at the ED ($T = 0$), after 10 min ($T = 1$), after 1 h ($T = 2$), after 3 h ($T = 3$) and after 24 h ($T = 4$)

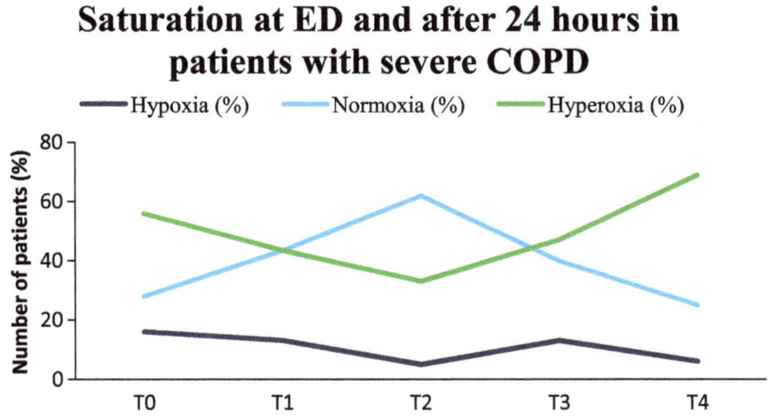

Fig. 4 Oxygen saturation COPD GOLD III and IV patients ($n = 25$). On arrival at the ED (T = 0), after 10 min (T = 1), after 1 h (T = 2), after 3 h (T = 3) en after 24 h (T = 4)

backgrounds. A limitation was that permission from the neurology department could not be obtained. There are several studies evaluating hyperoxia in neurology patients, however we could not include this subgroup in our study [10–15]. Education and feedback is needed to create more awareness of the importance of aiming for normoxia and applying this in clinical practice. Following the validation of the ideal target saturation, new guidelines for emergency oxygen therapy should be developed. To further assess primary and secondary outcome parameters, multicenter trials are required. Aiming for normoxia immediately after arrival in the hospital could prevent the potential harmful effects of hyperoxia, this could lead to health gains on short- and long term and reduced costs during hospital admission [16].

Conclusion

In this prospective cohort study we showed that it is feasible to attain normoxia in critically ill patients at the ED, demonstrating that it is possible to start titration of oxygen therapy immediately after arrival at the hospital. These study results can be a starting point for further research assessing the potential beneficial effects of normoxia compared to hyper- or hypoxia in the emergency department and the subsequent development of guidelines.

Abbreviations

COPD: Chronic obstructive pulmonary disease; ED: Emergency department; ICU: Intensive care unit; NRM: Non-rebreather mask; UMCG: University Medical Center Groningen; VM: VentiMask

Authors' contributions

JL and RS designed and critically revised the study. AD collected the data, interpreted and analyzed the data. AD was a major contributor in writing the manuscript. JM contributed to the study design and critically revised the study design and manuscript for important intellectual content. JM guided and supervised the study. All authors read and approved the final manuscript.

Competing interests

The authors declare that they have no competing interests.

Author details

[1]Emergency Department, Internal Medicine, University Medical Center Groningen (UMCG), Hanzeplein 1, 9700, RB, Groningen, The Netherlands. [2]BSc of Medicine, Faculty of Medicine, University of Groningen, Groningen, The Netherlands. [3]Emergency physician, Emergency Department, University Medical Center Groningen, Groningen, The Netherlands. [4]Internist acute medicine, Emergency physician, Emergency Department, University Medical Center Groningen, Groningen, The Netherlands.

References

1. O'Driscoll BR, Howard LS, Davison AG. BTS guideline for emergency oxygen use in adult patients. Thorax. 2008;63:1–68.
2. Stolmeijer Renate R. Oxygen therapy for sepsis patients in the emergency department: a little less? Eur J Emerg Med : official journal of the European Society for Emergency Medicine. 2014;21(3):233–5.
3. Moon RE. Oxygen in acute illness: more or less? Crit Care Med. 2015;43(7): 1547–8.
4. Sjöberg F, Singer M. The medical use of oxygen: a time for critical reappraisal. J Intern Med. 2013;274(6):505–28.
5. Girardis M, Busani S, Damiani E, Donati A, Rinaldi L, Marudi A, et al. Effect of conservative vs conventional oxygen therapy on mortality among patients in an intensive care unit: the oxygen-ICU randomized clinical trial. JAMA. 2016;316(15):1583–9.
6. de Graaff AE, Dongelmans DA, Binnekade JM, de Jonge E. Clinicians' response to hyperoxia in ventilated patients in a Dutch ICU depends on the level of FiO2. Intensive Care Med. 2011;37(1):46–51.
7. Young P, Bailey M, Bellomo R, Bernard S, Dicker B, Freebairn R, et al. HyperOxic therapy OR NormOxic therapy after out-of-hospital cardiac arrest (HOT OR NOT): a randomised controlled feasibility trial. Resuscitation. 2014; 85(12):1686–91.
8. Mechem CC. In: Post TW, editor. Pulse oximetry in adults. UpToDate Waltham, MA: UpToDate; 2016.
9. Helmerhorst HJ, Schultz MJ, van der Voort PH, Bosman RJ, Juffermans NP, de Jonge E, et al. Self-reported attitudes versus actual practice of oxygen therapy by ICU physicians and nurses. Ann Intensive Care. 2014;4:1–9.
10. Bitterman Haim H. Bench-to-bedside review: oxygen as a drug. Crit Care. 2009;13(1):1–8.
11. Helmerhorst HJ, Schultz MJ, van der Voort PH, de Jonge E, van Westerloo DJ. Bench to-bedside review: the effects of hyperoxia during critical illness. Crit Care. 2015;19:284.
12. Rincon Fred F. Association between hyperoxia and mortality after stroke: a multicenter cohort study. Crit Care Med. 2014;42(2):387–96.

13. Davis DP, Meade W, Sise MJ, Kennedy F, Simon F, Tominaga G, et al. Both hypoxemia and extreme hyperoxemia may be detrimental in patients with severe traumatic brain injury. J Neurotrauma. 2009;26(12):2217–23.
14. Rincon F, Kang J, Vibbert M, Urtecho J, Athar MK, Jallo J. Significance of arterial hyperoxia and relationship with case fatality in traumatic brain injury: a multicentre cohort study. J Neurol Neurosurg Psychiatry. 2014;85(7):799–805.
15. Asher SR, Curry P, Sharma D, Wang J, O'Keefe GE, Daniel-Johnson J, et al. Survival advantage and PaO2 threshold in severe traumatic brain injury. J Neurosurg Anesthesiol. 2013;25(2):168–73.
16. Decalmer S, O'Driscoll BR. Oxygen: friend or foe in peri-operative care? Anaesthesia. 2013;68(1):8–12.

10

Anxiety about anxiety: a survey of emergency department provider beliefs and practices regarding anxiety-associated low risk chest pain

Paul I. Musey Jr[1], John A. Lee[1,2], Cassandra A. Hall[1] and Jeffrey A. Kline[1*]

Abstract

Background: Approximately 80% of patients presenting to emergency departments (ED) with chest pain do not have any true cardiopulmonary emergency such as acute coronary syndrome (ACS). However, psychological contributors such as anxiety are thought to be present in up to 58%, but often remain undiagnosed leading to chronic chest pain and ED recidivism.

Methods: To evaluate ED provider beliefs and their usual practices regarding the approach and disposition of patients with low risk chest pain associated with anxiety, we constructed a 22-item survey using a modified Delphi technique. The survey was administered to a convenience sample of ED providers attending the 2016 American College of Emergency Physicians Scientific Assembly in Las Vegas.

Results: Surveys were completed by 409 emergency medicine providers from 46 states and 7 countries with a wide range of years of experience and primary practice environment (academic versus community centers). Respondents estimated that 30% of patients presenting to the ED with chest pain thought to be low risk for ACS have anxiety or panic as the primary cause but they directly communicate this belief to only 42% of these patients and provide discharge instructions to 48%. Only 39% of respondents reported adequate hospital resources to ensure follow-up. Community-based providers reported more adequate follow-up for these patients than their academic center colleagues (46% vs. 34%; $p = 0.015$). Most providers (82%) indicated that they wanted to have referral resources available to a specific clinic for further outpatient evaluation.

Conclusion: Emergency Department providers believe approximately 30% of patients seeking emergency care for chest pain at low risk for ACS have anxiety as a primary problem, yet fewer than half discuss this concern or provide information to help the patient manage anxiety. This highlights an opportunity for patient centered communication.

Keywords: Emergency department, Chest pain, Anxiety, Psychological conditions

Background

Chest pain is one of the most common chief complaints evaluated in the Emergency Department (ED), accounting for approximately 20% of all annual ED visits nationwide [1]. A small minority of these patients have a true cardiopulmonary emergency such as acute coronary syndrome (ACS) or pulmonary embolism (PE). Frequently, these patients have psychosomatic contributors to their symptoms, including panic or anxiety disorders. These disorders are present in up to 58% [2] of patients presenting with chest pain but remain undiagnosed in approximately 80% of these patients [3]. Many adults with chest pain undergo extensive ED evaluations to rule out cardiopulmonary emergencies. In some cases, these evaluations can last 48 h including multiple tests, radiation exposure, and high cost, only to yield no

* Correspondence: jefkline@iu.edu
[1]Department of Emergency Medicine, Indiana University School of Medicine, Indianapolis, IN 46202, USA
Full list of author information is available at the end of the article

named diagnosis [4]. A significant fraction of these patients go on to develop chronic chest pain and continue to seek medical attention despite negative cardiac evaluations [2]. Prior work has indicated emergency providers are hesitant to diagnose and discuss the role of anxiety [4] as a significant co-factor or etiology of their pain. However, the beliefs of ED providers regarding the prevalence of anxiety among patients with low risk chest pain and how they manage those patients both in the ED and at discharge have not been evaluated together.

Objective

We sought to evaluate ED provider beliefs regarding patients with low risk chest pain thought to be secondary to anxiety symptoms. Further, we wanted to evaluate if there was a discrepancy between these beliefs and their management practices.

Methods

This work was a hypothesis generating survey, conducted in accordance with guidelines by Mello et al., including both expert consensus and a modified Delphi technique [5, 6]. This protocol was deemed to be exempt by the IRB (protocol# 1601415405) at Indiana University School of Medicine. Authors PIM, JAL, CLH, and JAK initially determined that the objective of the hypothesis generating survey was to: evaluate the gap between ED provider beliefs regarding the approach and disposition of patients with low risk chest pain thought to be secondary to anxiety compared with their perceived practice patterns. The authors developed an initial set of themes which led to the generation of a 15-item survey which was test-administered to ED providers at Indiana University Department of Emergency Medicine. Responses from this test survey were analyzed along with feedback from participants by an advisory group who determined the final themes, domains, and survey architecture via a modified Delphi technique. This advisory group included individuals with expertise in both the subject areas as well as survey generation and administration in order to ensure face, content, and construct validity. The authors then generated a draft survey consisting of 26 items which were again vetted by the advisory group. Through an iterative process and consensus, edits were made and the items were reduced to a final survey consisting of 22 items. These included a mixture of multiple choice and visual analogue scale (0–100%) questions (Additional file 1: Appendix 1).

The survey was then administered to a convenience sample of Emergency Medicine (EM) providers visiting the exhibitor hall at the 2016 American College of Emergency Physicians Scientific Assembly (ACEP16) in Las Vegas, Nevada from October 16–19, 2016. This forum was chosen because it represents the largest annual gathering of EM providers [7]. Eligible survey participants included advanced practitioners (i.e.: nurse practitioners and physician's assistants), emergency medicine residents, as well as physicians at the fellow or attending level who were practicing in academic and/or community settings. The investigators obtained a booth in the ACEP16 exhibitor hall and invited all eligible participants passing by the vicinity of the booth to complete the survey. A description and invitation to the booth was printed in the ACEP16 program and the meeting's website. Additionally, the investigators handed out invitation cards at the meeting. To encourage participation, we provided a material incentive in the form of a raffle for a FitBit® activity monitor. The number of passers-by who were approached but declined participation was not tracked.

Participants first viewed a description and purpose of the survey prior to starting, and then completed the survey using either a laptop computer or electronic tablet. Study data were collected and managed using REDCap electronic data capture tools hosted at Indiana University [8]. Exported data were analyzed using Microsoft Excel for Mac, Version 15.14, and IBM SPSS Statistics for Mac, Version 22.0. The survey data was exported from REDCap into both software packages, and both univariate and multivariate analysis was completed. Where appropriate, 95% confidence intervals are reported. All visual analog-scale data were found to be non-normally distributed by both Kolmogorov-Smirnov and Shapiro-Wilk normality testing. All data generated or analyzed during this study are included in this published article as a supplemental excel dataset (The complete dataset generated from this survey and the basis for this manuscript is available from the authors upon request).

Results

Four-hundred-and-nine surveys were completed, representing approximately 5% of ACEP16 conference attendees. There was diversity in respondent geographic location (Fig. 1), years of experience, and primary practice environment. The majority of respondents practiced at academic centers (52%), had less than 10 years of experience (68%), and were male (72%) as shown in Table 1. Twenty-nine respondents (7.0%) identified their primary practice location as outside of the United States.

Current practice patterns

A majority of providers believed an "acceptable ACS miss rate" was either < 1% (52%) or 1–2% (44%) with only 4% of respondents willing to accept an ACS miss rate of 3–5% illustrated in Fig. 2. Providers estimated that 30% (95%CI 28–32) of patients presenting to the ED with chest pain, which they have stratified to be low risk by whatever method, have anxiety or panic as the

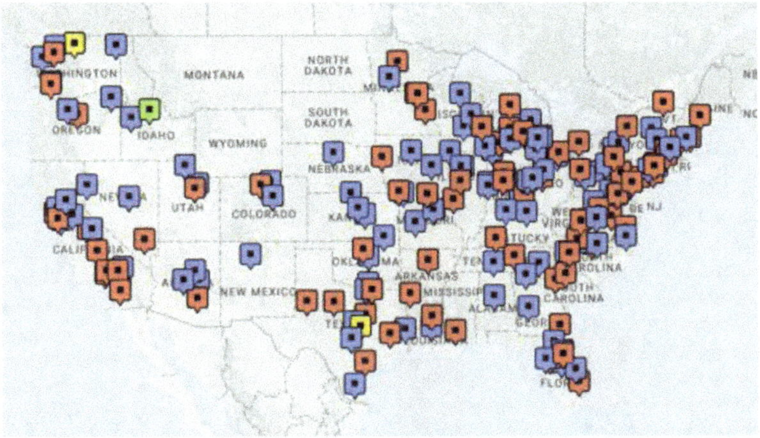

Fig. 1 Map of Providers by Practice Type and Location. Map of the continental United States with flags denoting the practice location and type of practice (academic, community, urgent care, or other) KEY: Red – Academic Practice, Blue – Community Practice, Green – Urgent Care Practice, Yellow – Other *Note: 2 responses from Alaska and 2 responses from Hawaii. An additional 29 responses were international (14 from Canada)

primary cause as shown in Table 2. Of those patients, the majority are female (38% male, 95%CI 36–39). For patients whom they believe anxiety or panic is the primary problem, respondents indicated that they directly communicate this belief to only 42% of these patients, and offer anxiolytic treatment to only 41% in the ED. Additionally, they offer discharge instructions and prescriptions for anxiolytics in 48 and 21%, respectively. Though 54% of respondents indicated they believe they have a professional responsibility to provide patients with an actual ICD-code diagnosis of anxiety when life threats are ruled out, providers report documenting a specific ICD-code diagnosis of "anxiety" or "panic" only 29% of the time (95%CI 27–32). Providers appeared more likely to diagnose anxiety in patients under age 25 (Additional file 2: Table S1).

Table 1 Provider gender, practice environment, and level of experience

	Male	Female	Other/No Response	
Practice Environment				
Academic	151	63	0	214 (52%)
Community	131	45	0	176 (43%)
Urgent/Other	12	5	2	19 (5%)
				409 (100%)
Experience				
Advanced Practitioner	12	12	1	25 (6%)
Current Resident	68	28	0	96 (24%)
Fellow/Attending 0-4 yrs	52	32	0	84 (20%)
Attending 5-9 yrs	53	20	0	73 (18%)
Attending 10 + yrs	109	21	1	131 (32%)
	294 (72%)	113 (28%)	2	409 (100%)

Addressing the problem of anxiety

Thirty-nine percent (161/407) of respondents reported adequate hospital resources to ensure follow-up for patients with low risk chest pain they suspect is secondary to anxiety. Community-based providers reported more adequate follow-up for these patients than their academic center colleagues (46% of community providers responded that they have adequate follow-up available, versus only 34% of academic center providers; 2-sided Fisher's exact test 0.015), (Table 3). When asked about possible strategies that could be used to improve management for patients with chest pain due to anxiety, most providers (82%) said that it would helpful to have a referral available to a specific clinic for further outpatient evaluation. In discussing what tools would make a provider more comfortable diagnosing and referring these patients (Table 4), practice patterns of colleagues (48%, 95%CI 45–50) and local hospital policy (56%, 95%CI 53–59) were found to be less helpful than a multicenter trial (74%, 95%CI 72–76) or professional organization practice guidelines (71%, 95%CI 69–73).

Discussion

This study incorporated both a diverse geographical representation, and a wide range of practice settings and experience. The main message of this work is that physicians believe that approximately 30% of patients seeking emergency care for low risk chest pain have anxiety or panic as a primary problem, yet fewer than half provide any treatment or information to help the patient manage anxiety. The authors recognize that the primary

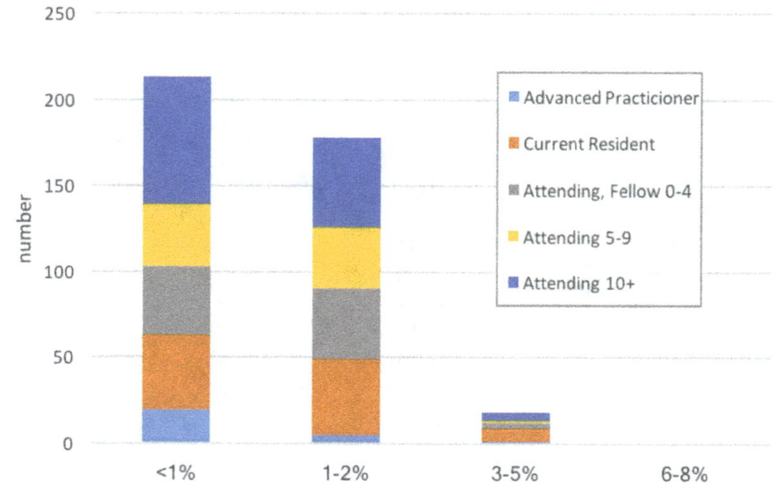

Fig. 2 Acceptable ACS Miss Rate by Experience. Stacked bar graph depicting participants selection of what they deem to be an acceptable ACS miss rate. Each colored stack in the bar corresponds to the provider position and/or experience level as noted on the graph

imperative of emergency care is to protect and intervene against threats to a patient's life. However, in patients without a serious cardiopulmonary disease, untreated anxiety can degrade quality of life and worsen perceptions of wellness [9, 10], contributing to systemic inflammation [11], which ironically creates the pathophysiology of coronary artery disease [12, 13]. Additionally, this is associated with an increased health resource burden [14–18]. We would argue that the most important of these to the emergency clinician is the detrimental effect on patient quality of life and unnecessary ED resource utilization and recidivism. Prior work in a large cohort of ED patients with chest pain discovered that only 0.2% were given an ICD9 diagnosis of anxiety; however, none of the 8% of patients who self-identified anxiety as likely the cause for their chest pain symptoms at follow-up were given this diagnosis even secondarily [4]. This low rate of anxiety diagnoses in patients with non-life threatening chest pain in the ED was further demonstrated in a national sample using the National Hospital Ambulatory Medical Care Survey, where only 2.3% received this diagnosis [19]. Whereas, a systematic review by Webster et al. incorporated nine studies and found the likely prevalence of diagnosable anxiety in patients with non-cardiac chest pain to be between 21 and 58% [2]. Our current work is consistent with that of Al-Ani et al., who found that 30% of chest pain patients who had been risk-stratified to be low-risk for ACS were identified as suffering from anxiety and 80% of those patients were untreated [20]. This highlights the fact that at least in this evaluation, EM provider gestalt regarding anxiety in the presence of low-risk anxiety is in line with objective measures shown previously. Taken together, these data indicate the need for a more patient-centered approach to communicating with and managing anxiety in patients with low risk chest pain. Helpful methods could include using formal anxiety risk stratification tools such as the Hospital Anxiety Depression Scale (HADS) or Generalized Anxiety Disorder scale (GAD-7). Both of these validated tools have been used to evaluate for the presence of anxiety in this patient population previously [21–23].

Furthermore, even after workup and provider reassurance, patients who present with possible cardiac symptoms are often left with "residual anxiety" despite normal test results [24]. Reassurance of negative test

Table 2 Attitudes and practices for patients with chest pain who are risk stratified as low risk for ACS (by whatever method)

	Mean (95% CI)		Mean (95% CI)
What % have anxiety or panic as primary cause of their symptoms?	30 (28–32)	How often do you provide anxiety/panic specific treatment in the ED for these patients?	41 (38–43)
Of these patients, what % are male?	38 (36–39)	How often do you provide any anxiety/panic specific prescriptions for these patients?	21 (19–24)
How often do you specifically tell these patients that you believe anxiety or panic may be the causing their symptoms?	42 (39–46)	How often do you discharge these patients with information or instructions about anxiety or panic?	48 (45–51)
		How often do you discharge these patients with and ICD diagnosis of "anxiety" or "panic"?	29 (27–32)

Table 3 Perceived ability to provide adequate follow-up

Do you believe you have adequate resources to ensure appropriate outpatient follow up for these patients?	# of Academic Providers [% of total]	# of Community/Urgent Care/ Other Providers [% of total]	Total
Yes	72 [17.6%]	89 [21.7%]	161
No/Unsure/No Response (Total)	113/28/1 (142) [34.7%]	82/23/1 (106) [25.9%]	248
Total	214	195	409

Our Fisher's Exact test revealed that the proportion of providers who do not believe or are unsure if they have adequate resources significantly differed by type of practice (academic vs. community), $p = 0.015$

results alone may not help reduce patient concerns about the potentially life-threatening causes of their chest pain [24–26]. Ackerman et al. defined the ideal content for ED discharge communication for patients with chest pain including directed follow-up suggestions and advice on self-care, [24] which are all important parts of the patient-provider interaction, particularly in the emergency department. Our data suggest these steps to be absent in current emergency care and may represent a missed opportunity to affect the trajectory of care [10]. This low rate of discharge communication is likely heavily influenced by the fact that the majority of respondents (61%) found their hospital resources for appropriate follow-up to be inadequate. Not surprisingly, 82% of providers wanted a specific clinic to direct their patients for further evaluation for anxiety.

Implications of these data are that patients could benefit from targeted interventions which minimize psychological distress, improve quality of life [9] and prevent futile emergency department visitation. There are a number of psychological interventions which are available for this patient population which include cognitive behavioral therapy (CBT), relaxation therapy, hyperventilation, hypnotherapy etc. [15]. Foremost and most well established is cognitive behavioral therapy (CBT), which has been shown to be both acceptable to patients and effective in reducing chest pain and improving quality of life [15, 27]. Even brief interventions have been successful as van Beek et al. randomized subjects with noncardiac chest pain and anxiety after psychological testing to usual treatment vs an abbreviated CBT course (6 sessions) showing a significant decrease in both depression and anxiety symptoms [28]. Unfortunately, CBT interventions are not a readily available resource for ED referral and can be expensive [29]. However, it appears the intervention need not be extensive or expensive, as simply providing self-help information explaining the connection between anxiety and chest pain can make a difference in both psychological and/or physical symptoms [18, 30, 31]. Other anxiety management strategies include training in breathing techniques and mindfulness-based exercises may show effectiveness in this patient population [32–35]. However, any intervention requires a frank conversation about anxiety and appropriate discharge instructions.

Table 4 Tools necessary to increase provider comfort with diagnosis

To what degree would each of the following increase your level of comfort in making a diagnosis of anxiety in patients with chest pain and providing a referral for treatment?	mean (95% CI)
Practice patterns of colleagues	48% (45–50)
Local hospital policy adoption	56% (53–59)
Multicenter trial	74% (72–76)
Professional organization practice guidelines	71% (69–73)

Limitations

The primary limitation of the work is that persons who completed our survey were self- selected by their decision to attend the national meeting, and their willingness to complete our survey. Additionally, we did not provide a formal definition or diagnostic criteria for anxiety to the provider as part of the survey. Thus, these results represent provider beliefs and gestalt based in large part on subjective assessments without the benefit of screening tests such as the HADS [21] or GAD-7 [22, 23] or formal evaluation using the Structured Clinical Interview for DSM Disorders (SCID) [36]. Thus, the objective reality of those beliefs were not assessed or quantified. However, we thought it important to explore as physician gestalt would likely be a trigger for further screening or referral for formal evaluation. Additionally, these screening tools and assessments are not regularly employed in this ED patient population and thus providers may not have been familiar.

Conclusions

ED providers believe 30% of patients seeking emergency care for chest pain stratified to be low risk for ACS have anxiety as a primary problem, yet fewer than half discuss this concern or provide information to help the patient manage anxiety. These data support the need for a more patient-centered approach to communication and management of anxiety in patients with low risk chest pain. Further investigation to elicit reasons why providers would be hesitant to discuss suspected anxiety in the setting of low risk chest pain and contributing biases is needed.

Abbreviation
ACEP16: 2016 American College of Emergency Physicians Scientific Assembly; ACS: Acute coronary syndrome; CBT: Cognitive behavior therapy; ED: Emergency department; EM: Emergency medicine; GAD-7: Generalized Anxiety Disorder – 7; HADS: Hospital Anxiety Depression Scale; PE: Pulmonary embolism; SCID: Structured Clinical Interview for DSM Disorders

Acknowledgements
Alexander B. Niculescu, MD, PhD, Professor of Psychiatry, Indiana University School of Medicine. Julie L. Welch, MD, Associate Professor of Clinical Emergency Medicine, Indiana University School of Medicine. Megan Palmer, PhD. Associate Dean for Faculty Affairs and Professional Development and Associate Professor in the Department of Emergency Medicine, Indiana University School of Medicine. Cherri D. Hobgood, MD, Chair, Department of Emergency Medicine, Indiana University School of Medicine.

Funding
None.

Authors' contributions
All four authors, PIM, JAL, CLH, and JAK were intimately involved in the conception, performance and writing of this manuscript. PIM and JAL performed the data analysis. All authors read and approved the final manuscript.

Competing interests
Paul Musey, MD - Research funding from Trevena, Inc. Jeffrey Kline, MD - Consultant to Janssen, Stago Diagnostica, Research funding from NIH, Mallingkrodt, Roche Diagnostics.

Author details
[1]Department of Emergency Medicine, Indiana University School of Medicine, Indianapolis, IN 46202, USA. [2]University of Virginia School of Medicine, Charlottesville, Virginia 22908, USA.

References
1. National Hospital Ambulatory Medical Care Survey: 2013 Emergency Department Summary Tables [https://www.cdc.gov/nchs/data/ahcd/nhamcs_emergency/2013_ed_web_tables.pdf]. Accessed 22 Oct 2017.
2. Webster R, Norman P, Goodacre S, Thompson A. The prevalence and correlates of psychological outcomes in patients with acute non-cardiac chest pain: a systematic review. Emerg Med J. 2012;29:267–73.
3. Foldes-Busque G, Marchand A, Chauny J-M, Poitras J, Diodati J, Denis I, Lessard M-J, Pelland M-E, Fleet R. Unexplained chest pain in the ED: could it be panic? Am J Emerg Med. 2011;29:743–51.
4. Musey PI Jr, Kline JA. Emergency department cardiopulmonary evaluation of low-risk chest pain patients with self-reported stress and anxiety. J Emerg Med. 2016;
5. Mello MJ, Merchant RC, Clark MA. Surveying emergency medicine. Acad Emerg Med. 2013;20:409–12.
6. Hsu C-C, Sandford BA. The Delphi technique: making sense of consensus. *Practical assessment, research & evaluation*. 2007;12:1–8.
7. Lloyd J. ACEP elects new officers. Washington, DC: American College of Emergency Physicians; 2016.
8. Harris PA, Taylor R, Thielke R, Payne J, Gonzalez N, Conde JG. Research electronic data capture (REDCap)–a metadata-driven methodology and workflow process for providing translational research informatics support. J Biomed Inform. 2009;42:377 81.
9. Webster R, Norman P, Goodacre S, Thompson AR, McEachan RRC. Illness representations, psychological distress and non-cardiac chest pain in patients attending an emergency department. Psychol Health. 2014;29:1265–82.
10. Webster R, Thompson AR, Norman P. 'Everything's fine, so why does it happen?' a qualitative investigation of patients' perceptions of noncardiac chest pain. J Clin Nurs. 2015;24:1936–45.
11. Khandaker GM, Zammit S, Lewis G, Jones PB. Association between serum C-reactive protein and DSM-IV generalized anxiety disorder in adolescence: findings from the ALSPAC cohort. Neurobiol Stress. 2016;4:55–61.
12. Roifman I, Beck PL, Anderson TJ, Eisenberg MJ, Genest J. Chronic inflammatory diseases and cardiovascular risk: a systematic review. Can J Cardiol. 2011;27:174–82.
13. Tona F, Serra R, Di Ascenzo L, Osto E, Scarda A, Fabris R, Montisci R, Famoso G, Tellatin S, Foletto M, et al. Systemic inflammation is related to coronary microvascular dysfunction in obese patients without obstructive coronary disease. Nutr Metab Cardiovasc Dis. 2014;24:447–53.
14. Jonsbu E, Dammen T, Morken G, Martinsen EW. Patients with noncardiac chest pain and benign palpitations referred for cardiac outpatient investigation: a 6-month follow-up. Gen Hosp Psychiatry. 2010;32:406–12.
15. Kisely SR, Campbell LA, Yelland MJ, Paydar A. Psychological interventions for symptomatic management of non-specific chest pain in patients with normal coronary anatomy. Cochrane Database Syst Rev. 2012;6:CD004101.
16. Jonsbu E, Martinsen EW, Morken G, Moum T, Dammen T. Illness perception among patients with chest pain and palpitations before and after negative cardiac evaluation. Biopsychosoc Med. 2012;6:19.
17. Kisely S, Guthrie E, Creed F, Tew R. Predictors of mortality and morbidity following admission with chest pain. J R Coll Physicians Lond. 1997;31:177–83.
18. Lewis C, Pearce J, Bisson JI. Efficacy, cost-effectiveness and acceptability of self-help interventions for anxiety disorders: systematic review. Br J Psychiatry. 2012;200:15–21.
19. Hsia RY, Hale Z, Tabas JA, National Study A. Of the prevalence of life-threatening diagnoses in patients with chest pain. JAMA Intern Med. 2016; 176:1029–32.
20. Al-Ani M, Winchester DE. Prevalence and overlap of noncardiac conditions in the evaluation of low-risk acute chest pain patients. Crit Pathw Cardiol. 2015;14:97–102.
21. Bjelland I, Dahl AA, Haug TT, Neckelmann D. The validity of the hospital anxiety and depression scale. An updated literature review. J Psychosom Res. 2002;52:69–77.
22. Ruiz MA, Zamorano E, Garcia-Campayo J, Pardo A, Freire O, Rejas J. Validity of the GAD-7 scale as an outcome measure of disability in patients with generalized anxiety disorders in primary care. J Affect Disord. 2011;128:277–86.
23. Spitzer RL, Kroenke K, Williams JB, Lowe B. A brief measure for assessing generalized anxiety disorder: the GAD-7. Arch Intern Med. 2006;166:1092–7.
24. McDonald IG, Daly J, Jelinek VM, Panetta F, Gutman JM. Opening Pandora's box: the unpredictability of reassurance by a normal test result. BMJ. 1996;313:329–32.
25. Ackermann S, Heierle A, Bingisser M-B, Hertwig R, Padiyath R, Nickel CH, Langewitz W, Bingisser R. Discharge communication in patients presenting to the emergency department with chest pain: defining the ideal content. Health Commun. 2016;31:557–65.
26. Serinken M, Zencir M, Karcioglu O, Sener S, Turkcuer I. Value of the timing of informing the emergency department patients on cardiac test results: a randomized controlled study. Eur J Emerg Med. 2009;16:74–9.
27. Webster R, Thompson AR, Norman P, Goodacre S. The acceptability and feasibility of an anxiety reduction intervention for emergency department patients with non-cardiac chest pain. Psychol Health Med. 2017;22:1–11.
28. van Beek MH, Oude Voshaar RC, Beek AM, van Zijderveld GA, Visser S, Speckens AE, Batelaan N, van Balkom AJ. A brief cognitive-behavioral intervention for treating depression and panic disorder in patients with noncardiac chest pain: a 24-week randomized controlled trial. Depress Anxiety. 2013;30:670–8.
29. Esler JL, Bock BC. Psychological treatments for noncardiac chest pain: recommendations for a new approach. J Psychosom Res. 2004;56:263–9.
30. Hirai M, Clum GA. A meta-analytic study of self-help interventions for anxiety problems. Behav Ther. 2006;37:99–111.
31. Arnold J, Goodacre S, Bath P, Price J. Information sheets for patients with acute chest pain: randomised controlled trial. BMJ. 2009;338:b541.
32. Hoge EA, Bui E, Marques L, Metcalf CA, Morris LK, Robinaugh DJ, Worthington JJ, Pollack MH, Simon NM. Randomized controlled trial of mindfulness meditation for generalized anxiety disorder: effects on anxiety and stress reactivity. J Clin Psychiatry. 2013;74:786–92.
33. Keng SL, Smoski MJ, Robins CJ. Effects of mindfulness on psychological health: a review of empirical studies. Clin Psychol Rev. 2011;31:1041–56.

11

Systematic reporting to improve the emergency medical response to major incidents

Sophie Hardy[1*], Sabina Fattah[2,3], Torben Wisborg[3,4,5], Lasse Raatiniemi[4,6,7], Trine Staff[8] and Marius Rehn[2,9,10]

Abstract

Background: Major incidents affect us globally, and are occurring with increasing frequency. There is still no evidence-based standard regarding the best medical emergency response to major incidents. Currently, reports on major incidents are non-standardised and variable in quality. This pilot study examines the first systematic reports from a consensus-based, freely accessible database, aiming to identify how descriptive analysis of reports submitted to this database can be used to improve the major incident response.

Methods: Majorincidentreporting.net is a website collecting reports on major incidents using a standardised template. Data from these reports were analysed to compare the emergency response to each incident.

Results: Data from eight reports showed that effective triage by experienced individuals and the use of volunteers for transport were notable successes of the major incident response. Inadequate resources, lack of a common triage system, confusion over command and control and failure of communication were reported failures. The following trends were identified: Fires had the slowest times for several aspects of the response and the only three countries to have a single dialling number for all three emergency services had faster response times. Helicopter Emergency Medical services (HEMS) were used for transport and treatment in rural locations and for triage and treatment in urban locations. In two incidents, a major incident was declared before the arrival of the first Emergency Medical Services (EMS) personnel.

Conclusion: This study shows that we can obtain relevant data from major incidents by using systematic reporting. Though the sample size from this pilot study is not large enough to draw any specific conclusions it illustrates the potential for future analyses. Identified lessons could be used to improve the emergency medical response to major incidents.

Keywords: Major incident, Disaster medicine, Uniform reporting, Standardised data

Background

Major incidents are a global issue that occur regardless of region or population affected. According to the Centre of Research on the Epidemiology of Disasters (CRED), disasters have become more frequent over the last 20 years [1]. Given the global and humanitarian impact of major incidents, learning lessons from them is essential. However, a Dutch study from 2010 that looked at reports from five consecutive national disasters suggests that we are not learning from them. It observed that, despite changes in protocol, legislation, organisation and funding, the same mistakes were being made each time [2]. Several studies have attempted to determine gold standards for various aspects of the emergency medical response to major incidents, but none have so far been successful [3, 4]. A failure to document, share and learn from our experiences of major incidents may be to blame [5, 6].

A literature review conducted on papers on emergency planning published between 1990 and 2010 found that the majority of publications came from North America and that given the large number of incidents that have occurred in Europe and Australasia, surprisingly few had

* Correspondence: sophiehardy50@doctors.org.uk
[1]Emergency Department, St George's Hospital, Tooting, London, UK
Full list of author information is available at the end of the article

been published from these areas. It concluded that the validity and generalisability of published literature on emergency planning has not been used to inform policy or change practice and that the type of evidence that would be useful to emergency planners in this respect needs to be identified [7].

Although a structured approach for responders exists [8], recent case reports on major incidents suggest that there is still much room for improvement, particularly in the areas of triage, treatment and transport of patients [9–11], communication [9, 12–14] and sufficient training of emergency medical responders [11].

Lately, many papers have highlighted the need to standardise research in this field so that a body of evidence can be assembled from the literature [5, 13, 15–18]. One way to approach this dilemma is to introduce a standardised method of reporting on major incidents (Fig. 1). Templates for reporting on major incidents have been developed globally, but none have been implemented or undergone feasibility testing [19]. This pilot study aims to evaluate whether common perceived successes and failures in major incident medical responses may be identified using a standardised template. A second aim is to investigate if this data can be used to identify trends in the major incident medical response and possible associations between actions and outcome.

Methods

In the majorincidentreporting.net database, an incident is defined as a major incident if it requires the mobilisation of extraordinary EMS resources and is identified as a major incident in that system [http://majorincidentreporting.net].

This was a retrospective pilot study based on an open access database available on http://www.majorincidentreporting.net [20, 21] (Fig. 2). Data was requested from EMS responders who were involved in a major incident and who had registered their data directly onto our database. Of the eight published major incident reports, the following themes were analysed: time from the occurrence of the major incident to declaration of a major incident, time from the occurrence of a major incident to the arrival of the first EMS, time from the occurrence of the major incident to the initial communication between emergency services, time from the arrival of the first EMS to the time that the major incident was declared, emergency contact number and response times, triage category numbers, effectiveness of communication, command and control and transportation. Whenever possible, these themes were compared between reports.

Data analysis

Quantitative data from each report was exported onto an Excel spreadsheet version 12.3.6 (©Microsoft Corporation, USA) and presented as frequencies with median and inter-quartile range (IQR). This was used to identify trends that, if consolidated with statistical data from a more significant number of reports, could change the way we respond to major incidents.

Perceived successes and failures were extracted as learning points in Fig. 3 to illustrate the potential of the database and data.

Ethics

Ethics approval for registering data on the website was granted by the Norwegian Data Protection Authority. All reports used in this analysis have been guaranteed by the author to comply with local ethics regulations prior to publication on the website [22].

Results

Eight reports on real life major incidents were published between April 2015 and March 2017 (Table 1). Key lessons in the published reports are summarised in Fig. 3.

Time intervals

A summary of important time intervals is presented in Table 2. Mexico, England and Finland were the only three countries in this study to have a single dialling number for all emergency services. Also, the reports from these countries represented the shortest time interval between the major incident being declared and the arrival of first EMS vehicles (6 min, 11 min and 12 min respectively). They also have the shortest time interval from the major incident being declared to the reported time of initial communication between different rescue organisations (1 min, 25 min and 17 min, respectively).

A summary of time intervals for each incident report is given in Table 2. In five reports, a major incident was declared after arrival of the first EMS and the time ranged from 10 to 30 min (median 18 min, IQR 15–25 min). In one report, the time interval was missing, and for the remaining two reports, a major incident was declared prior to arrival of the first EMS. One was declared 5 min before and the other 95 min before the arrival of the first EMS.

The two fires, a tunnel fire in Norway and a prison fire in Chile, reported the longest time interval, spanning from occurrence of the major incident to EMS arrival of 49 and 77 min, respectively. Both reports represented the longest time interval from major incident occurred to major incident declared (66 and 72 min., respectively) and the shortest time interval from major incident occurred to time of initial communication between different rescue organisations (61 and 90 min. respectively).

Triage

Triage systems divide casualties into green (delayed), yellow (urgent), red (immediate) and black (dead) categories. Figure 4 depicts triage categories for each incident.

EMS response data

20-1. Did the first medical team to arrive on-scene assume the role of medical commander? *	Yes
20-1.1. If possible, please provide the time the first medical team to arrive on-scene assumed the role of medical commander	2010-12-08
Hour	06
Minutes	17
20-1.2. Is the time given above exact or estimated? *	Exact
20-2. Did the first medical team to arrive on-scene begin to make an assessment of scene safety? *	Yes
20-3. Did the first medical team to arrive on-scene communicate a situation report to EMS coordinating centre? *	Yes
20-3.1. Was this done done according to a pre-existing system or mnemonic? (E.g. METHANE)? *	Yes
20-3.2. Please describe the mnemonic used in the report to EMS coordinating centre *	Similar to METHANE, not exact METHANE
20-4. Did the first medical team to arrive on-scene request additional resources? *	Yes
20-4.1. Please specify what type of resources where requested *	more ACLS, BLS ambulances; Physicians and Chief EMS
20-5. Did the first medical team to arrive on-scene initiate any safety related actions? *	No
20-6. Did the first medical team to arrive on-scene delegate responsibility for	No

Fig. 1 Excerpt from the EMS response subsection of the template. EMS: Emergency Medical Services. METHANE: M-Major incident declared? E-Exact location T-Type of incident H-Hazards A-Access. N-Number, Type, Severity of casualties E-Emergency services present and those required. ACLS: Advanced Cardiac Life Support. BLS: Basic Life Support

Three reports noted that the triage system used during major incidents was similar to the system they used on a daily basis. In relation to specific failures, three reports cited the lack of a common triage system between responders. In two reports it was highlighted that successful triage by skilled and experienced individuals prevented overcrowding of local hospitals.

Communication

Failure of communication both within the EMS response teams and between other emergency services (e.g. fire, police, military) was reported in five of the eight reports. Problems included inadequate radio systems with poor coverage, overloading and confusion over choice of communication group and difficulties in communication between two different incident sites resulting in a poor overview of the incident and separate response strategies.

In order to improve the emergency response, introduction of better communication systems with adequate coverage for more personnel and better systems for cooperating with other emergency services, was suggested.

Command and control

In two reports, confusion over who held which role in the command structure was reported. In one report,

- **What is majorincidentreporting.net?** A database that uses a standardised, consensus-based template to report on major incidents (*Figure 1*). These reports are peer-reviewed and published on the database
- **Who inputs data into the database?** Emergency medical providers who have been involved in a major incident
- **Who maintains the database?** Reports are regulated and updated by dedicated members of a non-profit, international steering group committee working on a voluntary basis
- **How is the database funded?** It was established in 2013 with funding from the Norwegian Air Ambulance Foundation
- **How is the validity of reports assessed?** It is the responsibility of submitting authors to ensure the validity of reports. Research into the reliability and inter-rater variability of reporting is ongoing
- **How much of the data is publically available?** Currently, all published reports are publicly available on the website
- **How is the reporting tool marketed?** Commentaries in medical journals, presentations at conferences, social media and through an animated video: https://www.youtube.com/watch?v=tisymgIwpXY

Fig. 2 Information on majorincidentreporting.net

delayed arrival of officers to their designated posts was reported to be due to long distances needed to travel. In two reports, they stated a need for more mandatory major incident training or exercises in order to improve MI command and control.

Transport

In one report, long distances from the incident site to the ambulance loading area was reported as a potential major incident EMS failure. A separate report praised their response for having a single port of access and egress to the incident for ambulances and other emergency vehicles. In two reports the use of volunteers for transporting of patients was suggested as one of their success criteria.

The Helicopter Emergency Medical Services (HEMS) was involved in five out of seven reports. In rural locations, HEMS was used both to transport and treat the patients on scene, while in the remaining reports, HEMS was involved only in triage or treatment on scene.

Discussion

The results show that we can obtain relevant data regarding common strengths and failures in major incident medical responses by using a consensus based template. Also, these data may be used to identify trends

Successes

- A single port of access and egress to the incident
- The use of volunteers for help with transport
- Triage by skilled and experienced individuals avoided overcrowding in local hospitals

Failures

- Resources inadequate (e.g. lack of fully equipped ambulances or appropriately skilled responders, failure to call in extra Emergency Operations Centre personnel)
- Resources sparsely located
- Communication failures within the EMS and between other emergency services (failure in technology and a failure in perception of the need to communicate)
- No national triage system used on a daily basis
- Lack of common triage system between responders
- Suboptimal safety measures with lack of safety planning
- Long distance to nearest ambulance
- Delayed access to casualties due to security issues
- Failure to establish a command structure or confusion over who held which position
- Delayed arrival of officers to their designated posts

Fig. 3 Successes and failures reported in published reports

Table 1 Details of the eight reports submitted to majorincidentreporting.net to date

Incident	Country	Type of incident	Environment	Number of people at risk
Prison fire	Chile	Fire	Urban	1900
School shooting	Finland	Shooting	Urban	200–299
Bus rollover	Norway	Transport accident	Rural	20
Truck & tunnel fire	Norway	Transport accident Fire	Rural	50
Terrorist mass-shooting	Norway	Shooting	Rural	600–699
Train collision	Norway	Transport accident Fire	Rural	86
Road traffic accident	United Kingdom	Transport accident Extreme weather	Rural	200–299
Hospital gas explosion	Mexico	Gas explosion	Urban	100–199

in major incident reporting and identify possible associations between actions and outcome. Moreover, an open-access webpage allows reports to be compared. To our knowledge, no study has been able to analyse a number of standardised reports on different major incidents. Despite the small number of reports, this study shows how results could be analysed to develop and later test hypotheses.

How results could affect major incident plans

The only three countries to use a single dialling number for EMS, police and fire had the fastest times from occurrence of incident to arrival of first EMS and occurrence of incident to initial communication between different rescue organisations. If later studies show a significant association between these factors, the emergency services should adapt for this.

Compared to the other six reports analysed, the two incidents involving fires took longer to be attended by EMS, longer to be declared as major incidents and longer to establish communication between rescue organisations. If studies later show that there is a positive association between incidents involving fires and longer response times, further studies could be initiated to establish the reason for this and major incident plans could be adapted accordingly.

Table 2 Time intervals for four aspects of the emergency response with time ranges, median time interval and IQR

Time Interval	Range (min)	Median (min)	IQR (min)
Major incident occurred to arrival of first EMS	6–95	15.5	11.5–63
Major incident occurred to major incident declared	16–72	51	25–66
Major incident occurred to time of initial communication between emergency services	1–90	42.5	17–61
Arrival of first EMS to major incident declared*	10–30	18	15–25

IQR Inter Quartile Range
* Does not include results for the two reports in which a major incident was declared before arrival of EMS

In most major incident plans, it is the role of the first EMS personnel who arrive on scene to declare or report a major incident [8]. In two out of seven reports, a major incident was declared before the arrival of the EMS. The appropriate declaration of a major incident should occur as early as possible. If later studies prove the hypothesis that declaration of a major incident by the Emergency Operations Centre before the arrival of the EMS is largely appropriate and effective, this information could be used to revise current major incident plans.

Recurring themes reinforce the need for change in current practice

The findings in this study are supported by others. Failure in communication and confusion over command structure is a recurring theme in major incident case reports [12–14, 23]. Similarly, making use of volunteers especially for transport of patients and resources, the camaraderie or "coming together" of people involved in the incident both from the rescue services and bystanders and their willingness to help beyond their means [24]. This reinforces the concept of "bystander-as-responder". That bystanders and volunteers should be used more effectively during major incidents and their role should be factored in to major incident plans [25] Also commonly mentioned was the use of highly skilled personnel for triage. This is echoed in a number of publications [23, 26] including a paper by Aylwin et al. which found that overtriage rates were reduced when trained and experienced pre-hospital teams carried out initial scene triage during the London bombings [10].

This study illustrates how a database such as majorincidentreporting.net could facilitate an evidence base for emergency response planning. Studies of a larger number of more homogeneous incidents may provide more valid analysis. Such research initiatives are welcomed.

Limitations

The number of reports analysed is small and heterogeneous. Additionally, potential subjective bias in the reports cannot be excluded. Most of the published reports

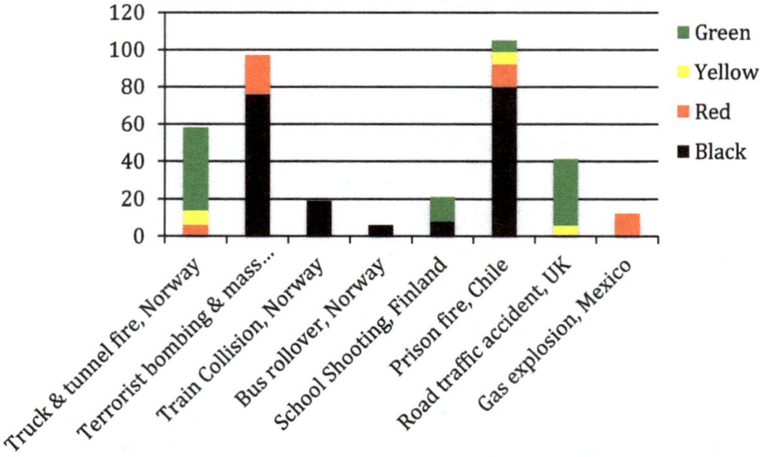

Fig. 4 Triage categories for each incident (category numbers marked as "unknown" on the report are not entered)

have been written by pre-hospital anaesthetists instead of a multi-professional team consisting of paramedics, dispatchers, medical incident commanders and physicians. To overcome this problem, the website could be updated to incorporate a different method of data input so that multiple authors can report on one incident. Furthermore, the reports have been submitted from different countries with different kinds of emergency medical services. Therefore, the comparison of the reports has to be interpreted with caution.

Conclusion

The findings of this study highlight the importance of identifying strengths and challenges in the major incident medical response through systematic reporting. Further, the identification of trends in the emergency response to major incidents could enable the formulation of hypotheses regarding the best approach to different aspects of the response. Systematic reporting of such data may be used to test hypotheses by comparing data before and after the introduction of new guidelines and policies. Ultimately, it can be used to compare major incidents to determine the optimal medical response. As we move towards a new era of collaborative consumption, anyone can help to develop and learn from a truly global and open access database.

Abbreviations

ACLS: Advanced Cardiac Life Support; BLS: Basic Life Support; CRED: Centre of Research on the Epidemiology of Disasters; EM-DAT: Emergency Events Database; EMS: Emergency Medical Services; HEMS: Helicopter Emergency Services; METHANE: M-Major incident declared? E-Exact location T-Type of incident H-Hazards A- Access N-Number, Type, Severity of casualties E-Emergency services present and those required

Acknowledgements

We acknowledge and thank all incident reporters for their willingness to participate and support this project, and for their continued dedication to improve major incident management. The authors thank Tormod Lunde Idsø for his contributions to the development of the website.

Funding

The www.majorincidentreporting.net webpage was sponsored by the Norwegian Air Ambulance. They have also contributed to the financial costs for editing and publishing this paper, but did not play any role in conducting the study.

Authors' contributions

MR and SF conceived the idea. SH analysed and interpreted the data and wrote the paper in collaboration with all authors. SF, MR and TW participated in developing the template and database. TS participated in developing the template. SH, SF, TS, MR and LR are editorial members of majorincidentreporting.net. All authors read and approved the final manuscript.

Competing interests

The authors declare that they have no competing interests.

Author details

[1]Emergency Department, St George's Hospital, Tooting, London, UK. [2]The Norwegian Air Ambulance Foundation, Drøbak, Norway. [3]Anaesthesia and Critical Care Research Group, Faculty of Health Sciences, University of Tromsø, Tromsø, Norway. [4]Hammerfest Hospital, Department of Anaesthesiology and Intensive Care, Finnmark Health Trust, Hammerfest, Norway. [5]Norwegian National Advisory Unit on Trauma, Division of Emergencies and Critical Care, Oslo University Hospital, Oslo, Norway. [6]Centre for Pre-Hospital Emergency Care/ FinnHEMS 50, Oulu University Hospital, Oulu, Finland. [7]Anaesthesia Research Group, MRC, University of Oulu, Oulu, Finland. [8]Paramedic Sciences, Oslo and Akershus University College, Oslo, Norway. [9]Department of Health Studies, University of Stavanger, Stavanger, Norway. [10]Division of Emergencies and Critical Care. Department of Anaesthesia, Oslo University Hospital, Oslo, Norway.

References

1. Centre for Research in the Epidemiology of Disasters (2015) The Human Cost of Natural Disasters 2015: A Global Perspective. http://emdat.be/human_cost_natdis (Accessed 8 June 2017).
2. Juffermans J, Bierens J. Recurrent medical response problems during five recent disasters in the Netherlands. Prehosp Disaster Med. 2010;25:127–36.
3. Rimstad R, Braut G. Literature review on medical incident command. Prehosp Disaster Med. 2015;30:205–15.

4. Johnsen AS, Fattah S, Sollid SJM, Rehn M. Utilisation of helicopter emergency medical services in the early medical response to major incidents: a systematic literature review. BMJ Open. 2016; https://doi.org/10.1136/bmjopen-2015- 010307.
5. Hardy S. Major incidents in England. BMJ. 2015; https://doi.org/10.1136/bmj.h1712.
6. Carley S, Mackway-Jones K, Donnan S. Major incidents in Britain over the past 28 years: the case for the centralised reporting of major incidents. J Epidemiol Community Health. 1998;52(6):392–8.
7. Challen K, Lee A, Booth A, Gardois P, Woods HB, Goodacre SW. Where is the evidence for emergency planning: a scoping review. BMC Public Health. 2012;12:542.
8. Advanced Life Support Group. Major incident medical management and support: the practical approach at the scene. 3rd ed. Manchester: Advanced Life Support Group; 2011.
9. Ardagh MW, Richardson SK, Robinson V. The initial health-system response to the earthquake in Christchurch, New Zealand, in February, 2011. Lancet. 2012;379(9831):2109–15.
10. Aylwin CJ, König TC, Brennan NW, et al. Reduction in critical mortality in urban mass casualty incidents: analysis of triage, surge, and resource use after the London bombings on July 7, 2005. Lancet. 2006;368:2219–25.
11. Biddinger PD, Baggish A, Harrington L, et al. Be prepared — the Boston Marathon and mass-casualty events. N Engl J Med. 2013;368(21):1958–9.
12. Philippe J, Brahic O, Carli P, Tourtier J, Riou B, Vallet B. French Ministry of Health's response to Paris attacks of 13 November 2015. Crit Care. 2016;20:85.
13. Koning SW, Ellerbroek PM, Leenen LPH. Indoor fire in a nursing home: evaluation of the medical response to a mass casualty incident based on a standardized protocol. Eur J Trauma Emerg Surg. 2015;41:167–78.
14. Howells NR, Dunne N, Reddy S. The casualty profile from the reading train crash, November 2004: proposals for improved major incident reporting and the application of trauma scoring systems. Emerg Med J. 2006;23:530–3.
15. Bradt DA, Aitken P. Disaster medicine reporting: the need for new guidelines and the CONFIDE statement. Emerg Med Australas. 2010;22:483–7.
16. Lennquist S. Protocol for reports from major accidents and disasters in the international journal of disaster medicine. Eur J Trauma Emerg Surg. 2008; 34(5):486–92.
17. WADEM/ Nordic Society for Disaster Medicine. Health disaster management: guidelines for evaluation and research in the "Utstein style". Prehosp Disaster Med. 2003;17(S):1–167.
18. Birnbaum M, Daily E, O'Rourke A, Loretti A. Disaster research/evaluation frameworks, part 1: an overview. Prehosp Disaster Med. 2014;29:1–12.
19. Fattah S, Rehn M, Reierth E, Wisborg T. Systematic literature review of templates for reporting prehospital major incident medical management. BMJ Open. 2013;3:e002658.
20. Fattah S, Rehn M, Lockey D, Thompson J, Lossius HM, Wisborg T. A consensus based template for reporting of pre-hospital major incident medical management. Scand J Trauma Resusc Emerg Med. 2014;22:5.
21. Hardy SEJ, Fattah S. Trials and tribulations: how we established a major incident database. Scand J Trauma Resusc Emerg Med. 2017;25:7.
22. Fattah S, Rehn M. Wisborg T, implementing a template for major incident reporting: experiences from the first year. Scand J Trauma Resusc Emerg Med. 2015;23:55.
23. Sollid SJ, Rimstad R, Rehn M, et al. Oslo government district bombing and Utoya island shooting July 22, 2011: the immediate prehospital emergency medical service response. Scand J Trauma Resusc Emerg Med. 2012;20:3.
24. Walls RM, Zinner MJ. The Boston marathon response, why did it work so well? JAMA. 2013;309:2441–2.
25. Jacobs LM, Wade D, McSwain NE, et al. Hartford consensus: a call to action for THREAT, a medical disaster preparedness concept. J Am Coll Surg. 2014; 218(3):467–75.
26. Turner CDA, Lockey DJ, Rehn M. Pre-hospital management of mass casualty civilian shootings: a systematic literature review. Crit Care. 2016;20:362.

12

Assessment of the Feasibility of automated, real-time clinical decision support in the emergency department using electronic health record data

Warren M. Perry[1,2], Rubayet Hossain[1,2] and Richard A. Taylor[1,2,3*]

Abstract

Background: The use of big data and machine learning within clinical decision support systems (CDSSs) has the potential to transform medicine through better prognosis, diagnosis and automation of tasks. Real-time application of machine learning algorithms, however, is dependent on data being present and entered prior to, or at the point of, CDSS deployment. Our aim was to determine the feasibility of automating CDSSs within electronic health records (EHRs) by investigating the timing, data categorization, and completeness of documentation of their individual components of two common Clinical Decision Rules (CDRs) in the Emergency Department.

Methods: The CURB-65 severity score and HEART score were randomly selected from a list of the top emergency medicine CDRs. Emergency department (ED) visits with ICD-9 codes applicable to our CDRs were eligible. The charts were reviewed to determine the categorization components of the CDRs as structured and/or unstructured, median times of documentation, portion of charts with all data components documented as structured data, portion of charts with all structured CDR components documented before ED departure. A kappa score was calculated for interrater reliability.

Results: The components of the CDRs were mainly documented as structured data for the CURB-65 severity score and HEART score. In the CURB-65 group, 26.8% of charts had all components documented as structured data, and 67.8% in the HEART score. Documentation of some CDR components often occurred late for both CDRs. Only 21 and 11% of patients had all CDR components documented as structured data prior to ED departure for the CURB-65 and HEART score groups, respectively. The interrater reliability for the CURB-65 score review was 0.75 and 0.65 for the HEART score.

Conclusion: Our study found that EHRs may be unable to automatically calculate popular CDRs—such as the CURB-65 severity score and HEART score—due to missing components and late data entry.

Keywords: Clinical decision support, Machine learning, Data quality, Electronic health records

* Correspondence: Richard.taylor@yale.edu
[1]Emergency Medicine Department, Yale School of Medicine, 464 Congress Avenue, Suite #260, New Haven, CT 06450, USA
[2]Emergency Department, Yale New Haven Hospital, 20 York Street, New Haven, CT 06510, USA
Full list of author information is available at the end of the article

Background

The use of big data and machine learning within clinical decision support systems (CDSSs) has the potential to transform medicine through better prognosis, diagnosis and automation of tasks [1, 2]. Real-time application of machine learning algorithms, however, is dependent on data being present and entered prior to, or at the point of, CDSS deployment [3]. While simple CDSSs may request the user to enter in data necessary to run the algorithm, this process becomes infeasible when tens or even hundreds of data elements are needed, thus requiring some form of automated capture and real-time integration of data from the electronic health record (EHR) [4].

The emergency department (ED), with a highly condensed time frame for decision making, represents a unique and challenging environment for CDSS deployment [5]. In the ED, patient medical problems are often acute with limited supporting information already present in the EHR, most of the information necessary for decision making is generated within a few hours, and recording of parts of this information in the form of provider notes may be delayed until well after the patient has left the department [6]. Currently, there is limited knowledge on when components necessary for calculation of CDSS in the ED are available in the EHR, what data type (structured vs unstructured) they exist in, and data completeness for specific algorithms [7].

Our study, therefore, aimed to examine the EHR data entry process for two common, simple clinical decision rules (CDRs) as a first step in assessing the potential feasibility of constructing more complex automated, real-time clinical decision support systems in the ED. Specifically, we examined whether the CDRs were calculable using EHR data, how the individual CDR components are recorded (structured versus unstructured data), and the timeliness of data entry.

Methods

Study design

This was a retrospective study of ED visits between 1/1/2015 and 1/1/2016. The study was approved by the institutional review board.

Study site

The study involved five different emergency department sites with combined annual visits > 250,000. All of the study sites are part of a larger hospital healthcare system with a single EHR vendor. The hospital system serves both an urban and suburban patient population. The sites are staffed with certified nursing assistants, midlevel providers, residents, and attending physicians.

Identification of clinical decision rules

The research team contacted the creators of the website, www.MDcalc.com, to acquire a list of the calculators used in the Emergency Medicine section. This table included the full list of calculators and the percentage each calculator composed of the total searches for all calculators in the 3 months prior to July 16, 2015. From this list of calculators, we ordered them from highest to lowest percentage of searches. We defined a clinical decision rule as a "clinical tool that quantifies the individual contributions that various components of the history, physical examination, and basic laboratory results make toward the diagnosis, prognosis, or likely response to treatment in a patient" [8]. A calculator from the list was eligible for selection if it met this definition and excluded if it was not created for the purpose of being a CDR, was targeted to a population less than 18 years of age, had no diagnostic significance, no prognostic significance for a condition or treatment, or cannot be calculated in the emergency department. From this definition, the research team identified the top 10 clinical decision rules, and randomly selected two from the list to investigate, the CURB-65 score and HEART score.

Patient chart selection and review

The calculated sample size of each CDR, assuming 70% structured data, 95% confidence intervals for a 7.5% margin of error was 140 charts. We selected 145 charts to review for both the CURB-65 score and HEART score. In order to identify charts where the CDRs would be used, the team performed a keyword search to make a list of ICD-9 codes that corresponded with the diagnoses targeted by each CDR (Additional file 1: Table S1). From this list, the team performed a database query for all emergency department diagnoses within the study period that matched the ICD-9 codes identified for each CDR. Prior to full review, the team randomly selected and reviewed 10 separate charts from each CDR list to ensure the chosen ICD-9 codes appropriately selected patients with medical presentations applicable to their corresponding CDR.

Data collection

Patient charts were stored in a database (FileMaker, Inc., FileMaker International) as multiple iterations with noted timestamps to document changes made to the patient chart (i.e. every time a chart was modified a new timestamped instance was generated). The team excluded a chart if the chart had more iterations than is supported by the query text field and was therefore truncated. In the analysis, the charts were reviewed to categorize the individual CDR components as structured or unstructured data. The team defined structured data as any data with designated fields containing discrete data elements within the electronic health record. All other data was considered unstructured. Each element documented, had its corresponding timestamp of when it appeared in the EHR documented as well. The team documented the portion of charts with all structured data components required to calculate each corresponding CDR. Furthermore, the total time from triage to disposition, and the portion of charts with all data components entered as structured data prior to the patient's departure from the emergency department were obtained. All chart reviewers had at least 5 months of experience using EPIC and went through training to ensure all members understood what data is structured versus unstructured. The team agreed on a guide of instructions for both the CURB-65 score and HEART score CDRs to standardize the review (Additional file 2: Appendix B).

Data analysis

Results were analyzing using standard descriptive statistics. Box plots were generated for time to date entry of the various components and operational metrics. A kappa score was calculated to assess the interrater reliability among reviewers. All analysis was performed in R (**R** Core Team (2017). **R**: A language and environment for statistical computing).

Results

A total of 83 calculators were received from the creators of www.MDcalc.com. Seventeen calculators were excluded to reach our final list of ten emergency medicine clinical decision rules. To view a full list of these calculators and why each one was excluded, please refer to Additional file 3: Appendix C. One hundred and forty-five charts were reviewed for the CURB-65 rule and HEART score, each. In the HEART score group, 2 charts had either missing or errant data from the review process and were excluded in the data analysis. The demographic information for the patients is demonstrated in Table 1. The Kappa statistic was 0.75 and 0.65 for the CURB-65 and HEART score respectively. Overall, the HEART score was able to be calculated 67.8% of the time and the CURB-65 rule 26.8% of the time from the provided structured data.

Percentage documentation of structured and unstructured date elements for the HEART and CURB-65 score are presented in Table 2. Median times and interquartile ranges for each unstructured and structured data components of each rule are presented in Table 3 and Figs. 1 and 2. The median time from triage to a disposition was 280 (IQR 195–386] and 248 (IQR 170–381] minutes for the CURB-65 score and HEART score, respectively. Approximately 21% of the CURB-65 score patients and 11% of the HEART score patients had all their CDR components entered prior to their departure from the emergency department.

Table 1 Study demographics

	CURB-65[a] Score	HEART[b] Score
N	145	143
Median age	64.00	51.00
Male n (%)	68 (46.9)	54 (37.8)
Ethnicity n (%)		
Hispanic or Latino	26 (17.9)	28 (19.6)
Non-Hispanic	118 (81.4)	115 (80.4)
Unknown	1 (0.7)	0 (0.0)
Race n (%)		
Asian	3 (2.1)	0 (0.0)
Black or African American	21 (14.5)	34 (23.8)
Hispanic/Latino	1 (0.7)	2 (1.4)
Not documented	1 (0.7)	2 (1.4)
Other	26 (17.9)	23 (16.1)
Patient refused	2 (1.4)	1 (0.7)
White or Caucasian	91 (62.8)	81 (56.6)

[a]Confusion, Urea, Respiratory rate, Blood pressure, Age ≥ 65
[b]History, Electrocardiogram, Age, Risk factors, Troponin

Discussion

Automated real-time CDSSs integrating machine learning algorithms trained on big data have the potential to transform healthcare, however necessary data for the algorithms must be present at the time of use, and little is known about how data availability impacts the feasibility of these systems in general, and more specifically within the emergency department. This study examines the data entry process for two popular clinical decision rules, CURB-65 score and HEART score as a first step in assessing the feasibility of more complex CDSSs. Our findings demonstrate that, even for these simple CDRs, the HEART score and CURB-65 rule were only able to be calculated prior to ED departure in 21, and 11% of visits, respectively. For structured data only, regardless of timing, the HEART score was able to be calculated in 67.8% of visits and the CURB-65 rule in 26.8% of visits. Data components that depended on historical information (confusion, risk factors, etc.) or provider entry of data were entered frequently after ED departure.

Prior studies have noted the need for EHR integration of CDSSs, however previous studies examining the ability of CDRs to be automated are limited [7, 9–11]. Aakre et al. [10] investigated the programmability of clinical decision rules in an EHR based on the ability of their components to be extracted from structured data sources or retrieved using advanced technology such as natural language processing (NLP) and Boolean logic text search. Out of the 168 CDRs investigated in this study, only 26 (15.5%) were programmable exclusively using structured objective data elements. If additional advanced technology, such as NLP and Boolean logic

Table 2 Portion of data elements documented as structured vs. Unstructured

CURB-65[a] Score			HEART[b] Score		
Elements	Structured [c]	Unstructured [c]	Elements	Structured [c]	Unstructured [c]
Confusion	141 (97.2)	22 (15.2)	Age	143 (100.0)	75 (52.4)
Blood urea nitrogen	117 (80.7)	3 (2.1)	Risk factors	127 (88.8)	87 (60.8)
Respiratory rate	145 (100.0)	9 (6.2)	History	128 (89.5)	128 (89.5)
Blood pressure	144 (99.3)	10 (6.9)	Electrocardiogram	66 (46.2)	141 (98.6)
Age	145 (100.0)	88 (60.7)	Troponin	120 (83.9)	54 (37.8)
All structured elements documented (%)	26.8		67.8		
All structured elements documented prior to ED[d] departure (%)	21		11		
Kappa statistic	0.75		0.65		

[a]Confusion, Urea, Respiratory rate, Blood pressure, Age ≥ 65
[b]History, Electrocardiogram, Age, Risk factors, Troponin
[c]Results reported as n (%)
[d]Emergency department

text search, were utilized to extract both the structured and unstructured subjective components, this theoretical number increased to 43 (25.6%). This study did not examine the data completeness or timeliness of these CDRs within an existing EHR. Sheehan et al. [7], examined through qualitative analysis the Pediatric Emergency Care Applied Research Network (PECARN) clinical prediction rules for children with minor blunt head trauma and found the need for seamless integration, flowsheets to facilitate data entry, among other workflow, organizational, and human factors impeding automization. Our study adds to this knowledge about the difficulty and planning necessary for CDSSs.

Our findings have important implications for CDSS implementation within the ED. If CDDSs are to be effectively utilized, the data must be available at the point in time the CDSS provides value in the decision-making process. The fact that in our study the CDRs were often unable to be calculated from structured data indicates that for CDSSs to be effective structured fields must be built within the EHR that are designed to capture the components of the CDSSs and/or natural language processing should be utilized. In addition, CDSSs, must take into consideration the timing of data entry. For the two CDRs in this study, most of the delay in calculability resulted from data components collected through the history and physical or were dependent on provider entry of data (e.g. EKG interpretation). This is not surprising as ED providers often get behind in documentation during a shift or wait until after their shifts to complete documentation [6]. This lack of timeliness implies that the performance of CDSSs within the ED will be hampered by data entry and future efforts at CDSSs should consider more effective methods of timely data entry such as speech recognition with natural language processing pipelines.

Limitations

Our study has several limitations. We only chose two clinical decision rules to examine. While it is possible that other CDRs would have better data-entry, we believe that the themes derived from our results (late entry of historical/physical findings, and overall poor ability to calculate in a timely fashion) would be the same. It is possible that emergency physicians at our site could have used other CDRs relevant to our patient population, but the research team did not observe other CDRs documented as

Table 3 Median times and interquartile ranges for elements documentation[a]

CURB-65[b] Score			HEART[c] Score		
Elements	Structured	Unstructured	Elements	Structured	Unstructured
Confusion	383.00 [343.50, 451.00]	407.00 [376.25, 475.75]	Age	10.00 [6.00, 17.25]	350.00 [297.00, 426.00]
Blood area nitrogen	88.00 [66.00, 120.00]	431.00 [426.50, 2401.00]	Electrocardiogram	354.00 [315.00, 418.00]	7.00 [3.00, 17.00]
Respiratory rate	7.00 [3.00, 14.00]	410.00 [350.00, 422.00]	Risk factors	342.00 [301.50, 404.50]	357.00 [318.00, 433.00]
Blood pressure	7.00 [3.00, 14.50]	401.50 [372.25, 445.25]	History	347.50 [310.75, 418.25]	346.00 [304.75, 415.75]
Age	9.00 [4.00, 18.00]	371.00 [338.00, 449.00]	Troponin	87.50 [54.00, 129.75]	504.50 [390.00, 665.25]
Time to departure	280.00 [195.00, 386.00]		248.00 [170.00, 381.00]		

[a]All items are reported in minutes, median time [interquartile range time]
[b]Confusion, Urea, Respiratory rate, Blood pressure, Age ≥ 65
[c]History, Electrocardiogram, Age, Risk factors, Troponin

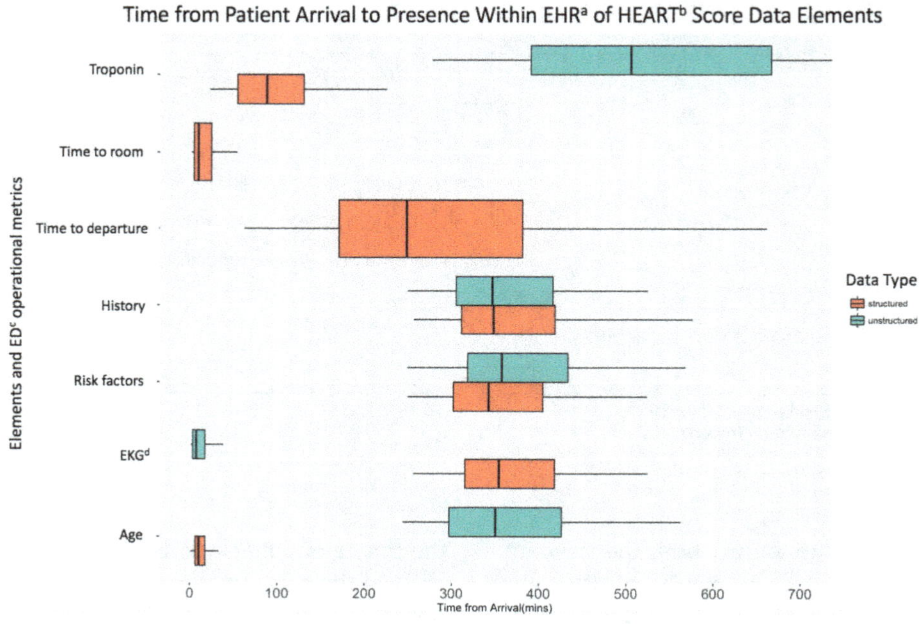

Fig. 1 Time from Arrival to Presence Within EHR[a] of HEART[b] Score Data. The above figure is a box and whiskers plot representation of Table 3 data from the HEART score. [a] electronic health record. [b] History, Electrocardiogram, Age, Risk Factors, Troponin. [c] emergency department. [d] electrocardiogram

unstructured data in the patient chart. Some of the clinicians may not believe in the value of our selected CDRs; however, we chose our CDRs randomly from a reliable source of the top searched emergency medicine calculators. The guidelines for presence of the data components we used in our study were not strict, but this method optimized the number of components that satisfied our criteria and provided a best-case scenario. Even with these relaxed parameters, the findings show that all components are not documented for the CURB-65 and HEART scores. Lastly, our study had a small sample size of patients and thus we were unable to determine the effects of different ED environments for documentation (e.g., effect of provider type, presence or absence of dictation software).

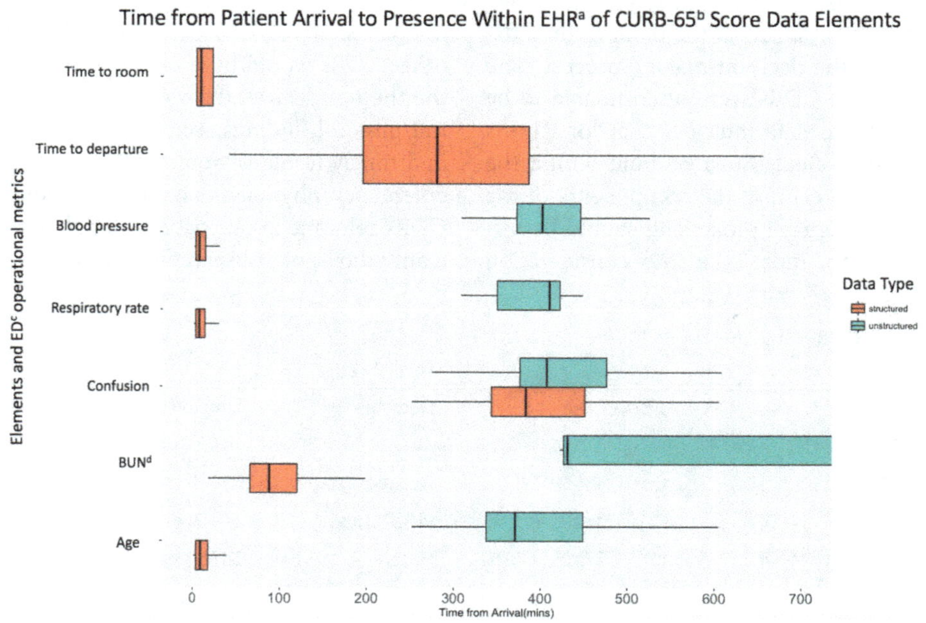

Fig. 2 Time from Arrival to Presence Within EHR[a] of CURB-65[b] Score Data. The above figure is a box and whiskers plot representation of Table 3 data from the CURB-65 score. [a] electronic health record. [b] Confusion, Urea, Respiratory Rate, Blood Pressure, Age ≥ 65. [c] emergency department. [d] blood urea nitrogen leve

Conclusion

Our study assessing the potential feasibility of constructing more complex automated, real-time CDSSs in the ED through examination of the EHR data entry process for two common, simple CDRs demonstrates that the CDRs cannot be calculated reliably during the emergency department visit because of problems with data completeness and timeliness of entry.

Abbreviations

CDR: Clinical Decision Rule; CDSSs: Clinical decision support systems; ED: Emergency department; EHR: electronic health records

Funding

There was no funding for the study.

Authors' contributions

WP and RAT designed the study. WP, RH and RAT performed chart review. RAT analyzed the results. WP drafted the manuscript. All authors contributed to revisions. All authors have read and approved the manuscript.

Competing interests

The are no competing interests to disclose.

Author details

[1]Emergency Medicine Department, Yale School of Medicine, 464 Congress Avenue, Suite #260, New Haven, CT 06450, USA. [2]Emergency Department, Yale New Haven Hospital, 20 York Street, New Haven, CT 06510, USA. [3]Yale School of Medicine, Yale New Haven Hospital, 464 Congress Avenue, Suite #260, New Haven, CT 06450, USA.

References

1. Obermeyer Z, Emanuel EJ. Predicting the future - big data, machine learning, and Clinical Medicine N. Engl J Med. 2016;375:1216–9.
2. Murdoch TB, Detsky AS. The inevitable application of big data to health care. JAMA. 2013;309:1351–2.
3. Bates DW, Kuperman GJ, Wang S, et al. Ten commandments for effective clinical decision support: making the practice of evidence-based medicine a reality. J Am Med Inform Assoc. 2003;10:523–30.
4. Amarasingham R, Patzer RE, Huesch M, Nguyen NQ, Xie B. Implementing electronic health care predictive analytics: considerations and challenges. Health Aff (Millwood). 2014;33:1148–54.
5. Bennett P, Hardiker NR. The use of computerized clinical decision support systems in emergency care: a substantive review of the literature. J Am Med Inform Assoc. 2017;24:655–68.
6. Perry JJ, Sutherland J, Symington C, Dorland K, Mansour M, Stiell IG. Assessment of the impact on time to complete medical record using an electronic medical record versus a paper record on emergency department patients: a study. Emerg Med J. 2014;31:980–5.
7. Sheehan B, Nigrovic LE, Dayan PS, et al. Informing the design of clinical decision support services for evaluation of children with minor blunt head trauma in the emergency department: a sociotechnical analysis. J Biomed Inform. 2013;46:905–13.
8. McGinn TG, Guyatt GH, Wyer PC, et al. Users' guides to the medical literature: xxii: how to use articles about clinical decision rules. JAMA. 2000;284:79–84.
9. Ebell M. AHRQ White Paper: Use of clinical decision rules for point-of-care decision support. Med Decis Mak. 2010;30:712–21.
10. Aakre C, Dziadzko M, Keegan MT, Herasevich V. Automating clinical score calculation within the electronic health record. A Feasibility Assessment. Appl Clin Inform. 2017;8:369–80.
11. Green SM. When do clinical decision rules improve patient care? Reply. Ann Emerg Med. 2014;63:373.

13

A cross-sectional exploratory study of knowledge, attitudes, and practices of emergency health care providers in the assessment of child maltreatment in Maputo, Mozambique

Liliana Pinto[1], Adriana Lein[2], Raquel Mahoque[3], David W. Wright[4], Scott M. Sasser[5] and Catherine A. Staton[2,6,7*]

Abstract

Background: In Mozambique, and other low-income countries (LICs), there is little information on the burden of child maltreatment (CM). Emergency care services (ECS) play an important role in recognizing, treating, and intervening in situations of CM. We aim to identify knowledge, attitudes, and practices regarding CM among health care providers in ECS at Mavalane General Hospital in Maputo, Mozambique.

Methods: This exploratory cross-sectional study evaluates the knowledge, attitudes, and practices of health care providers to diagnose and treat cases of CM. A 25 min, pilot-tested verbal interview questionnaire was administered to 49 physicians and nurses working in ECS at Mavalane General Hospital. Interviews were completed between October–November 2010. Data were managed and analyzed in SPSS 14.0 and descriptive statistics were generated.

Results: Of 49 health care providers, 83.6% reporting receiving no, or very little CM education or training. Only 61.2% had knowledge of physical abuse as a main form of child maltreatment and 38.8% were able to identify corresponding symptoms of physical abuse. Sexual abuse as a main form of CM was mentioned by 26.5 and 2% cited its symptoms. While 87.7% of health care providers strongly agreed or agreed that they hold an important role in preventing CM, 51.1% also strongly disagreed or disagreed that they feel confident diagnosing and treating CM cases. In regards to follow-up, 14.3% strongly disagreed or disagreed that they know where to refer victims for further follow-up and an additional 14.3% did not know whether they agreed or disagreed.

Conclusion: This study revealed knowledge gaps in emergency health care provider knowledge of the main forms of CM and their symptoms. The fact that a majority of health care providers in our sample did not receive information specific to CM in their medical education and training could explain this gap, as well as their unawareness of where to refer victims. Given that health care providers believe they play an important role in identifying and treating CM, future research should focus on raising physician awareness of CM and developing education and training materials grounded in cultural contexts to build response capacity in Mozambique and other LICs.

Keywords: Child maltreatment, Emergency care services, Health care providers, Mozambique-Africa, Human rights abuses

* Correspondence: catherine.staton@duke.edu
[2]Duke Global Health Institute, Duke University, 310 Trent Drive, Durham, North Carolina 27710, USA
[6]Division of Emergency Medicine, Department of Surgery, Duke University Medical Center, 2301 Erwin Road, Durham, North Carolina 27710, USA
Full list of author information is available at the end of the article

Background

Child maltreatment (CM), the physical, sexual and emotional abuse, neglect, or exploitation of under 18 populations carries a heavy social cost and is a serious human rights and public health issue [1–3]. Distinct from other forms of violence against children, child maltreatment CM refers specifically to acts perpetrated by parents or caregivers [4]. CM is alarmingly pervasive; globally, an estimated 60% of children aged 2–14 experience frequent physical punishment and as many as 70% are victims of psychological abuse from their caregivers [5]. Rates of CM are the highest in low-income countries, particularly in the African region where the heaviest burden is observed [5–7]. Studies from Africa have found that between 75 and 94.4% of children experienced physical abuse from caregivers in the past year and 58.3–64% experienced emotional abuse [6, 8, 9]. The highest prevalence of child sexual abuse is also seen in Africa, with 34.4% of children experiencing a form before the age of 18 [10]. CM causes a range of long-term physical and mental sequelae, including neurological, cognitive, affective, and social disorders [11, 12], and is associated with poor school performance [13] and internalized acceptance towards gender-based violent attitudes in girls [14].

CM is closely tied to the social and cultural context. Numerous studies from Africa point towards poor knowledge of what constitutes abuse and accepting attitudes of abusive behaviors in cultures where corporal punishment and other forms of harsh discipline are entrenched in traditions and commonly practiced as main drivers [15–18].CM is also associated with poverty and socioeconomic status [8, 19, 20] and exposure to other forms of violence, namely domestic violence, within the household [14, 21]. Due to the normalization of CM, cases are rarely reported and it's often termed a silent phenomenon [4, 22–25]. Literature from high-income countries suggests that training health care providers to be aware of abusive behaviors, recognize warning signs, and refer suspected cases to appropriate services might be one effective form of intervention and prevention [26–29]. This is due to the fact emergency departments are often critical entry points into crisis response systems [30]. Despite the potential for emergency care services (ECS) to act as a first line of defense against CM, studies of this population from Sub-Saharan Africa are limited.

Existing studies from the region related to CM management in a hospital tend to focus on the profile of injuries, rather than health care providers. One study of physicians in the region found poor knowledge in correctly diagnosing cases of CM [31]. Yet, studies from ECS in Africa have found the burden of intentional injuries to be higher, between 18 and 21.3% [32, 33]. Training health care providers to recognize warning signs of CM is critical for timely intervention and prevention [27, 34]. Given the cultural context, knowledge of symptoms of CM alone may be insufficient. Thus, there is a need for reliable studies from Africa that take a holistic approach to examining barriers to diagnosis and intervention in suspected CM, which may include limited knowledge [31, 34], negative attitudes towards their role to intervene [23], and uncertainty in diagnosing and confusion about their responsibility to report cases [35, 36]. Consequently, there is a need for reliable studies to better understand current deficiencies and their determinants in the diagnosis and case management of child maltreatment victims in emergency departments.

In Mozambique, a low-income country in Southeast Africa, 5696 cases of violence against children were reported to police authorities and 190,000 cases were reported to the Child Help Line (*A Linha Fala Criança*) in 2015 alone [33].The actual prevalence of CM is likely underestimated due to fragmented surveillance, limited legal infrastructure, and the absence of children's rights protections [22]. While the Ministry of Health has recently adopted a new approach centered on education and preparedness, the capacity to identify and treat CM in emergency care services in Mozambique (ECS) is still unknown. This study aims to advance current understandings of ECS providers' knowledge, attitudes, and practices in identifying and intervening in situations of CM. Findings will assist in highlighting key areas to focus policies and trainings to support response capacity for this first line of defense.

Methods

Study design and ethical approval

This is an exploratory cross-sectional study of knowledge, attitudes, and practices of health care providers working in ECS in relation to cases of CM at Mavalane General Hospital (MGH). Ethical approval for this study was obtained from Mozambique's National Committee for Bioethics for Health (*Comité Nacional de Bioética para Saúde*).

Setting

This study was carried out at MGH located in the federal capital of Maputo. MGH is a tertiary care facility with a catchment area of 19 neighborhoods, a covered population of 521,333 inhabitants (47.6% of the population of Maputo). MGH is the only primary hospital in its region and offers 24-h ECS, contracting approximately 40 physicians and 20 nurses. Hospital infrastructure for ECS consists of three triage rooms, each staffed by three general physicians and organized around three shifts of morning, afternoon, and night. Patients are first triaged prior to receiving treatment.

Participants

Sixty health care providers working in ECS at MGH were selected through a purposive sample and invited to participate in this study. Under time and resource constraints, this number was considered sufficient for data collection. Study eligibility was based on 1) status as a current clinical health care provider in ECS at MGH, and 2) voluntary agreement and written informed consent. Participants were also informed that they could withdraw participation or choose not to respond to questions at any point in the study without repercussions. Of the 60 health care providers invited to participate in the study, 49 consented to participate (82%).

Data collection

This study relied on primary data collected through direct interviews with participants by interviewers trained in administration by the study's principal investigator. Interviews occurred in the emergency department of MGH at the time and location preferred by participants to not interfere with work schedules and maximize privacy. Data collection between October and November 2010.

Survey

The data collection instrument for this study was a survey created through a content analysis of a similar study conducted by the United Nations Children's Fund (UNICEF) in Nepal [23]. The original study contained open-ended questions related to health care providers' knowledge, attitudes, and practices in the assessment of and response to CM. Qualitative data were systematized and analyzed through to facilitate the classification and development of items to measure the three thematic categories of knowledge, attitudes, and practices.

Prior to the initiation of the study, a pilot test was carried out at José Macamo General Hospital, also in Maputo. This hospital was selected for its similar location and capacity to MGH and adjustments were made to the survey following the pilot to account for the context of Mozambique.

Our survey consisted of a combination of demographic, multiple-choice (E.g. "Identify which of the below are forms of child maltreatment") yes-no (E.g. "Does child maltreatment cause long-term adverse effects on child development?"), and Likert-type scale items (E.g. "Indicate your level of agreement with the statement that 'health care providers have an important role in treating CM", organized in the following four sections: 1) sociodemographic characteristics, 2) health care provider knowledge of CM, 3) health care provider attitudes of CM, and 4) health care provider practices in recognizing and responding to CM. In total, there were seven demographic questions, 18 questions to measure knowledge, 20 questions to measure attitudes, and eight questions to measure practices.

Surveys, containing both qualitative short answer as well as quantitative Likert scale questions, were administered by an interviewer trained by the study's principal investigator. Interviews were conducted individually, maintaining confidentiality and anonymity of responses by storing data by a study number only without participants' identifying information.

Data analysis

Following data collection, previously coded surveys were reviewed to verify and validate responses. Descriptive statistics (frequencies and percentages) were used to report and characterize responses. Responses to the demographic, multiple choice, and Likert-type scale items were included in our analysis.

Results

Of the 60 health professionals identified as eligible, 49 (81.6%) consented to participate and were interviewed. Physicians made up 60% of health professionals interviewed. The final sample was composed primarily of women (69.4%). The mean respondent age was 32 years and most respondents were between 25 and 45 years (81.6%). Generalist physicians made up 57.1% of respondents. Table 1 details the sociodemographic characteristics and professional classifications of study participants.

Data on previous education and training specific to CM was also collected to characterize health care providers' background (Table 2). On identifying or responding to CM, 83.6% of respondents disclosed having received no education/training or almost no education/training. Only 14.3% of respondents indicated having received some education/training specific to CM. Regarding knowledge, health care providers interviewed were asked to cite the main forms of CM (Table 3); 61.2% of

Table 1 Sociodemographic characteristics and professional classifications of study participants

Sociodemographic characteristics	Frequency (n)	Percent (%)
Sex		
Male	15	30.6
Female	34	69.4
Age		
<25 years	7	14.3
25–45 years	40	81.6
> 45 years	2	4.1
Professional classifications		
Generalist physician	28	57.1
Nurse	19	38.7
Pediatrician	1	2.0
Surgeon	1	2.0

Table 2 Level of education and training specific to child maltreatment

Category	Frequency (n)	Percent (%)
No education nor training	35	71.4
Almost no education nor training	6	12.2
Some education and training	7	14.3
Does not know	1	2.0

respondents cited physical violence/aggression as being a main form of CM, 26.5% cited sexual abuse, and 12.2% cited emotional/psychological abuse. Although the majority of respondents reported physical violence/aggression as the main form of CM, 8.2% of respondents did not identify any of the forms of CM.

Knowledge of health care providers to recognize CM was also measured based on awareness of typical physical symptoms. Approximately 38.8% of the health care providers surveyed identified scarring and bruising at different stages of healing, 32.6% identified marks on the body in the form of objects such as a belt or cigarette burn, 4.1% identified burns, and 2.0% identified the presence of a sexually transmitted infection. Additional symptoms were mentioned by 20.4% of respondents; including malnutrition, scratches, ecchymosis, abrasions, and redness of the lips, lacerations in the case of sexual abuse, swelling, fear, ulceration, and depression. It is important to note that 8.2% of health care providers revealed that they did not know the typical physical symptoms of CM.

In relation to attitudes, 87.7% of respondents strongly agreed or agreed that health care providers hold an important role in the prevention of CM. Only 8.2% disagreed that health care providers hold an important role in the prevention of CM. Respondents were also asked their level of agreement with the attitude that "victim follow-up is not required because it is not important." A majority of respondents (86.2%) strongly disagreed or disagreed with that statement; only 10.2% strongly agreed or agreed. In contrast, health care providers expressed low confidence diagnosing and treating CM (Table 4). Over half (51.1%) strongly disagreed or disagreed that they felt confident diagnosing and treating CM.

To examine practices, participants were asked about the existence of a standard protocol for the care of victims of CM. Just 55.1% of respondents correctly stated that there is not a care protocol for cases of CM, while 24.5% incorrectly referred to an existing care protocol, and 16.3% did not know if such a protocol is in place. Respondents were then asked if they know where to refer for further treatment (Table 5). Most respondents (69.3%) strongly agreed or agreed that they know where to refer victims; 14. 3% strongly disagreed or disagreed and 14.3% of respondents admitted that they do not know.

Discussion

Our study is one of the first evaluations in a LIC of the knowledge and practice deficiencies in diagnosing and treating CM in an emergency department. Health care providers in ECS are the front line of the health system and can reduce harm by identifying CM when and before it happens. This study adds much needed literature on Sub-Saharan Africa, where rates are among the highest in the world [5–7]. The latest global guidelines for the prevention of CM emphasize the vital role of the health sectors of LMICs and our study offers evidence to guide the creation of new policies and investment in human resources in this context [25]. We found a significant gap in health care providers' knowledge of the forms of CM and their symptoms beyond physical violence. The attitudes expressed by health care providers overwhelmingly suggest agreement with their role to intervene. However, our findings reveal a disconnect between the attitudes held by health care providers and the training they receive; one plausible explanation for this discrepancy is a lack of consensus and blurred

Table 3 Knowledge of the main forms of child maltreatment[a]

Category	Frequency (n)	Percent (%)
Physical violence/aggression	30	61.2
Sexual abuse	13	26.5
Negligence	5	10.2
Exploitation	5	10.2
Emotional/psychological abuse	6	12.2
Others	11	22.4
Does not know	4	8.2

[a]Participants were asked to identify all responses that applied and responses are not mutually exclusive

Table 4 "I feel confident diagnosing and treating cases of child maltreatment"

Category	Frequency (n)	Percent (%)
Strongly disagree	3	6.2
Disagree	22	44.9
Neutral	4	8.2
Agree	15	30.6
Strongly agree	1	2.0
Does not know	3	6.1
Did not respond	1	2.0

Table 5 "I know where to refer cases of child maltreatment for further follow-up"

Category	Frequency (n)	Percent (%)
Strongly disagree	2	4.1
Disagree	5	10.2
Neutral	0	0
Agree	32	65.3
Strongly agree	2	4.1
Does not know	7	14.3
Did not respond	1	2.0

boundaries around what constitutes CM amid a context in which the harsh punishment of children in normalized and widespread.

A slight majority (61.2%) of participants identified physical violence as a main form of CM. Yet, only 26.5% cited sexual violence and even fewer (12.2 and 10.2%, respectively) referred to psychological abuse and exploitation. Conformingly, bruises/scarring and marks on the body were the most frequently mentioned symptoms, and responses pointing to symptoms of sexual abuse were virtually absent. These findings of health care providers having knowledge predominantly of physical abuse are consistent with those of CM studies in international literature [37, 38]. A central challenge in the correct diagnosis of CM is that fact that most pediatric injuries globally (90%) are in fact unintentional and occur without malice [39]. Accordingly, future interventions to educate health care providers and increase knowledge should focus on individual-level risk factors for CM and encourage consideration of patient history and demographics in the assessment. Moreover, there is a need to better understand and treat negligence and emotional abuse as forms of CM, as well as provide long-term support to victims [26, 37, 38, 40].

Despite a limited knowledge base, the attitudes expressed in our study show strong agreement that health care providers have an important role in preventing CM, as 87.7% of respondents agreed. Similar attitudes regarding a responsibility to document, report, and treat suspected CM have been affirmed in some previous studies of diverse health care providers [37, 41]. Likewise, attitudes indicated a strong commitment to appropriately managing cases of CM, with an overwhelming majority of participants disagreeing that victim follow-up is not important. At the same time, over half of our participants did not feel confident in diagnosing and treating CM; only 2.1% strongly agreed that they felt confident. This is not surprising as 71.4% of participants did not receive any education or training specific to CM. Health care providers who have received training specific to CM have been found to have significantly greater knowledge of reporting procedures, compared to physicians who did not receive training specific to CM [27]. Although, it is important to consider the extent to which the presence of training within the medical curricula of countries may be indicative of broader social and cultural infrastructure concerned with and understanding of CM, rather than a targeted intervention. Regardless, the attitudes present in our study suggest that these health care providers would be open to education and training to build awareness and understanding around CM and increase knowledge and adherence of best practices.

What our findings do communicate is an apparent gap between attitudes and current practices. Responses implied a limited understanding of protocols and laws. For example, slightly half of participants correctly indicated that the hospital does not have an existing care protocol for cases of CM and approximately one-third stated that they did not know the referral process for suspected cases of CM. Lack of training specific to CM and its symptoms may be partially responsible for this disconnect; however, the cultural context might have more of an influence. Globally, in high-income and LMIC alike, training to recognize and follow CM protocols in medical curriculums is minimal and only a small part of overall education [27, 31, 42]. For example, in the United States, only one state mandates that physicians complete the Identification and Reporting of Child Abuse and Maltreatment course before licensing [42]. Yet, poor knowledge of what constitutes CM and lack of best reporting practices are not observed uniformly across countries; studies from other countries have found baseline physician knowledge and reporting to be higher, although still limited in some respects [27, 29, 43, 44]. Health care providers in our sample are operating within a context where the harsh punishment of children is normalized; in the region, there has been found to be poor societal knowledge of what constitutes abuse and accepting attitudes towards such behaviors in community-based surveys [15]. Consequently, a major barrier to improving the capacity of health care providers to intervene is not a lack of concern or acceptance of CM, but rather the difficulty in training physicians to recognize normalized and accepted behaviors as in fact acts of CM within their community threshold. To accomplish this, awareness around definitions of CM and risk factors should be the focal point of training, rather than purely knowledge-based instruction around symptoms. These interventions in health care providers are needed jointly with administrative reforms in the hospital to strengthen coordination between the health system and the legal authorities. MGH where our study was based currently does not have a care protocol specific to CM, although health care providers in Mozambique are obligated by law to report suspected CM to the police [45].

Limitations

The main limitations of this study are its small sample size of 60 health care providers and its use of purposive sampling. Given the study size and sampling methods, findings are not statistically generalizable to the greater population of health care providers in Mozambique. However, the study's objectives were concerned with health care providers working in emergency services and studies of subpopulations of health care providers, such as pediatricians or family physicians, have utilized comparable sampling approaches [28, 35]. Another point of consideration stemming from the methodology of survey administration is the potential for social desirability bias. While the generally low levels of knowledge and adherence to best practices reported makes this unlikely, it is important to consider that positive attitudes may be overstated. Future surveys administered electronically or in other anonymizing manners would allow for comparisons and minimize the influence of social desirability bias.

Although the interpretation of our results is confined to one hospital, MGH is the largest hospital in the federal capital and serves almost half of the area's population. As is common in LMICs, city hospitals are tasked with providing care to both urban and peri-urban populations and may be the only source of specialized care for those living in rural areas who may have to travel long distances [41, 46]. Therefore, studying urban hospitals in LMICs has the potential to yield significant benefits for the health system as a whole due to their large catchment populations and their tendency to possess greater resources for service delivery. The size and location of MGH make it one of the country's most-equipped hospitals and inadequacies suggest that more research should also be focused on smaller and more rural hospitals in the country that likely experience increased deficiencies.

Conclusion

Child maltreatment is a leading public health problem internationally. Health care providers in ECS play an important role in the prevention and management of cases of CM through appropriate services and referrals. This study found that ECS providers working at Mavalane General Hospital in Maputo, Mozambique, have limited knowledge of the forms of child maltreatment and their associated symptoms beyond physical abuse and most have not received training on the topic. Attitudes expressed by health care providers suggest a strong commitment to their role and openness to CM training. Thus, investing in programs to raise awareness to confront sociocultural attitudes and recognize warning signs integrated with education and training to build skills and confidence have the potential to strengthen response capacity to improve care for victims of CM in Mozambique and other LICs.

Abbreviations

CM: Child maltreatment; ECS: Emergency care services; LIC: Low-income country; LMIC: Low- and middle-income country; MGH: Mavalane General Hospital

Acknowledgements

The investigators would like to acknowledge the University of Eduardo Mondlane Faculty of Medicine especially Dr. Baltazar Chilundo, Dra. Fatima Cuembelo and Dra Alda Mariano. A warm thank you to Emory University School of Medicine mentors including Dr. Debra Houry. Similarly, we would like to thank Abel Muiambo who supported this project. Finally and possibly most importantly, thank you to Jose de Sousa Pinto, Maria Isabel and Jeronimo Francisco da Fonseca for your support of Dr. Pinto during this process.

Funding

This project was supported by the Fogarty International Center, National Institutes of Health, grant D43 TW007262. Dr. Staton would like to acknowledge salary support funding from the Fogarty International Center (Staton, K01 TW010000-01A1). Funders had no role in the data collection nor the analysis or interpretation of results.

Authors' contributions

LP, AL and CAS conceived of the project. RM, DWW and SMS advised on the development of the project idea. LP collected the data. LP and AL analyzed the data. LP, AL, RM and CAS interpreted the data. AL and LP created the first draft of the manuscript. All authors edited and approved of the final manuscript.

Competing interests

The authors declare that they have no competing interests.

Author details

[1]Ordem dos Médicos de Moçambique (Mozambique Medical Council), Maputo, Mozambique. [2]Duke Global Health Institute, Duke University, 310 Trent Drive, Durham, North Carolina 27710, USA. [3]World Health Organization, Rua Pereira Marinho 280, CP 377 Maputo, Mozambique. [4]Emory Department of Emergency Medicine, 531 Asbury Circle, Annex Building, Suite N340, Atlanta, GA 30322, USA. [5]Department of Emergency Medicine, Greenville Health System, University of South Carolina School of Medicine Greenville, Greenville, SC 29605, USA. [6]Division of Emergency Medicine, Department of Surgery, Duke University Medical Center, 2301 Erwin Road, Durham, North Carolina 27710, USA. [7]Division of Global Neurosurgery and Neurology, Department of Neurosurgery, Duke University Medical Center, 2301 Erwin Road, Durham, North Carolina 27710, USA.

References

1. Devakumar D, Osrin D. Child homicide: a global public health concern. PLoS Med. 2016;13:e1002004.
2. Baccarat de Godoy Martins C, Prado de Mello Jorge MH. Abuso sexual na infância e adolescência: perfil das vítimas e agressores em município do sul do Brasil. Texto & Contexto Enfermagem. 2010;19:2.
3. World Health Organization: Child Maltreatment. http://www.who.int/topics/child_abuse/en/ (2018) Accessed 30 Jan 2018.
4. Leeb RT, Paulozzi LJ, Melanson C, Simon TR, Arias I. Child Maltreatment Surveillance. Uniform Definitions for Public Health and Recommended Data Elements Version 1.0: Centers for Disease Control and Prevention, National Center for Injury Prevention and Control. https://www.cdc.gov/violenceprevention/pdf/cm_surveillance-a.pdf; 2008. Accessed 30 Jan 2018
5. United Nations Children's Fund, Hidden in Plain Sight: A statistical analysis of violence against children. UNICEF, New York. http://files.unicef.org/publications/files/Hidden_in_plain_sight_statistical_analysis_EN_3_Sept_2014.pdf (2014) Accessed 30 Jan 2018.

6. Akmatov MK. Child abuse in 28 developing and transitional countries—results from the multiple Indicator cluster surveys. Int J Epidemiol. 2010;40(1):219–27. https://doi.org/10.1093/ije/dyq168.
7. Hillis S, Mercy J, Amobi A, Kress H. Global prevalence of past-year violence against children: a systematic review and minimum estimates. Pediatrics. 2016;137(3):e20154079. https://doi.org/10.1542/peds.2015-4079.
8. Clarke K, Patalay P, Allen E, Knight L, Naker D, Devries K. Patterns and predictors of violence against children in Uganda: a latent class analysis. BMJ Open. 2016; 6(5):e010443. https://doi.org/10.1136/bmjopen-2015-010443.
9. Hecker T, Hermenau K, Salmen C, Teicher M, Elbert T. Harsh discipline relates to internalizing problems and cognitive functioning: findings from a cross-sectional study with school children in Tanzania. BMC Psychiatry. 2016; 16:118. https://doi.org/10.1186/s12888-016-0828-3.
10. Pereda N, Guilera G, Forns M, Gómez-Benito J. The prevalence of child sexual abuse in community and student samples: a meta-analysis. Clin Psychol Rev. 2009;29(4):328–38. https://doi.org/10.1016/j.cpr.2009.02.007.
11. Gilbert R, Widom CS, Browne K, Fergusson D, Webb E, Janson S. Burden and consequences of child maltreatment in high-income countries. Lancet. 2009;373:68–81.
12. Ramos D, Amaral F, Spinola F, Lobo G, Silva H, Costa Í, Silva J, Chaves L, Junior T, Miranda V. A violência contra a criança e o adolescente: uma abordagem histórica e clinica. Gazeta Médica da Bahia. 2008;78
13. Sherr L, Hensels IS, Skeen S, Tomlinson M, Roberts KJ, Macedo A. Exposure to violence predicts poor educational outcomes in young children in South Africa and Malawi. Int Health. 2016;8(1):36–43. https://doi.org/10.1093/inthealth/ihv070.
14. Ameli V, Meinck F, Munthali A, Ushie B, Langhaug L. Associations between adolescent experiences of violence in Malawi and gender-based attitudes, internalizing, and externalizing behaviors. Child Abuse Negl. 2017;67:305–14. https://doi.org/10.1016/j.chiabu.2017.02.027.
15. Abeid M, Muganyizi P, Massawe S, Mpembeni R, Darj E, Axemo P. Knowledge and attitude towards rape and child sexual abuse–a community-based cross-sectional study in rural Tanzania. BMC Public Health. 2015;15(1):428. https://doi.org/10.1186/s12889-015-1757-7.
16. Bridgewater G. Physical and sexual violence against children in Kenya within a cultural context. Community Pract. 2016;89(2):30–4.
17. Lansford JE, Godwin J, Tirado LM, Zelli A, Al-Hassan SM, Bacchini D, et al. Individual, family, and culture level contributions to child physical abuse and neglect: a longitudinal study in nine countries. Dev Psychopathol. 2015; 27(4pt2):1417–28. https://doi.org/10.1017/S095457941500084X.
18. Mudany MA, Nduati R, Mboori-Ngacha D, Rutherford GW. Perceptions of child discipline and its contributions to child abuse in a low-income community in Nairobi, Kenya. Paediatr Int Child Health. 2013;33(4):228–32. https://doi.org/10.1179/2046905513Y.0000000071.
19. Meinck F, Cluver LD, Boyes ME. Household illness, poverty and physical and emotional child abuse victimisation: findings from South Africa's first prospective cohort study. BMC Public Health. 2015;15(444) https://doi.org/10.1186/s12889-015-1792-4.
20. Ward C, Sanders MR, Gardner F, Mikton C, Dawes A. Preventing child maltreatment in low- and middle-income countries: Parent support programs have the potential to buffer the effects of poverty. Child Abuse Negl. 2016;54:97–107. https://doi.org/10.1016/j.chiabu.2015.11.002.
21. Devries KM, Knight L, Child JC, Kyegombe N, Hossain M, Lees S, et al. Witnessing intimate partner violence and child maltreatment in Ugandan children: a cross-sectional survey. BMJ Open. 2017;7(2):e013583. https://doi.org/10.1136/bmjopen-2016-013583.
22. United Nations Children's Fund. Situation analysis of children in Mozambique 2014: United Nations Children's Fund (UNICEF); 2014.
23. Shrestha AD, Thapa K, Janardan KC. Violence against children in Nepal: health Practitioners' knowledge, attitude and practice on child abuse and sexual abuse in Nepal: United Nations Children's Fund (UNICEF); 2006.
24. Pinheiro PS. World report on violence against children. 2006.
25. World Health Organization. Development of Guidelines for the health sector response to child maltreatment http://www.who.int/violence_injury_prevention/violence/child/child_maltreatment_guidelines/en/. Accessed 1 June 2017.
26. Dakil SR, Cox M, Lin H, Flores G. Physical abuse in US children: risk factors and deficiencies in referrals to support services. J Aggress Maltreat Trauma. 2012;21:555–69.
27. Regnaut O, Jeu-Steenhouwer M, Manaouil C, Gignon M. Risk factors for child abuse: levels of knowledge and difficulties in family medicine. A mixed method study. BMC Res Notes. 2015;8:620.
28. Schols MW, De Ruiter C, Öry FG. How do public child healthcare professionals and primary school teachers identify and handle child abuse cases? A qualitative study. BMC Public Health. 2013;13:807.
29. Starling SP, Heisler KW, Paulson JF, Youmans E. Child abuse training and knowledge: a national survey of emergency medicine, family medicine, and pediatric residents and program directors. Pediatrics. 2009;123:e595–602.
30. Newton AS, Zou B, Hamm MP, Curran J, Gupta S, Dumonceaux C, Lewis M. Improving child protection in the emergency department: a systematic review of professional interventions for health care providers. Acad Emerg Med. 2010;17(2):117–25. https://doi.org/10.1111/j.1553-2712.2009.00640.x.
31. Miller AJ, Barlup Toombs K. Educating physicians internationally in the diagnosis of child sexual abuse: evaluation of a brief educational intervention in Malawi. J Child Sex Abus. 2014;23(3):247–55. https://doi.org/10.1080/10538712.2014.888120.
32. Youssef MR, Galal YS. Causes and outcome predictors of traumatic brain injury among emergency admitted pediatric patients at Cairo University hospitals. J Egypt Public Health Assoc. 2015;90(4):139–45. https://doi.org/10.1097/01.EPX.0000473569.10092.e7.
33. Yahaya I, De Leon AP, Uthman OA, Soares J, Macassa G. Individual and community-level socioeconomic position and its association with adolescents experience of childhood sexual abuse: a multilevel analysis of six countries in Sub-Saharan Africa. J Inj Violence Res. 2014;6(1):21–30. https://doi.org/10.5249/jivr.v6i1.316.
34. Garbin CA, Saliba Rovida TA, Colturato Joaquim R, Mendes de Paula A, Dossi de Guimarães e Queiroz AP. Violência denunciada: ocorrências de maus tratos contra crianças e adolescentes registradas em uma unidade policial. Revista Brasileira de Enfermagem 2011; 64.
35. Al-Moosa A, Al-Shaiji J, Al-Fadhli A, Al-Bayed K, Adib SM. Pediatricians' knowledge, attitudes and experience regarding child maltreatment in Kuwait. Child Abuse Negl. 2003;27:1161–78.
36. Cho O-H, Cha K-S, Yoo Y-S. Awareness and attitudes towards violence and abuse among emergency nurses. Asian Nurs Res. 2015;9:213–8.
37. Andrade EM, Nakamura E, de Paula CS, do Nascimento R, Bordin IA, Martin D. A visão dos profissionais de saúde em relação à violência doméstica contra crianças e adolescentes: um estudo qualitativo. Saúde e Sociedade. 2011;20(1):147–55.
38. Kraus C, Jandl-Jager E. Awareness and knowledge of child abuse amongst physicians–a descriptive study by a sample of rural Austria. Wien Klin Wochenschr. 2011;123:340–9.
39. Sminkey L. World report on child injury prevention. Injury Prevention. 2008; 14(1):69. https://doi.org/10.1136/ip.2007.018143.
40. Butchart A, Phinney Harvey A, Mian M, Furniss T, Kahane T. Preventing child maltreatment: a guide to taking action and generating evidence: World Health Organization; 2006.
41. Tansley G, Schuurman N, Amram O, Yanchar N. Spatial access to emergency services in low-and middle-income countries: a GIS-based analysis. PLoS One. 2015;10:e0141113.
42. Flaherty EG, Sege R. Barriers to physician identification and reporting of child abuse. Pediatr Ann. 2005;34(5):349–56.
43. Alnasser Y, Albijadi A, Abdullah W, Aldabeeb D, Alomair A, Alsaddiqi S, Alsalloum Y. Child maltreatment between knowledge, attitude and beliefs among Saudi pediatricians, pediatric residency trainees and medical students. Ann Med Surg. 2017;16:7–13. https://doi.org/10.1016/j.amsu.2017.02.008.
44. Menoch M, Zimmerman S, Garcia-Filion P, Bulloch B. Child abuse education: an objective evaluation of resident and attending physician knowledge. Pediatr Emerg Care. 2011;27(10):937–40. https://doi.org/10.1097/PEC.0b013e3182307ae5.
45. Lei Sobre a Violência Doméstica Praticada Contra a Mulher [Domestic Violence Against Women Law], Lei n° 29/2009. Maputo.
46. Nesbitt RC, Gabrysch S, Laub A, Soremekun S, Manu A, Kirkwood BR, Amenga-Etego S, Wiru K, Höfle B, Grundy C. Methods to measure potential spatial access to delivery care in low-and middle-income countries: a case study in rural Ghana. Int J Health Geogr. 2014;13:25.

14

Ambulance use is not associated with patient acuity after road traffic collisions

Yonas Abebe[1*], Tolesa Dida[1], Engida Yisma[2,3] and David M. Silvestri[4]

Abstract

Background: Africa accounts for one sixth of global road traffic deaths—most in the pre-hospital setting. Ambulance transport is expensive relative to other modes of pre-hospital transport, but has advantages in time-sensitive, high-acuity scenarios. Many countries, including Ethiopia, are expanding ambulance fleets, but clinical characteristics of patients using ambulances remain ill-defined.

Methods: This is a cross-sectional study of 662 road traffic collisions (RTC) patients arriving to a single trauma referral center in Addis Ababa, Ethiopia, over 7 months. Emergency Department triage records were used to abstract clinical and arrival characteristics, including acuity. The outcome of interest was ambulance arrival. Secondary outcomes of interest were inter-facility referral and referral communication. Descriptive and multivariable statistics were computed to identify factors independently associated with outcomes.

Results: Over half of patients arrived with either high (13.1%) or moderate (42.2%) acuity. Over half (59.0%) arrived by ambulance, and nearly two thirds (65.9%) were referred. Among referred patients, inter-facility communication was poor (57.7%). Patients with high acuity were most likely to be referred (aOR 2.20, 95%CI 1.16–4.17), but were not more likely to receive ambulance transport (aOR 1.56, 95%CI 0.86–2.84) or inter-facility referral communication (aOR 0.98, 95%CI 0.49–1.94) than those with low acuity. Nearly half (40.2%) of all patients were referred by ambulance despite having low acuity.

Conclusions: Despite ambulance expansion in Addis Ababa, ambulance use among RTC patients remains heavily concentrated among those with low-acuity. Inter-facility referral appears a primary contributor to low-acuity ambulance use. In other contexts, similar routine ambulance monitoring may help identify low-value utilization. Regional guidelines may help direct ambulance use where most valuable, and warrant further evaluation.

Keywords: Ethiopia, Africa, Trauma, Road traffic collisions, Road traffic accident, Road traffic injury, Ambulance, Pre-hospital, Triage acuity, Referral

* Correspondence: yonbbb@gmail.com
[1]Department of Emergency and Critical Care Nursing, St. Paul's Hospital Millennium Medical College, Addis Ababa, Ethiopia
Full list of author information is available at the end of the article

Background

Worldwide, road traffic collisions (RTC) are a leading cause of preventable morbidity and mortality. Each year, more than 1.2 million people die from RTC globally—one every thirty seconds—and as many as 50 million more incur non-fatal injuries [1, 2]. This burden is borne disproportionately by low- and middle-income countries (LMIC). Although Africa has just 2% of the world's vehicles, it accounts for 16% of global road traffic deaths [1].

The World Health Organization has highlighted several key interventions for the prevention of RTC, including notably laws and regulations to improve driver, vehicle, and road safety [1]. Nevertheless, in conjunction with such prevention efforts, quick and effective emergency health systems are needed to limit resultant morbidity and mortality after RTC. This starts with rapid and appropriate pre-hospital care and transport. In LMIC, it is estimated that 80% of road traffic deaths occur before patients even reach a hospital [3]. Although much of this mortality may be attributed to rural regions, where collision speeds are often higher and transport times longer [4], pre-hospital delays remain a significant contributor to excess road traffic mortality in urban contexts as well, despite increased ambulance availability [5].

As pre-hospital systems become more widely available in LMIC, attention is needed to ensure appropriate use of limited ambulance services. Many types of pre-hospital care and transport systems have been described in low-income contexts [6]. Care by formally trained pre-hospital personnel and transport by equipped ambulances is relatively expensive and remains scarce compared to other lower-resource approaches (e.g., modified motorcycles), but has advantages in certain time-sensitive and high-acuity scenarios [6]. In sub-Saharan Africa, a minority of urban RTC patients arrive by ambulance [7, 8], but the precise populations receiving such pre-hospital care and transport remain ill-defined.

To address this important research gap, we aim to describe the characteristics of RTC patients arriving by ambulance at a single urban public trauma center in Addis Ababa, Ethiopia. Addis Ababa is the capital and largest city in Ethiopia, Africa's second most populous nation. As elsewhere in Africa, RTC are a growing problem in Ethiopia, causing nearly 3500 fatalities annually and costing 1% of gross domestic product [1]. The distribution of injuries, interventions, and outcomes of RTC patients in Addis Ababa have been described [8]. Although many of these patients arrive from the scene, a large percent are referred from primary health centers or hospitals without specific trauma care capabilities. Understanding which patients receive ambulance transport, including those referred for higher levels of care, may help identify opportunities for targeted trauma system resource allocation.

Methods

Study design, setting, and population

We performed a retrospective chart review of all adult and pediatric patients arriving after RTC to Addis Ababa Burn Emergency and Trauma (AaBET) Hospital from August 22nd 2015 to March 9th 2016 (7 months). AaBET Hospital is a newly established 250-bed and 12 ICU-bed teaching and public referral hospital in Addis Ababa, Ethiopia, affiliated with St. Paul's Hospital Millennium Medical College (SPHMMC). AaBET Hospital provides 24/7 specialty services in emergency medicine, critical care, trauma and acute care surgery, orthopedics, neurosurgery, and forensic medicine; patients presenting with complaints requiring additional specialty services (e.g., cardiology, gastroenterology) are stabilized and transferred to nearby SPHMMC.

All patients presenting to the AaBET Hospital emergency department (ED) pass through a single point of triage, where trained emergency triage nurses record essential clinical and demographic information and assign a triage acuity designation according to the South African Triage Scale (SATS) [9]. The SATS has been validated for use in diverse low-income urban adult and pediatric ED settings, [10–13] and has high reported inter-rater reliability among emergency nurses ($\kappa = 0.92$), [14, 15] and in trauma settings [16]. It is currently used in all public EDs in Addis Ababa. Patients are categorized into five priority levels (emergent, very urgent, urgent, routine, dead on arrival) based on clinical instability, vital signs, and presenting complaint [10].

Data collection and analysis

Patient triage records were included for analysis if they were complete or partially complete. AaBET Hospital employs a hand-written triage and medical record system. All information was entered electronically into a standardized abstraction form by trained transcriptionists clinically trained in emergency care nursing and blinded to the intended analysis, in accordance with recommended best practice for retrospective chart reviews [17]. Subsequently, an audit was performed to ensure a low rate of data entry error.

Variables abstracted for analysis from triage records included patient age and sex, date of arrival to ED (weekday, weekend), patient origin (Addis Ababa, outside Addis), mode of arrival to ED (ambulance, taxi or private car, ambulatory or carried), triage acuity, referral status and source of referral (government hospital, health center, private institution), and whether communication had been received from referring institutions prior to patient arrival. Descriptive statistics were calculated for all variables. Triage acuity scores were grouped into three categories: low (routine), moderate (urgent), or high (very urgent, emergent, dead on arrival). Children were considered less than 13 years, in conjunction SATS validation [13]. We used simultaneous multivariable logistic regression to identify factors (selected a priori) independently associated with arrival by ambulance, the primary outcome of interest. Subsequent regressions were performed to determine factors associated with inter-facility referral and inter-facility referral communication, which were secondary outcomes of interest. Missing data were accounted for using multiple imputation, and all statistical analysis was performed using SPSS version 21.0.0 (IBM Corporation, 2012).

Results

Population characteristics

During the seven-month study period, a total of 2062 patients were evaluated after trauma in AaBET Hospital ED. RTC accounted for 662 patients (32%), of which all had complete or partially complete triage records and were included in analysis. Two thirds of RTC patients were male (66.2%), with a median age of 27 years (Table 1). Children less than 13 accounted for a minority (4.8%) of all RTC cases. Most patients (72.4%) were seen on weekdays, with over half originating from outside Addis Ababa city limits (60.6%). Nearly half were assigned low (routine) triage acuity upon arrival (44.7%), while 42.2% were designated as moderate and another 13.1% as high acuity—9.0% as very urgent, 3.8% as emergent, and two patients (0.3%) dead on arrival.

Inter-facility referral

Most RTC patients (65.9%) were referred to AaBET Hospital from outside institutions (Table 1), with government hospitals comprising the single largest source of referral (42.5% of all RTC patients and 64.5% of total RTC referrals) and outpatient health centers referring one fifth (20.3%) of all RTC patients. As might be expected, the frequency of referral differed when accounting for patient origin. Among patients arriving from Addis Ababa, over half (138/249; 55.4%) arrived from the scene without any prior referral, whereas 80% (292/365) of patients from outside Addis Ababa were referred via another institution (Table 2). In fact, independent of other characteristics, patients arriving from within Addis Ababa were nearly five times less likely to be referred than peers originating from outside the city (aOR 0.22, 95%CI 0.15–0.32). Sicker patients were independently more likely to have been referred to AaBET Hospital after RTC. Patients with high and moderate triage acuity were more likely to be referred compared to those with low acuity (High: aOR 2.20, 95%CI 1.16–4.17; Moderate: aOR 1.55, 95% 1.05–2.28). Neither patient age nor sex was associated with increased odds of referral.

Table 1 Characteristics of patients presenting after RTC to AaBET Hospital, Addis Ababa

Characteristic	Total ($n = 662$)
Patient sex, n (%)[a]	
Female	224 *(33.8)*
Male	438 *(66.2)*
Patient age, n (%)[a]	
< 13	31 (4.8)
13–24	214 (32.9)
25–40	252 (38.8)
> 40	153 (23.5)
Patient origin, n (%)[a]	
Addis Ababa	259 *(39.4)*
Outside Addis	398 *(60.6)*
Date of Arrival, n (%)[a]	
Weekday	467 *(72.4)*
Weekend	178 *(27.6)*
Triage Acuity, n (%)[a,b,c]	
Low acuity	289 *(44.7)*
Moderate acuity	273 *(42.2)*
High acuity	85 *(13.1)*
Referral status/source, n (%)[a]	
Not referred (from scene)	211 *(34.1)*
Referred from government hospital	263 *(42.5)*
Referred from health center	126 *(20.3)*
Referred from private institution	19 *(3.1)*
Ref. communication, n (%)[a,d]	
Yes (before arrival)	224 *(57.7)*
No	164 *(42.3)*
Mode of arrival[a]	
Ambulance	366 *(59.0)*
Taxi or private car	234 *(37.7)*
Walking or being carried	20 *(3.2)*

[a]Percent of non-missing data reported. Missing data per variable as follows: sex ($n = 0/662$; 0%), age ($n = 12/662$; 1.8%), patient origin (5/662; 0.8%), date of arrival (17/662; 2.6%), triage acuity (15/662; 2.3%), referral status/source (43/662; 6.5%), referral communication (20/408; 4.9%), mode of arrival (42/662; 6.3%)
[b]South Africa Triage Scale acuity designations
[c]High acuity includes very urgent (58/647; 9.0%), Emergent (25/647; 3.8%) and Dead on arrival (2/647; 0.3%). Dead on arrival grouped within very urgent or emergent due to presumed scene/pre-hospital acuity
[d]Subset of referred patients only

Inter-facility communication

Despite the high frequency of RTC referrals, overall communication from referring institutions to AaBET Hospital was poor. Among all RTC patients referred from other health institutions, more than two in five (164/388; 42.3%) arrived with no prior notification

Table 2 RTC patient factors associated with referral to AaBET Hospital, Addis Ababa

Characteristic	Referral status		Adjusted odds of referral
	Referred (*n* = 408)	Not Referred (*n* = 211)	
	N (%)[a]	*N (%)*[a]	*aOR (95%CI)*
Patient sex			
Female	138 *(33.8)*	78 *(37.0)*	1.0 *(ref)*
Male	270 *(66.2)*	133 *(63.0)*	1.11*(0.76–1.63)*
Patient age			
< 13	23 *(5.7)*	8 *(3.9)*	1.03 (0.39, 2.67)
13–24	122 (30.2)	78 (38.2)	0.62 (0.38, 1.03)
25–40	162 (40.1)	74 (36.3)	0.86 (0.53, 1.42)
> 40	97 (24.0)	44 (21.6)	1.0 (ref)
Patient origin			
Addis Ababa	111 *(27.5)*	138 *(65.4)*	0.22 *(0.15, 0.32)*
Outside Addis	292 *(72.5)*	73 *(34.6)*	1.0 *(ref)*
Date of Arrival			
Weekday	290 *(72.9)*	141 *(68.8)*	1.02 *(0.68, 1.54)*
Weekend	108 *(27.1)*	64 *(31.2)*	1.0 *(ref)*
Triage Acuity[b,c]			
Low Acuity	157 *(39.6)*	119 *(57.2)*	1.0 *(ref)*
Moderate Acuity	178 *(44.9)*	73 *(35.1)*	1.55 *(1.05, 2.28)*
High Acuity	61 *(15.4)*	16 *(7.7)*	2.20 *(1.16, 4.17)*
Referral status/source			
Not referred (from scene)	N/A	211 *(100)*	N/A
Referred from government hospital	263 *(64.5)*	E N/AEN	N/A
Referred from health center	126 *(30.9)*	NE N/A N	N/A
Referred from private institution	19 *(4.7)*	NE N/A N	N/A

[a]Percent of non-missing data reported
[b]South Africa Triage Scale acuity designations
[c]High acuity includes very urgent, emergent, and dead on arrival. Dead on arrival grouped within very urgent or emergent due to presumed scene/pre-hospital acuity

from the referring facility (Table 1). Communication was most likely to occur on weekdays (aOR 1.74, 95%CI 1.06–2.85), when health facility staffing is highest. Rates of communication were similar between patients referred from within (64/104; 61.5%) and from outside (156/279; 55.9%) Addis Ababa, and did not significantly differ according to the type of referring institution. Interestingly, despite higher acuity among referred RTC patients than those not referred, communication from transferring facilities was no higher among the most ill than the least (aOR 0.98, 95%CI 0.49–1.94), nor among those sent by ambulance (aOR 1.46, 95%CI 0.88–2.43) (Table 3).

Table 3 RTC patient factors associated with inter-facility referral communication, AaBET Hospital, Addis Ababa

Characteristic	Referral communication		Adjusted odds of communication
	Yes (*n* = 224)	No (*n* = 164)	
	N (%)[a]	*N (%)*[a]	*aOR (95%CI)*
Patient sex			
Female	82 *(36.6)*	50 *(30.5)*	1.0 *(ref)*
Male	142 *(63.4)*	114 *(69.5)*	0.69 *(0.43, 1.12)*
Patient age			
< 13	11 *(5.0)*	12 *(7.3)*	0.73 *(0.27, 1.97)*
13–24	66 (30.0)	50 (30.5)	0.98 *(0.54, 1.79)*
25–40	93 (42.3)	61 (37.2)	1.38 (0.78, 2.45)
> 40	50 (22.7)	41 (25.0)	1.0 *(ref)*
Patient origin			
Addis Ababa	64 *(29.1)*	40 *(24.5)*	1.32 *(0.79, 2.20)*
Outside Addis	156 *(70.9)*	123 *(75.5)*	1.0 *(ref)*
Date of Arrival			
Weekday	171 *(77.7)*	104 *(65.4)*	1.74 *(1.06, 2.85)*
Weekend	49 *(22.3)*	55 *(34.6)*	1.0 *(ref)*
Triage Acuity[b,c]			
Low Acuity	85 *(38.8)*	61 *(38.9)*	1.0 *(ref)*
Moderate Acuity	102 *(46.6)*	69 *(43.9)*	1.11 *(0.68, 1.79)*
High Acuity	32 *(14.6)*	27 *(17.2)*	0.98 *(0.49, 1.94)*
Referral source			
Referred from government hospital	130 *(58.0)*	121 *(73.8)*	0.55 *(0.18, 1.68)*
Referred from health center	80 *(35.7)*	38 *(23.2)*	1.15 *(0.36, 3.72)*
Referred from private institution	14 *(6.2)*	5 *(3.0)*	0 *(ref)*
Mode of arrival (transport)			
Ambulance	136 *(66.0)*	121 (77.6)	0 *(ref)*
No ambulance	70 *(34.0)*	35 (22.4)	1.46 *(0.88, 2.43)*

[a]Percent of non-missing data reported
[b]South Africa Triage Scale acuity designations
[c]High acuity includes very urgent, emergent, and dead on arrival. Dead on arrival grouped within very urgent or emergent due to presumed scene/pre-hospital acuity

Mode of arrival

The vast majority (96.7%) of RTC patients arrived at AaBET hospital by vehicle, including over half (59.0%) by ambulance (Table 1). Regardless of other characteristics, patients were more likely to arrive by ambulance if coming from another government hospital than from the scene itself (aOR 4.23, 95%CI 2.63–6.78; Table 4). However, ambulance use did not differ significantly based on the day of patients' arrival, nor whether they originated from within or outside Addis Ababa. Importantly, patients with highest acuity were not more likely to arrive by ambulance than those with lowest severity

Table 4 RTC patient factors associated with ambulance arrival, AaBET Hospital, Addis Ababa

Characteristic	Arrival by ambulance		Adjusted odds of ambulance use
	Yes (*n* = 366)	No (*n* = 254)	
	N (%)[a]	*N (%)*[a]	*aOR (95%CI)*
Patient sex			
Female	139 *(38.0)*	74 *(29.1)*	1.0 *(ref)*
Male	227 *(62.0)*	180 *(70.9)*	0.63 (0.43, 0.91)
Patient age			
< 13	19 (5.3)	12 (4.8)	0.77 (0.32,1.86)
13–24	115 (31.9)	83 (33.3)	1.21 (0.75, 1.95)
25–40	145 (40.2)	93 (37.3)	1.15 (0.73, 1.82)
> 40	82 (22.7)	61 (24.5)	1.0 *(ref)*
Patient origin			
Addis Ababa	121 *(33.4)*	119 *(46.9)*	0.78 (0.53, 1.13)
Outside Addis	241 *(66.6)*	135 *(53.1)*	1.0 *(ref)*
Date of Arrival			
Weekday	257 *(72.6)*	177 *(70.8)*	1.05 (0.71, 1.55)
Weekend	97 *(27.4)*	73 *(29.2)*	1.0 *(ref)*
Triage Acuity[b,c]			
Low Acuity	145 *(41.1)*	132 *(52.2)*	1.0 *(ref)*
Moderate Acuity	155 *(43.9)*	97 *(38.3)*	1.34 (0.92, 1.95)
High Acuity	53 *(15.0)*	24 *(9.5)*	1.56 (0.86, 2.84)
Referral status/source			
Referred from government hospital	191 *(54.6)*	55 *(23.9)*	4.23 (2.63, 6.78)
Referred from health center	68 *(19.4)*	51 *(22.2)*	1.61 (0.97, 2.69)
Referred from private institution	7 *(2.0)*	9 *(3.9)*	0.88 (0.29, 2.69)
Self-Referral/Scene	84 *(24.0)*	115 *(50.0)*	1.0 *(ref)*

[a]Percent of non-missing data reported
[b]South Africa Triage Scale acuity designations
[c]High acuity includes very urgent, emergent, and dead on arrival. Dead on arrival grouped within very urgent or emergent due to presumed scene/pre-hospital acuity

injuries (aOR 1.56, 95%CI 0.86–2.84). Interestingly, males were less likely to arrive by ambulance after RTC than their female counterparts (aOR 0.63, 95%CI 0.43–0.91), independent of other factors.

Discussion

Road traffic collisions are a leading cause of morbidity and mortality worldwide and particularly in sub-Saharan Africa, where growth in motorization has outpaced efforts to implement and enforce RTC prevention interventions [1]. Estimated annual African RTC fatality rates (26 per 100,000 population) are twice those in the United States and three times greater than in Europe [1]. In Ethiopia, RTC fatality rates are among the continent's highest [18].

The alarming burden of RTC has attracted mounting international attention in recent years. The United Nations General Assembly declared 2011–2020 the Decade of Action for road safety [2], while the body's Sustainable Development Goals (SDGs), ratified unanimously in 2015, called for 50% fewer RTC deaths and injuries by 2020 [19]. A number of national and local policy efforts have been implemented toward this end [20, 21]. These have mostly included legislative regulations, educational interventions, law enforcement, infrastructural reform, and community-based prevention programs [21]. At the same time, a growing number of sub-Saharan African trauma registries have aimed to provide clinicians, researchers, and administrators clearer data regarding local burden of traumatic illness [18, 22, 23].

Despite positive trends in growing global attention to RTC, surprisingly little focus has been placed on evaluating and improving formal pre-hospital trauma systems in low-income settings. Most trauma deaths occur in the pre-hospital setting, and the percent who die before reaching a hospital is highest in low-income settings where formal pre-hospital systems are weakest [24]. Most studies evaluating ambulance use after RTC have described the frequency of use [25–29], rather than independent predictors of use. Knowing which patients currently receive ambulance transport after RTC is essential to developing policies to direct its use given relative scarcity and cost compared to other modes of transport.

In our study of over six hundred RTC patients arriving to a single tertiary trauma referral hospital in Addis Ababa, Ethiopia, a higher percentage of patients arrived by ambulance (59%) compared to other published studies from elsewhere across Africa [7, 8, 25–27]. Such disparities in ambulance utilization are likely multifactorial. Our methodological decision to focus exclusively on RTC rather than all trauma patients resulted in our exclusion of large numbers of violent trauma victims transported by police, accounted for in other studies [7]. In addition, Ethiopian governmental efforts to coordinate and concentrate specialty care across city public hospitals in Addis Ababa means AaBET Hospital is one of only two major trauma centers citywide, receiving a higher proportion of regional trauma referrals than reported elsewhere [25–27]. Finally, as one of the first African countries to prioritize emergency care specialization and specialty training [28–30], Ethiopia has also placed comparatively large emphasis on formal pre-hospital infrastructure and training. Large ambulance provisions by the federal government have supplemented private and non-governmental pre-hospital organizations already in practice [31], while a regional emergency medical dispatch phone line enables easy public ambulance access. These factors may have contributed to increased ambulance availability.

Even accounting for higher rates of ambulance use, our findings highlight several important yet concerning trends that warrant further attention in other settings. Importantly, we found that ambulance use among RTC patients arriving to AaBET Hospital was not significantly associated with triage acuity. This is in contrast to prior work among both trauma and non-trauma patients in Ghana [32], and suggests that ambulance adoption in lower-income urban settings may not always naturally align with patient clinical needs. RTC patients with high acuity need time-sensitive stabilization and are at greatest risk of mortality, disability, or hospital admission, yet in our population were no more likely to receive ambulance transport than those with minimal injury burden. There are several possible explanations for this. While these findings may reflect persistent pervasive public unawareness regarding ambulance services or public ambulance avoidance due to fear of financial liability, we instead suspect they represent a discrepancy in the extent to which patient acuity influences ambulance selection among referred and non-referred populations.

To better test this hypothesis, we performed separate subgroup analyses assessing ambulance use among referred and non-referred populations (i.e., effect modification). Results did not change among patients referred to AaBET from another institution; patients with high and moderate acuity were no more likely to be transported by ambulance than those with low acuity (Additional file 1: Table S1). Similarly, among patients arriving directly from the scene, those with high acuity were not more likely to receive ambulance transport than those with low acuity (Additional file 2: Table S2). However, those with moderate acuity from the scene were nearly three times more likely to arrive by ambulance than those with low acuity (aOR 2.97, 95%CI 1.50–5.86). This finding is important, and suggests that transportation decisions made at the scene may be influenced by patient acuity. In light of this, lower rates of ambulance transportation among high-acuity patients at the scene may reflect lay first responders' preferential selection of immediate on-site (lay) transportation for the sickest patients deemed unable to wait for ambulance arrival. By contrast, we found no evidence to suggest that acuity influenced ambulance decisions made by referring providers—consistent as well with poor inter-facility communication (58%), even for the sickest patients.

In low-income countries, ambulances remain scare resources but possess key benefits over pre-hospital lay transportation in the appropriate clinical settings. Given the relative expense of ambulances in such settings, maximizing their value is essential, and will depend on judicious use in accordance with patient clinical needs. When assessed alongside contrasting work from Ghana [32], our findings suggest heterogeneity in post-traumatic ambulance utilization patterns in sub-Saharan Africa, and highlight the need for locally-driven assessments to ensure value-directed care. Furthermore, our data suggest that in promoting appropriate ambulance use, training of healthcare providers may be equally important as ongoing lay education. Inappropriate inter-facility ambulance use for patients deemed low-acuity after clinician evaluation offers few benefits over lay transportation, while limiting ambulance availability in higher-acuity settings elsewhere. When ambulances are free to respond in a timely fashion to high-acuity patients, a greater proportion of these patients may be brought directly from the scene to trauma centers like AaBET Hospital, bypassing outside institutions with little or no trauma expertise and improving mortality [33]. In our study, 103 low-acuity patients received ambulance transport from another facility (40% of all referred patients transported by ambulance), while one third (40) of high- and moderate-acuity patients arrived from the scene by other means (Additional file 1: Table S1 and Additional file 2: Table S2).

We suggest that countries like Ethiopia that seek to develop formal pre-hospital ambulance transportation systems should develop measures to ensure this scarce pre-hospital resource is available to be used when and where it is of highest value. Such measures could include guidelines on inter-facility ambulance use in specific clinical settings (e.g., trauma), auditing of referring providers and institutions to identify variability and opportunities for targeted intervention, or regional regulations. Such measures might be best implemented by different stakeholders, including institutions, ambulance providers, or regional governments. In some cases, it may be necessary to modify existing guidelines, including those that may inadvertently pressure providers to refer lower-acuity trauma patients [32]. Once ambulances are freed from lower-acuity referral demand, clinical and geospatial dispatch algorithms might be employed to best allocate them among patients arriving from the scene [34].

Limitations

Our study has several limitations. As a single-center cross-sectional assessment, our findings may not generalize to other settings, including to rural or district-level hospitals, private facilities, and those that are not regional referral or specialty centers of excellence. Moreover, the high rates of referral among RTC patients and the relative abundance of ambulances we observed may limit replicability where pre-hospital and emergency health systems are organized differently or at different stages of development.

Because we employed ED triage records, we are inherently constrained in the inferences we are able to draw. Specifically, we are unable to draw conclusions regarding specific types of injuries, treatments obtained, clinical outcomes, or costs of care. In addition, we are unable to examine reasons underlying ambulance use decisions among providers or patients/laypersons, nor can we deduce appropriateness of referral decision in the first place. Several of these questions might be best explored through future survey-based and qualitative designs [35]. Nevertheless, our findings suggest considerable opportunities for improvement in local regional trauma system coordination, and highlight the utility of ED triage data as a feasible, low-cost, and efficient means of monitoring local pre-hospital use and referral patterns.

Conclusions

As urban trauma and pre-hospital care systems mature across sub-Saharan Africa, regional governments and health policymakers should regularly and critically evaluate whether limited resources are being directed to those patients most likely to benefit. In Addis Ababa, ambulance use does not appear to parallel clinical acuity among patients presenting after RTC. Further studies should explore ambulance use in other contexts, as well as factors influencing ambulance selection for low-acuity patients. Reducing ambulance use among low-acuity inter-facility referrals may represent a targetable opportunity to increase ambulance value where they are scarcest.

Abbreviations

AaBET: Addis Ababa Burn Emergency and Trauma (Hospital); aOR: Adjusted odds ratio; CI: Confidence interval; ED: Emergency department; ICU: Intensive care unit; LMIC: Low- and middle-income; RTC: Road traffic collisions; SATS: South Africa triage scale; SDGs: Sustainable development goals; SPHMMC: St. Paul's Hospital Millennium Medical College; SPSS: Statistical Package for the Social Sciences

Acknowledgements

Authors are grateful to St. Paul's Hospital Millennium Medical College for technical and financial support, and to AaBET hospital senior managements and triage officers for facilitating data collection.

Funding

This study was funded by St. Paul's Hospital Millennium Medical College, Addis Ababa, Ethiopia. The college didn't involve in the study design, data collection, analysis and reporting.

Authors' contributions

YA and TD designed the study. YA collected study data. YA and EY analyzed the data. All authors participated in data interpretation. YA and DS wrote the manuscript. All authors contributed critical revisions to the report, and all approved the final version.

Competing interests

The authors declare that they have no competing interests.

Author details

[1]Department of Emergency and Critical Care Nursing, St. Paul's Hospital Millennium Medical College, Addis Ababa, Ethiopia. [2]School of Allied Health Sciences, College of Health Sciences, Addis Ababa University, Addis Ababa, Ethiopia. [3]Robinson Research Institute, School of Medicine, The University of Adelaide, Adelaide, Australia. [4]National Clinician Scholars Program and Department of Emergency Medicine, Yale School of Medicine, New Haven, USA.

References

1. World Health Organization. Global status report on road safety. Geneva, Switzerland: WHO; 2015.
2. World Health Organization. Global plan for the decade of action for road safety 2011–2020 Geneva, WHO.
3. Merchant A, Outhay M, Gonzaléz-Calvo L, Moon TD, Sidat M, Taibo CLA, McQueen K. Training laypersons and hospital personnel in basic resuscitation techniques: an approach to impact the global trauma burden in Mozambique. World J Surg. 2015;39(6):1433–7.
4. Benie Bi Vroh J, Tiembre I, Ekra DK, Ano Ama MN, Ka OM, Ncho Dagnan S, Tagliante-Saracino J. Determinants of fatal road traffic injuries in cote d'Ivoire from 2002 to 2011. Sante Publique. 2016;28(5):647–53.
5. Chandrasekharan A, Nanavati AJ, Prabhakar S, Prabhakar S. Factors impacting mortality in the pre-hospital period after road traffic accidents in urban India. Trauma Mon. 2016;21(3):e22456.
6. Kobusingye OC, Hyder AA, Bishai D, Hicks ER, Mock C, Joshipura M. Emergency medical systems in low- and middle-income countries: recommendations for action. Bull World Health Organ. 2005;83(8):626–31.
7. Hsia RY, Ozgediz D, Mutto M, Jayaraman S, Kyamanywa P, Kobusingye OC. Epidemiology of injuries presenting to the national hospital in Kampala, Uganda: implications for research and policy. Int J Emerg Med. 2010;3(3):165–72.
8. Seid M, Azazh A, Enquselassie F, Yisma E. Injury characteristics and outcome of road traffic accident among victims at adult emergency Department of Tikur Anbessa specialized hospital, Addis Ababa, Ethiopia: a prospective hospital based study. BMC Emerg Med. 2015;15(1):10.
9. Bruijns SR, Wallis LA, Burch VC. A prospective evaluation of the cape triage score in the emergency department of an urban public hospital in South Africa. Emerg Med J. 2008;25(7):398–402.
10. Twomey M, Wallis LA, Thompson ML, Myers JE. The South African triage scale (adult version) provides reliable acuity ratings. Int Emerg Nurs. 2012;20(3):142–50.
11. Dalwai MK, Twomey M, Maikere J, Said S, Wakee M, Jemmy J-P, Valles P, Tayler-Smith K, Wallis L, Zachariahi R. Reliability and accuracy of the south African triage scale when used by nurses in the emergency Department of Timergara Hospital, Pakistan. S Afr Med J. 2014;104:372–5.
12. Rominski S, Bell SA, Oduro G, Ampong P, Oteng R, Donkor P. The implementation of the south African triage score (SATS) in an urban teaching hospital, Ghana. Afr J Emerg Med. 2014;4(2):71–5.
13. Twomey M, Cheema B, Buys H, Cohen K, de Sà A, Louw P, Ismail M, Finlayson H, Cunningham C, Westwood A. Vital signs for children at triage: a multicentre validation of the revised south African triage scale (SATS) for children. S Afr Med J. 2013;103:304–8.
14. Twomey M, de Sá A, Wallis LA, Myers JE. Inter-rater reliability of the south African triage scale: assessing two different cadres of health care workers in a real time environment. Afr J Emerg Med. 2011;1(3):113–8.
15. Lowsby R, Kamara C, Kamara M, Nyhus H, Williams N, Bradfield M, Harrison H-L. An assessment of nurse-led triage at Connaught hospital, Sierra Leone in the immediate post-Ebola period. Afr J Emerg Med. 2017;7(2):51–5.
16. Gardner A, Forson PK, Oduro G, Stewart B, Dike N, Glover P, Maio RF. Diagnostic accuracy of the Kampala trauma score using estimated abbreviated injury scale scores and physician opinion. Injury. 2017;48(1):177–83.
17. Nagurney JT, Brown DFM, Sane S, Weiner JB, Wang AC, Chang Y. The accuracy and completeness of data collected by prospective and retrospective methods. Acad Emerg Med. 2005;12(9):884–95.
18. Adeloye DTJ, Akanbi MA, et al. The burden of road traffic crashes, injuries and deaths in Africa: a systematic review and meta-analysis. Bull World Health Organ. 2016;94:510–21A.
19. United Nations. Resolution adopted by the General Assembly on 25 September 2015: Transforming our world: the 2030 Agenda for Sustainable Development. Washington; United Nations; 2015. [undocs.org/A/RES/70/1].
20. LaGrone LRK, Joshipura M, et al. Uptake of the World Health Organization's trauma care guidelines: a systematic review. Bull World Health Organ. 2016;94:585–98C.

21. Staton C, Vissoci J, Gong E, Toomey N, Wafula R, Abdelgadir J, Zhou Y, Liu C, Pei F, Zick B, et al. Road traffic injury prevention initiatives: a systematic review and Metasummary of effectiveness in low and middle income countries. PLoS One. 2016;11(1):e0144971.
22. Boughton O, Jones GG, Lavy CBD, Grimes CE. Young, male, road traffic victims: a systematic review of the published trauma registry literature from low and middle income countries. SICOT-J. 2015;1:10.
23. Vissoci JRN, Shogilev DJ, Krebs E, Ld A, Vieira IF, Toomey N, Portero Batilana A, Haglund M, Staton CA. Road traffic injury in sub-Saharan African countries: a systematic review and summary of observational studies. Traffic Inj Prev. 2017;18(7):767–73.
24. Mock CN, Jurkovich GJ, nii-Amon-Kotei D, Arreola-Risa C, Maier RV. Trauma mortality patterns in three nations at different economic levels: implications for global trauma system development. J Trauma Acute Care Surg. 1998;44(5):804–14.
25. Ahidjo KA, Olayinka SA, Ayokunle O, Mustapha AF, Sulaiman GAA, Gbolahan AT. Prehospital transport of patients with spinal cord injury in Nigeria. J Spinal Cord Med. 2011;34(3):308–11.
26. Ibrahim NA, Ajani AWO, Mustafa IA, Balogun RA, Oludara MA, Idowu OE, Solagberu BA. Road traffic injury in Lagos, Nigeria: assessing prehospital care. Prehosp Disast Med. 2017;32(4):424–30.
27. Mowafi H, Oranmore-Brown R, Hopkins KL, White EE, Mulla YF, Seidenberg P. Analysis of prehospital transport use for trauma patients in Lusaka, Zambia. World J Surg. 2016;40(12):2868–74.
28. Azazh A, Teklu S, Woldetsadi A, Seyoum N, Geremew H, Busse H, Tefera G, Wubben R, Rankin P, Tupesis JP, et al. Emergency medicine and its development in Ethiopia with emphasis on the role of Addis Ababa University, School of Medicine, emergency medicine department. Ethiop Med J. 2014;(Suppl 2):1–12.
29. Busse H, Azazh A, Teklu S, Tupesis JP, Woldetsadik A, Wubben RJ, Tefera G. Creating change through collaboration: a twinning partnership to strengthen emergency medicine at Addis Ababa University/Tikur Anbessa specialized hospital—a model for international medical education partnerships Generación Cambios a través de la Colaboración: un Acuerdo de Asociación para Fortalecer la Medicina de Urgencias y Emergencias de la Universidad de Addis Ababa y el Hospital Especializado Tikur Anbessa. Acad Emerg Med. 2013;20(12):1310–8.
30. W/Tsadik A, Azazh A, Teklu S, Seyum N, Geremew H, Rankin P, Erschen MJ. Development of emergency medicine and critical care masters program for nurses at Addis Ababa University, School of Medicine. Ethiop Med J. 2014;(Suppl 2):21–6.
31. Directorate MS: Emergency medical services: timely delivery of life saving medical interventions. Federal Ministry of Health 16th National Annual Review Meeting Group Discussion. ARM16-doc 12/14. 2014.
32. Nee-Kofi Mould-Millman C, Rominski S, Oteng R. Ambulance or taxi? High acuity prehospital transports in the Ashanti region of Ghana. Afr J Emerg Med. 2014;4(1):8–13.
33. Boschini LP, Lu-Myers Y, Msiska N, Cairns B, Charles AG. Effect of direct and indirect transfer status on trauma mortality in sub Saharan Africa. Injury. 2016;47(5):1118–22.
34. Ohshige K, Kawakami C, Mizushima S, Moriwaki Y, Suzuki N. Evaluation of an algorithm for estimating a patient's life threat risk from an ambulance call. BMC Emerg Med. 2009;9(1):21.
35. Chandran A, Ejaz K, Karani R, Baqir M, Razzak J, Hyder AA. Insights on the effects of patient perceptions and awareness on ambulance usage in Karachi, Pakistan. Emerg Med J. 2014;31:990-993.

15

Value of early change of serum C reactive protein combined to modified Alvarado score in the diagnosis of acute appendicitis

Mohamed Amine Msolli[1,4*], Kaouther Beltaief[1,4], Wahid Bouida[1,4], Nahla Jerbi[2,4], Mohamed Habib Grissa[1,4], Hamdi Boubaker[1,4], Riadh Boukef[3,4] and Semir Nouira[1,4]

Abstract

Background: The aim of this study is to test the diagnostic value of baseline and early change of C-reactive protein (CRP) concentrations, evaluated separately or in combination with the modified Alvarado score (MAS), in patients with clinically suspected acute appendicitis.

Methods: This is a prospective observational study including all patients presenting to the emergency department with an equivocal diagnosis of acute appendicitis. After inclusion, clinical and demographic data are recorded and blood samples were taken at baseline and 3 h after for serum CRP measurements (3 h CRP). The MAS is also calculated for all patients. The ultimate diagnosis of appendicitis was based on the histologic findings of the excised appendix in operated patients and clinical follow-up in emergency department discharged patients. Diagnostic accuracy of admission CRP, early change of CRP 3 h CRP minus admission CRP, MAS and the combination of these parameters was expressed by sensitivity, specificity, positive predictive value, negative predictive value and area under receiver operating characteristics curve.

Results: Five hundred patients were included from January 2010 to December 2013. Overall, 387 patients were operated the negative appendectomy rate was 8,3%. CRP concentrations were higher in patients with acute appendicitis. However, the diagnostic value of admission CRP, delta CRP and MAS was moderate with area under ROC curve respectively equal to 0.63, 0.53 and 0.6. Combining admission CRP and delta CRP values to MAS did not result in a better performance. The area under ROC curve did not exceed 0.7 with the different combinations.

Conclusion: Early change of CRP has a moderate diagnostic value in patients with clinically suspected acute appendicitis. Combining CRP values to MAS did not improve diagnostic accuracy.

Keywords: C-reactive protein, Acute appendicitis, Alvarado score

Background

Acute appendicitis is the most common surgical emergency and the most common source of community-acquired intra-abdominal infections [1]. Clinical diagnosis of acute appendicitis is still difficult. It has been estimated that the diagnostic accuracy of acute appendicitis is between 70 and 85% [2], and that up to 50% of patients hospitalized for possible appendicitis have normal appendices [3]. Misdiagnosing acute appendicitis is responsible of two types of outcomes: in one hand, a delay to surgical treatment can that lead to perforation and peritonitis in up to 15% of the cases [4] and, in the other hand, negative appendectomy which is associated with post-operative complications such as wound infection and adhesions [3]. Several approaches have been introduced to improve the diagnostic accuracy of acute appendicitis and therefore to reduce complications. Imaging techniques, especially abdominal ultrasonography [5] and CT scans [6], have been shown to be particularly accurate with a sensitivity and specificity overcoming 90% [7]. However, doubts have been

* Correspondence: m.amine.msolli@gmail.com
[1]Emergency Department, FattoumaBourguiba University Hospital Monastir, 5000 Monastir, Tunisia
[4]Research Laboratory (LR12SP18), University of Monastir, 5000 Monastir, Tunisia
Full list of author information is available at the end of the article

raised about their usefulness in patients with high clinical probability of acute appendicitis associated with the need for qualified staff and medical facilities contributing to the increase of healthcare costs [8, 9]. Diagnostic scoring systems have been developed in an attempt to improve the diagnostic accuracy of acute appendicitis. The most prominent of those scores is that developed by Alvarado [10, 11]. The modified Alvarado score (MAS) is a more simplified and practical version of the original one and has been widely accepted after it was successfully tested in different studies [12, 13]. Modified Alvarado score is based on three symptoms, three signs, and one laboratory investigation and ranged from 1 to 9 (Table 1).

However, prospective studies have suggested that Alvarado score and MAS alone are inadequate as a diagnostic test for appendicitis [12–14]. During the evaluation of patients with possible appendicitis in the emergency department (ED), repeated physical examination of the abdomen may provide further information to help decision making. Repeated laboratory tests were also proposed to this issue without proven benefit [15].

C-reactive protein (CRP) is an acute phase protein that is often relied-on by many surgeons as a diagnostic marker of acute appendicitis [16]. Actually, there is no strong evidence supporting its use in the diagnosis of acute appendicitis and related clinical data are controversial [2]. The purpose of this study was to investigate the diagnostic performance of initial serum CRP measurement at admission and its early variation, evaluated both separately and in combination to the MAS in patients presenting to the ED with clinically suspected appendicitis.

Methods

This was a prospective observational study. We prospectively included all patients aged more than 10 years and admitted to our ED for clinically suspected acute appendicitis. The clinical suspicion of appendicitis was made based on the presence of direct tenderness in the right lower quadrant, percussion and rebound tenderness, pyrexia, anorexia, nausea and vomiting. Patients using warfarin or heparin, pregnant women, and patients using antibiotics during the study period were excluded. All patients were initially evaluated by the ED physician and demographic, clinical and biological findings were recorded on a specific data form. Blood samples were obtained immediately after admission and analyzed for while blood cell (WBC) count and admission CRP concentrations. Three hours after, a second CRP measurement (3 h CRP) was carried out in patients with an equivocal diagnosis of acute appendicitis. The CRP concentration was measured by immune turbidimetry (Beckman Collin, CA). The normal range of CRP concentrations, in our hospital, is between 0 and 6 mg/ml and concentrations >6 mg/L were considered abnormal. At the term of this evaluation, the MAS was calculated for all the included patients. A score above 4 was considered highly suggestive of acute

Table 1 Modified Alvarado Score

Symptoms	Score
Migratory right iliac fossa pain	1
Nausea/Vomiting	1
Anorexia	1
Signs	
Tenderness in right iliac fossa	2
Rebound tenderness in right iliac fossa	1
Elevated temperature	1
Laboratory findings	
Leukocytosis	2
Total	9

Table 2 Baseline characteristics of the patients enrolled in the study

	Appendicitis $n = 323$ (64.6%)	No appendicitis $n = 177$ (34.4%)	p
Sex (male: female)	181: 142	74: 103	0.002
Age (y); mean (SD)	28 (13)	26 (12)	0.17
Pain duration n (%)			0.12
< 6 h	24 (7,4)	21 (11,8)	
6–12 h	72 (22,2)	43 (24,2)	
12–24 h	138 (42,7)	68 (38,4)	
24–48 h	69 (21,3)	37 (20,9)	
> 48 h	20 (6,2)	8 (4,5)	
Associated symptoms, n (%)			
Nausea and vomiting	145 (44,8)	69 (38,9)	0.20
Anorexia	29 (8,9)	15 (8,4)	0.84
Temperature at presentation, n (%)			0.016
Afebrile	12 (3,7)	13 (7,3)	
37–37.9	187 (57,8)	118 (66,6)	
38–38.9	112 (34,6)	38 (21,4)	
> 39 °C	12 (3,7)	8 (4,5)	
Physical examination, n (%)			
RLQ tenderness	268 (82,9)	132 (74,5)	0.025
Rebound tenderness	227 (70,2)	91 (51,4)	0.036
RLQ defense	74 (22,9)	21 (11,8)	0.003
Modified Alvarado score, n (%)			< 0.001
≤ 4	142 (44)	115 (65)	0.014
s> 4	181 (56)	62 (35)	

RLQ: right lower quadrant of the abdomen

appendicitis. Surgical decision was made at the discretion of senior surgeons based on medical history, clinical examination and initial blood cell count only. All appendectomies were performed by conventional methods and surgeons were blinded about the CRP values. In patients for whom the surgical treatment was decided within the 2 weeks of ED presentation, the ultimate diagnosis of appendicitis was based on histologic examination of the excised appendix. Appendicitis was defined as ulcerative, suppurative, phlegmonous, gangrenous or perforated appendicitis. Absence of appendicitis was considered if, in home discharged patients, initial symptoms has subsisted within the 2-week follow-up at the outpatient clinic; and, in operated patients, a normal appendix was found at the histopathological examination. All patients gave their written informed consent to participate in the study which was approved by our institutional ethics committee.

Statistical analysis

Data were presented as mean ± SD (standard deviation) or as percentages. The clinical data were compared using the student-t test for the continuous variables and the Chi-square test for categorical variables. The admission CRP and delta CRP (3 h CRP − admission CRP) diagnostic performance was evaluated alone and in combination to the MAS by the calculation of the sensitivity, specificity, positive and negative predicted values for each category and the calculation of the area under curve (AUC) of the receiver operating characteristic (ROC) presentation. The closer AUC is to 1, the better is the overall performance of the test. An AUC =0.5 means that the test is not better than a random one. All p values < 0.05 were considered statistically significant.

Results

During the study period, 551 patients were eligible from them 542 patients were admitted. 42 patients did not undergo a second CRP measurement and a total of 500 patients with clinically suspected appendicitis were included in the study. The patients mean age was 28 ± 3 years with extremes ranging from 8 to 85. Young subjects aged under 30-year-old and males were the most frequent (Table 2). Most of the patients (n = 385) underwent appendectomy within the first 24 h of ED admission. In the operated group, negative appendectomy rate was 8,3% (64 cases). Histologic findings included 155 (40%) ulcerative, 37 (9.6%) suppurative, 60 (15.5%) phlegmonous, 41 (10.6%) gangrenous and 28 (7.2%) perforated appendices. Only two patients (1.7%) in the non-operated group had been diagnosed with acute appendicitis during their 2-week follow-up (Fig. 1). Mean WBC count, mean level of admission CRP and 3 h CRP and mean delta CRP between patients with and without appendicitis are shown in Table 3. In patients with acute appendicitis mean WBC and CRP measurements were significantly higher than in the patients with normal appendix (both p < 0.01). The delta CRP was positive in 73% patients with appendicitis and in 46% patients with normal appendix; the difference was significant (P < 0.001).

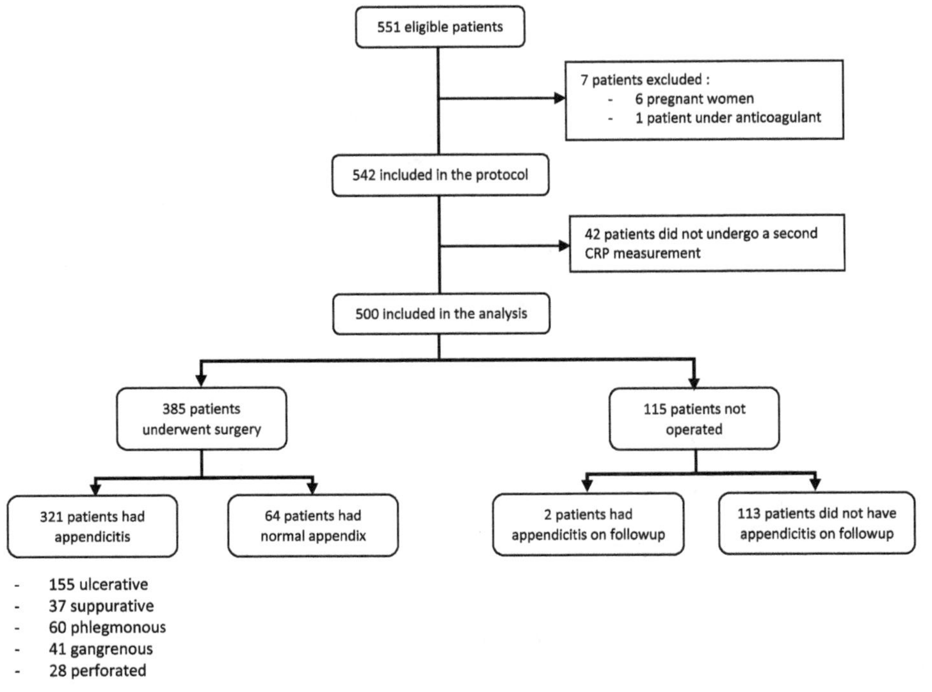

Fig. 1 Patients flow chart

Table 3 Comparison of C-reactive protein values and modified Alvarado score between patients with and without appendicitis

	Appendicitis, n (%) $n = 323$ (64.6%)	No appendicitis, n (%) $n = 177$ (35.4%)	p
White blood cell count, 1000/mm^3	14.6 (5.9)	12.1 (4.1)	0.002
Admission CRP mg/L, mean (SD)	40.4 (30.5)	20.3 (42.9)	< 0.001
Admission CRP mg/L, median (IQ range)	16.3 (5.4–60)	4,8 (1.1–14.9)	
3 h CRP mg/L, mean (SD)	48.4 (31.9)	21.9 (23.5)	< 0.001
3 h CRP mg/L, median (IQ range)	26.9 (8.3–77.9)	7.9 (1.6–24.3)	
Delta CRP mg/L, mean (SD)	+ 9.7 (23.3)	+ 1.8 (28.5)	0.001
Delta CRP mg/L, median (IQ range)	3.7 (0.5–11.9)	1.1 (0.06–4.6)	
Modified Alvarado score, mean (SD)	4.5 (1.5)	3.8 (1.6)	< 0.001

CRP: C-reactive protein
Delta CRP: admission CRP minus 3 h CRP

The diagnostic performance of both CRP and delta CRP in predicting acute appendicitis were further analyzed by using the ROC curves (Fig. 2). The AUC for admission CRP and 3 h CRP was respectively 0.63 and 0.65. However, for delta CRP it was only 0.53. The performance (sensitivity, specificity, PPV and NPV) of admission CRP and delta CRP analyzed separately and in combination to the MAS, in the diagnosis of acute appendicitis were shown in Table 4. Both admission CRP and delta CRP had a better sensitivity than MAS alone (73, 84 and 56% respectively). Combining admission CRP or delta CRP to MAS was associated with a reduced sensitivity and a moderate increase of specificity compared to MAS alone. Moreover, applying admission CRP and delta CRP to each of MAS risk category (MAS ≤ 4 versus MAS > 4) did not improve the diagnostic performance (Table 5).

Discussion

The accurate diagnosis of acute appendicitis in the ED remains a challenge for the emergency physician [17]. Good clinical approach with detailed physical examination is keystone in the diagnosis of appendicitis. However, atypical clinical presentations and nonspecific findings are frequent which could delay the diagnosis leading to complications, more often perforation; or carry misdiagnosis and lead to unnecessary surgical interventions. To overcome these difficulties, many diagnostic strategies were developed including short period admission for observation, serial laboratory tests and imaging investigations [18]. Although the utility of repeated laboratory examinations may seem helpful, diagnostic yield of serial tests has not been studied thoroughly enough to be validated in this condition. Also, it is unclear which serum inflammatory markers should be used and how well the early levels changes can function as a discriminator factor in patients with a suspected diagnosis of acute appendicitis [19]. In this prospective study we analyzed 500 patients with suspected appendicitis, and evaluated the utility of early changes in serum CRP concentrations in the diagnosis of acute appendicitis.

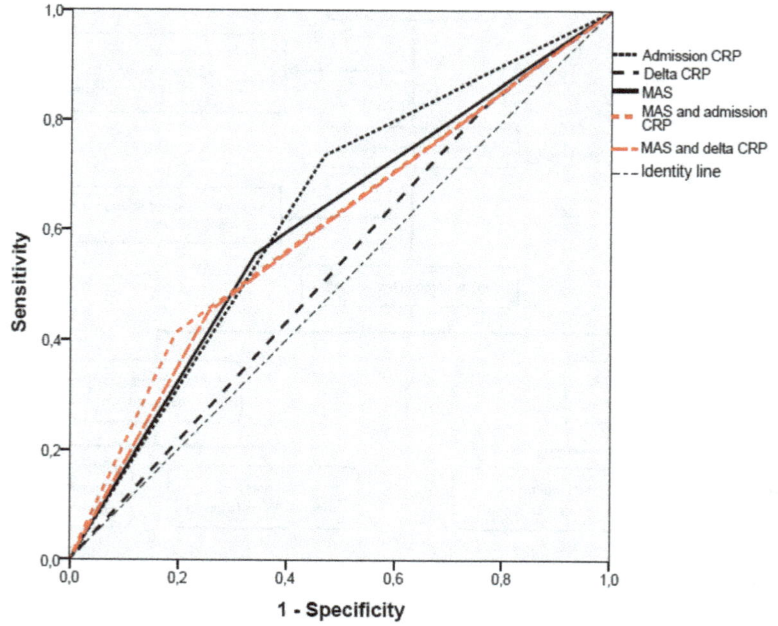

Fig. 2 Area under ROC curve of admission CRP (0.63), delta CRP (0.53), modified Alvarado score (0.6), MAS combined to admission CRP (0.6) and MAS combined to delta CRP (0.59). Delta CRP = admission CRP minus 3 h CRP

Table 4 Performance of C-reactive protein values, MAS and their combinations in the diagnosis of acute appendicitis

	Sensitivity (95% CI)	Specificity (95% CI)	PPV (95% CI)	NPV (95% CI)	LR+ (95% CI)	LR- (95% CI)
MAS > 4 alone	56 (50–61)	64 (57–71)	74 (68–79)	44 (38–51)	1.55 (1.16–2.1)	0.68 (0.54–0.87)
Elevated admission CRP	73 (68–78)	53 (45–60)	74 (69–78)	52 (44–59)	1.55 (1.23–1.95)	0.50 (0.36–0.71)
Positive delta CRP	84 (79–87)	19 (13–26)	66 (61–71)	38 (27–50)	1.03 (0.90–1.17)	0.84 (0.50–1.61)
MAS combined with admission CRP	41 (36–47)	80 (73–85)	79 (72–85)	42 (37–48)	2.05 (1.33–3.13)	0.73 (0.62–0.87)
MAS combined with delta CRP	42 (37–48)	76 (69–82)	76 (69–82)	42 (36–47)	1.75 (1.19–2.66)	0.76 (0.63–0.91)

MAS: Modified Alvarado Score
Delta CRP: admission CRP minus 3 h CRP

We demonstrated that both CRP markers were not of significant utility either alone or in combination to MAS in the diagnosis of appendicitis. Our findings contrast with some previous studies suggesting that repeated serum inflammation tests may increase the diagnostic accuracy of acute appendicitis. Recently, Han-ping et al. found that the change between primary and repeated serum inflammatory markers may improve diagnostic accuracy in pediatric appendicitis [20]. ROC analysis showed that a cut-off value of serum CRP more than 4.5 mg/L on day 2, or the increase in CRP above 15.0 mg/L on day 3 were good predictors of acute appendicitis in children. In the same way, Wu HP et al. concluded that the change in the serum parameters could point for simple appendicitis when the increase in CRP is more than 118 mg/L; and that appendicitis could be excluded when the increase in CRP is less than 10 mg/L. For perforated appendicitis, the authors concluded that changes in CRP values was not helpful for the diagnosis [21]. In our study the second measurement of the CRP concentrations was made only 3 h which could explain our negative results. Indeed, several studies have reported that serum CRP increase is delayed 12 to 24 h from the onset of inflammation symptoms [22]. In Practice, repeating serum analysis more than 12 h after ED admission would be very late especially in acute appendicitis context where complications are potentially life-threatening. Our findings highlight the need for other new biomarkers with faster expression and kinetics.

A variable combination of clinical signs has been used together in association with laboratory tests in several scoring systems for evaluating the probability of acute appendicitis. The Alvarado score is the most widely studied score. Because counting the neutrophils as a parameter of the Alvarado score is not routine in many laboratories, a simplified version was proposed (MAS) by omitting the neutrophil count and demonstrated similar diagnostic performance [23]. Some studies have shown enhanced diagnostic potential and utility when scoring systems and inflammatory markers are combined [24]. However, our results did not confirm these findings which suggest that alternative diagnostic approach are needed. Combination of inflammatory markers or the use of novel ones combined to available scores could be of greater promise [25].

As far as we know, this is the largest study to prospectively evaluate the diagnostic value of early variation of CRP concentrations in subjects presenting to the ED with clinically suspected appendicitis. Although the important sample size we acknowledge that this trial has some limitations. First, our study is monocentric, which could lead to a potential selection bias. Moreover, some subjects discharged home with a false diagnosis of non-appendicitis may have presented to other hospitals as for some patients contact information was lacking for follow-up. Finally, in our study, the diagnosis of acute appendicitis was a compromise between patient statement, physical examination and laboratory findings and no

Table 5 Diagnostic performance of CRP 1 and delta CRP depending on modified Alvarado score risk category

	Low risk (MAS ≤ 4) *n* = 257 (95% CI)					High risk (MAS > 4) *n* = 243 (95% CI)				
	Se	Sp	PPV	NPV	AUC	Se	Sp	PPV	NPV	AUC
Elevated admission CRP	73 (65–80)	58 (49–67)	68 (60–76)	63 (53–72)	0.66	74 (67–80)	43 (30–56)	79 (72–85)	36 (25–48)	0.58
Delta CRP > 1 mg/L	83 (76–89)	23 (15–32)	57 (50–64)	53 (38–67)	0.53	81 (74–86)	25 (14–38)	76 (69–82)	30 (17–45)	0.53

Delta CRP: 3 h CRP minus admission CRP
Se sensitivity
Sp specificity
PPV positive predictive value
NPV negative predictive value
AUC area under receiver operating characteristics curve

imaging tests were performed which could explain the relatively high rate of normal appendices findings at the histological examination.

Conclusion

Based on our findings, we conclude that CRP levels at admission and its early change 3 h later, in patients with clinically suspected acute appendicitis, has a moderate diagnostic value. Combining values to the MAS added no more diagnostic utility. Other diagnostic approaches should be considered in this context.

Abbreviations

CRP: C - reactive protein; ED: Emergency Department; MAS: Modified Alvarado Score

Acknowledgements

The authors would like to gratefully acknowledge all of our colleagues at the Emergency Department of University Hospital Fattouma Bourguiba Monastir who contributed greatly to this study.

Authors' contributions

MAM designed the study, performed data analysis, and wrote the manuscript. KB, WB, NJ, HB and MHG performed data collection and reviewed the manuscript. RB interpreted the data and critically reviewed the manuscript. SN revised the intellectual content of the manuscript. All authors read and approved the final manuscript.

Competing interests

The authors declare that they have no competing interests.

Author details

[1]Emergency Department, FattoumaBourguiba University Hospital Monastir, 5000 Monastir, Tunisia. [2]Emergency Department, Mahdia University Hospital, 5100 Mahdia, Tunisia. [3]Emergency Department, Sahloul University Hospital, 4011 Sousse, Tunisia. [4]Research Laboratory (LR12SP18), University of Monastir, 5000 Monastir, Tunisia.

References

1. Sartelli M, Catena F, Ansaloni L, et al. Complicated intra-abdominal infections in Europe: preliminary data from the first three months of the CIAO study. World J Emerg Surg. 2012;7:15.
2. Hallan S, Asberg A. The accuracy of C-reactive protein in diagnosing acute appendicitis–a meta-analysis. Scand J Clin Lab Invest. 1997;(5):373–80.
3. Jones K, Peña AA, Dunn EL, et al. Are negative appendectomies still acceptable? Am J Surg. 2004;(6):748–54.
4. Bixby SD, Lucey BC, Soto JA, et al. Perforated versus nonperforated acute appendicitis: accuracy of multidetector CT detection. Radiology. 2006;(3): 780–6.
5. Puylaert JB. Acute appendicitis: US evaluation using graded compression. Radiology. 1986;(2):355–60.
6. Balthazar EJ, Megibow AJ, Siegel SE, et al. Appendicitis: prospective evaluation with high-resolution CT. Radiology. 1991;(1):21–4.
7. Rao PM, Boland GW. Imaging of acute right lower abdominal quadrant pain. Clin Radiol. 1998;(9):639–49.
8. Ford RD, Passinault WJ, Morse ME. Diagnostic ultrasound for suspected appendicitis: does the added cost produce a better outcome? Am Surg. 1994;11:895–8.
9. Sivit CJ. Imaging children with acute right lower quadrant pain. Pediatr Clin N Am. 1997;(3):575–89.
10. Andersen DK. Maingot's abdominal operations, 8th edition, Vol. 1 & 2. Ann Surg. 1986;5:607–8.
11. Alvarado A. A practical score for the early diagnosis of acute appendicitis. Ann Emerg Med. 1986;(5):557–64.
12. Macklin CP, Radcliffe GS, Merei JM, et al. A prospective evaluation of the modified Alvarado score for acute appendicitis in children. Ann R Coll Surg Engl. 1997;3:203–5.
13. Al-Hashemy AM, Seleem MI. Appraisal of the modified Alvarado score for acute appendicits in adults. Saudi Med J. 2004;9:1229–31.
14. Ohmann C, Yang Q, Franke C. Diagnostic scores for acute appendicitis. Abdominal pain study group. Eur. J Surg Acta Chir. 1995;4:273–81.
15. Ng K-C, Lai S-W. Clinical analysis of the related factors in acute appendicitis. Yale J Biol Med. 2002;1:41–5.
16. Clyne B, Olshaker JS. The C-reactive protein. J Emerg Med. 1999;6:1019–25.
17. Pal KM, Khan A. Appendicitis: a continuing challenge. JPMA. 1998;7:189–92.
18. Rosengren D, Brown AFT, Chu K. Radiological imaging to improve the emergency department diagnosis of acute appendicitis. EMA. 2004;(5–6):410–6.
19. Groselj-Grenc M, Repše S, Vidmar D, et al. Clinical and laboratory methods in diagnosis of acute appendicitis in children. Croat Med J. 2007;3:353–61.
20. Lin CY, Wu H-P. Predictive value of C-reactive protein at different cutoff levels in acute appendicitis. Am J Emerg Med. 2005;(4):449–53.
21. Wu H-P, Chang C-F, Lin C-Y. Predictive inflammatory parameters in the diagnosis of acute appendicitis in children. Acta Paediatr Taiwan. 2003;4:227–31.
22. Paajanen H, Mansikka A, Laato M, et al. Novel serum inflammatory markers in acute appendicitis. Scand J Clin Lab Invest. 2002;(8):579–84.
23. Golden SK, Harringa JB, Pickhardt PJ, et al. Prospective evaluation of the ability of clinical scoring systems and physician-determined likelihood of appendicitis to obviate the need for CT. Emerg Med J. 2016;(7):458–64.
24. Shogilev DJ, Duus N, Odom SR, et al. Diagnosing appendicitis: evidence based review of the diagnostic approach in 2014. West J Emerg Med. 2014;(7):859–71.
25. Kharbanda AB, Cosme Y, Liu K, et al. Discriminative accuracy of novel and traditional biomarkers in children with suspected appendicitis adjusted for duration of abdominal pain. Acad Emerg Med Off J Soc Acad Emerg Med. 2011;(6):567–74.

16

High inter-observer agreement of observer-perceived pain assessment in the emergency department

Martin Høhrmann Hangaard[1*], Brian Malling[2] and Christian Backer Mogensen[3]

Abstract

Background: Triage is used to prioritize the patients in the emergency department. The majority of the triage systems include the patients' pain score to assess their level of acuity by using a combination of patient reported pain and observer-perceived pain; the latter therefore requires a certain degree of inter-observer agreement. The aim of the present study was to assess the inter-observer agreement of perceived pain among emergency department nurses and to evaluate if it was influenced by predetermined factors like age and gender.

Method: A project assistant randomly recruited two nurses, who were not allowed to interact with each other, to assess patient pain intensity on the numeric ranking scale. The project assistant afterwards entered the pain scores in a predesigned electronic questionnaire.
We used weighted Fleiss-Cohen (quadratic) kappa statistics, Bland-Altman statistics and logistic regression analysis to assess the inter-observer agreement.

Results: One hundred and sixty-two patients were included. They had a median age of 38 years and 45% were females. 30% of the patients were acute surgical patients and 70% acute orthopedic patients. The average time between the pain assessments were 1,7 min. The Bland Altman analysis found a mean difference in pain score of 0.2 and 95% limits of agreement of +/− 3 point. When the NRS scores were translated to commonly used pain categories (no, mild, moderate or severe pain) we found a 70% agreement with a mean difference in categories of 0.05 and 95% limits of agreement of +/− 1 category. Patient age, gender, localization of pain, examination room or presence of a significant other did not affect the inter-observer agreement.

Conclusion: We found 70% agreement on pain category between the nurses and it is justified that nurse-perceived pain assessment is used for triage in the emergency department.

Background

Pain is one of the most common complaints in the emergency department (ED) [1]. Primarily a subjective perception, it is not easily quantified and depends on various factors, including age, gender, surroundings, and previous experience with pain [2, 3]. Previous studies have found that nurses tend to underestimate patients' pain intensity [4–6]. The discrepancy between the patient's self-reported pain and nurses' estimations is higher when assessing abdominal pain compared to bone fracture pain [4] and in younger than older patients [7, 8].

Pain assessment is an integrated part of many triage systems, which determine the patient's level of acuity and, thus, their treatment priority. Using patient-reported pain assessments creates risks of misclassification, either as over-triage, which binds resources unnecessarily, or under-triage, where a serious condition risks going unrecognized.

Some triage systems have tried to compensate for this risk of misclassification by using observer-perceived pain assessment, either instead of or in combination with the patient-reported pain assessment. In the Danish Emergency Process Triage (DEPT), which has been implemented in most Danish EDs [9], patient-reported pain is

* Correspondence: herbivori@hotmail.com
[1]Upper GI Section, Department of Surgery, Odense University Hospital, Sdr. Boulevard 29, DK-5000 Odense C, Denmark
Full list of author information is available at the end of the article

validated by a nurse to ensure that it is neither over nor underreported, resulting in a patient receiving a higher triage priority than warranted or, alternatively, that a patient might be overlooked in the ED. [10]

However, observer-perceived pain assessments in the triage process require a certain level of agreement between ED nurses when rating patient pain. Thus far, no studies have examined the inter-observer agreement of perceived pain among nurses in an ED setting, which is the primary aim of this study. As a secondary aim we assessed whether patient location (emergency room or a ward room), type of pain or the presence of a significant other would affect this inter-observer agreement.

Methods

This was a cross-sectional, single-center study conducted at the ED in the Hospital of Southern Jutland, Denmark, between October 23 and November 26, 2013. The ED consisted of "emergency rooms" equipped with facilities for resuscitations and surgical procedures and "ward rooms" with only a hospital bed and facilities for monitoring.

All of the patients with musculoskeletal pain or abdominal pain assessed in the ED were invited to participate in the study if they were able to speak Danish, German, or English. Patients with obvious life- or limb-threatening conditions and patients who were unable to provide informed consent were excluded, as were patients with no pain complaint. We did not include patients with chest pain, as this group always receives high-level triage according to most triage systems, including the DEPT.

Two project assistants identified the patients who met the inclusion criteria and received the informed consent to participate. All of the ED nurses participated in the study. Among the staff on duty, two available nurses were recruited to assess patient pain intensity on the numeric ranking scale (NRS) in the same way that they would normally according to the DEPT instructions. The first nurse went to the patient, secured privacy, and asked them to assess their pain on a 10-point NRS scale. The nurse then assessed the patient's pain on the same scale without informing the patient of the result, went out, and immediately reported the patient's score and the nurse score to the project assistant.

The second nurse then went to the patient and performed the same procedure. The nurses were not allowed at any time to discuss or compare their results with each other. The project assistants entered the scores into a predesigned electronic questionnaire together with the time, patient age, gender, main complaint, the presence of a significant other, if the patients had received analgesics, and if the pain assessment was in an emergency room or a ward room.

The data was collected on random days, including weekends, from 9 am to 6 pm, which was the time with the highest patient flow.

The study was powered to detect a mean difference of 2 NRS points between observers, giving a sample size of 44 paired observations, based on a power of 90% and a confidence interval of 95%. For the kappa statistics, a kappa value of 0.60 was expected and the study was powered to detect a difference in positive proportion in a dichotomous test between observers of 10% with a 95% confidence interval not larger than kappa +/− 0.11, resulting in a sample size of 164 patients.

The data from the electronic questionnaire was transferred to Stata 14 for statistical analysis.

We used weighted Fleiss-Cohen (quadratic) kappa statistics, which accounts for a situation where there were constantly two raters but their identity varied and the rating was in ordered categories. We also calculated the Bland-Altman statistics to assess the agreement between the two rating nurses. We then transferred the NRS assessment to four categories of pain in accordance with the definitions in the DEPT: No pain 0, mild pain as NRS 1–3; moderate pain as 4–6 and severe pain as 7–10 [11] and repeated the same statistical analysis. Finally, we performed a logistic regression analysis to identify if gender, age, location of pain in the ED, and presence of significant other would influence the inter-observer agreement.

Since the study only involved an assessment of the patients' pain, no acceptance from an ethical committee was required according to Danish legislation. The study was registered with the Danish Data Protection Agency.

Results

A total of 163 patients participated in the study. One patient received analgesics between the nurses' respective assessments and was therefore excluded. The remaining 162 patients had a median age of 38 years (p25–p75: 20–61 years) and 73 were females (45%), 48 of the patients (30%) had abdominal pain and 114 (70%) musculoskeletal pain. The mean time between the two pain assessments was 1.7 min (95% CI: 1.2–2.3 min). The data was primarily collected during working days (76%). The inclusion time was from 9 am to 6 pm, with 57% of the inclusions performed before 2 pm.

The mean NRS scores between Nurse 1 (3.8, 95% CI: 3.4–4.1) and Nurse 2 (3.6, 95% CI: 3.3–3.9) did not differ significantly (p: 0.18), with a Kappa-value of 0.55 (95% CI: 0.48–0.57), i.e. a moderate agreement [12]. The Bland Altman analysis revealed that the mean difference in pain score was 0.2 (95% CI: -0.1–0.4), and the 95% prediction interval for the Nurse 2 score was from −2.8–3.1 on the NRS scale, i.e. the second nurse would score within 3 points higher or lower compared to

Nurse 1. This is reflected in the Bland-Altman plot in Fig. 1.

Table 1 shows the distribution of pain assessments in the categories between the two nurse observations of the same patient. There was an overall agreement of 70% (95% CI: 63–77%), with a Kappa-value of 0.55 (0.51–0.65), moderate agreement. The difference between the nurses was greater than one category for only two of the patients (1%). The Bland-Altman analysis showed a mean difference of 0.05 categories with a 95% prediction interval of +/1 category (Fig. 2).

Table 2 reflects the inter-observer agreement depending on age, gender, pain localization, examination room, and the presence of a significant other during the assessment. The only difference was a significantly higher agreement between the nurses among the patients aged 61–80 (OR 2.9, 95% CI 1.0–8.4), but this was not found after adjustments.

Table 1 Two nurses perceptions of 162 patients pain categories

Second nurse pain assessment						
		no	mild	moderate	severe	Total
First nurse pain assessment	no	1	3	0	0	4
	mild	2	60	15	0	77
	moderate	2	15	47	3	67
	severe	0	0	8	6	14
Total		5	78	70	9	162

Discussion

We found that when two nurses independently assessed the same patient, the inter-observer agreement had a kappa value of 0.55, which correlates to a moderate agreement.

Transferred to commonly used pain categories of no, mild, moderate or severe pain, a 70% agreement among the nurses was found, with a 95% prediction interval of +/− 1 pain category. This was independent of age, gender, presence or absence of a significant other, whether the patient was assessed in an emergency room or ward room, or if the patient complained of abdominal or musculoskeletal pain. The nurses were disagreeing more than one out of four pain categories in only 1% of the assessments.

Few studies have compared the inter-observer variation of pain assessment among nurses, and none of these studies have been in emergency departments. We are thus unable to compare our results directly with others in similar work environments. Studies based on theoretical pain cases revealed that there was a certain variation between nurses' assessments, which could be attributed to the patient's age, type and stage of illness, as well as the nurses' professional experience and personal experiences of pain [13, 14]. Furthermore, pain assessment tools have been developed and validated for pain assessment in patients who are unable to express their sense of pain due to dementia or other mental distortions. The validation of these tools showed an acceptable agreement between the nurses [15, 16].

Our results have some clinical implications. The inter-observer agreement was lower than we had expected in a group of experienced ED nurses, who were well trained in using the NRS scale, but we found high inter-observer agreement when pain scores were transferred to commonly used pain categories. Also, the assessment of patient pain intensity where not influenced by different patient groups, age, gender, or other circumstances. Thus, our results justifies that nurse-perceived pain assessment is used for triage in the emergency department.

The advantage of our study was that it is the first to evaluate the inter-observer agreement of perceived pain of patients in an ED setting and the study has a reasonable size. However, the study is weakened by a number of factors. It was performed in an ED where all of the nurses had been trained in the use of NRS scales and had a considerable clinical ED experience, on average more than 2 years. A more heterogeneous nursing staff might have produced different results. Furthermore, we

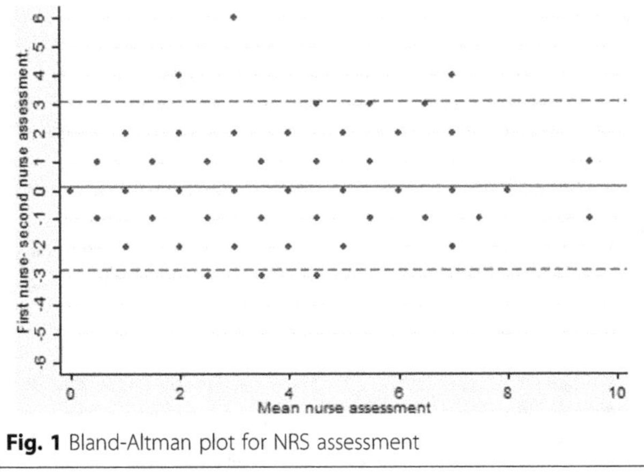

Fig. 1 Bland-Altman plot for NRS assessment

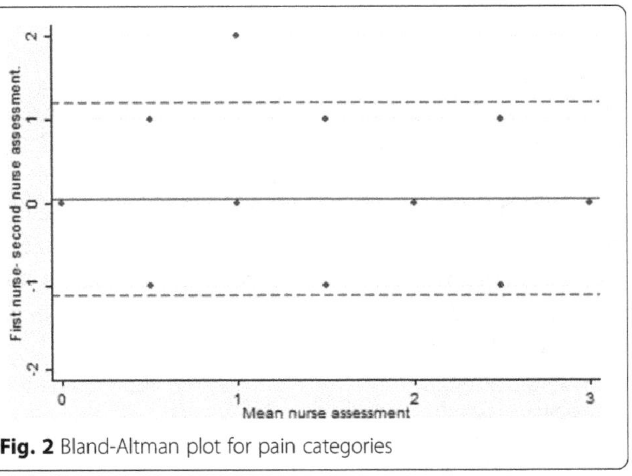

Fig. 2 Bland-Altman plot for pain categories

Table 2 Variables influencing the agreement among nurses in percieved pain categories of 162 patients

			univariat analysis		multivariat analysis (1)	
Variable	no. of agreements	% of agreements	OR	95% CI	OR	95% CI
gender						
female	50	68%	1			
male	64	72%	1.2	0.6-2.3		
age group						
< 20 yrs	23	58%	1			
20-40 yrs	35	74%	2.1	0.9-5.4	2.0	0.6-7.1
41-60 yrs	24	75%	2.2	0.8-6.1		
61-80 yrs	28	80%	2.9	1.0-8.4		
>= 80 yrs	4	50%	0.7	0.2-3.4		
specialty						
surgical	37	77%	1			
ortopaedic	77	68%	0.6	0.3-1.4		
significant other						
not present	61	76%	1			
present	53	65%	0.6	0.3-1.1		
room						
emergency room	80	68%	1			
ward room	34	77%	1.6	0.7-3.6		

(1) adjustment for gender, age, specialty, relative present and examination room

did not include patients with chest pain, and our results should not be extended to this group of patients. Moreover, we did not include patients who did not complain about pain. This might be considered as a bias, but for the evaluation of the clinical use of a triage system, which uses pain as a variable, it does not make sense to assess patients who were not complaining of pain or had no pain-associated reason for referral to the ED. Finally, since the nurses first asked the patients for their own pain assessment and first made their own assessment thereafter, the pain score was not absolutely independent. As this is how the currently used DEPT and other triage systems are used, our study reflects the pragmatic usage of the triage.

Conclusion

This is the first study to validate inter-observer pain agreement in an emergency department. We found 70% agreement on pain category between the nurses, and the pain assessment was unaffected by age, gender, localization of pain, examination room, or whether or not a significant other was present. This justifies that nurse-perceived pain assessment is used for triage in the emergency department.

Abbreviations

DEPT: Danish Emergency Process Triage; ED: Emergency Departments; NRS: Numeric Ranking Scale

Acknowledgements

None.

Funding

None.

Authors' contributions

BM and MHH identified the patients who met the inclusion criteria and received their informed consent to participate. BM and MHH overlooked the pain assessment to make sure it went by protocol. All authors contributed to data analysis. MMH was the main writer of the manuscript. All authors read, contributed and approved the final manuscript.

Competing interests

The authors declare that they have no competing interests. CBM works as an Associate Editor for BMC Emergency Medicine.

Author details

[1]Upper GI Section, Department of Surgery, Odense University Hospital, Sdr. Boulevard 29, DK-5000 Odense C, Denmark. [2]Department of Diagnostic Radiology, Rigshospitalet, Blegdamsvej 9, DK-2100 København Ø, Denmark. [3]Emergency Department, Hospital of Southern Jutland, Kresten Philipsensvej 15, DK-6200 Aabenraa, Denmark.

References

1. Cordell WH, Keene KK, Giles BK, Jones JB, Jones JH, Brizendine EJ. The high prevalence of pain in emergency medical care. Am J Emerg Med. 2002; 20(3):165–9.
2. Body R, Foex BA. Optimising well-being: is it the pain or the hurt that matters? Emerg Med J. 2012;29(2):91–4.
3. McGrath PA. Psychological aspects of pain perception. Arch Oral Biol. 1994; 39:Suppl:55s–62s.
4. Duignan M, Dunn V. Congruence of pain assessment between nurses and emergency department patients: a replication. Int Emerg Nurs. 2008;16(1):23–8.

5. Puntillo K, Neighbor M, O'Neil N, Nixon R. Accuracy of emergency nurses in assessment of patients' pain. Pain Manag Nurs. 2003;4(4):171–5.
6. Guru V, Dubinsky I. The patient vs. caregiver perception of acute pain in the emergency department. J Emerg Med. 2000;18(1):7–12.
7. Marco CA, Kanitz W, Jolly M. Pain scores among emergency department (ED) patients: comparison by ED diagnosis. J Emerg Med. 2013;44(1):46–52.
8. Marco CA, Nagel J, Klink E, Baehren D. Factors associated with self-reported pain scores among ED patients. Am J Emerg Med. 2012;30(2):331–7.
9. Lindberg SO, Lerche la Cour J, Folkestad L, Hallas P, Brabrand M. The use of triage in Danish emergency departments. Dan Med Bull. 2011;58(10):A4301.
10. Bible D. Pain assessment at nurse triage: a literature review. Emerg Nurse. 2006;14(3):26–9.
11. Breivik H, Borchgrevink PC, Allen SM, Rosseland LA, Romundstad L, Hals EK, Kvarstein G, Stubhaug A. Assessment of pain. Br J Anaesth. 2008;101(1):17–24.
12. Viera AJ, Garrett JM. Understanding interobserver agreement: the kappa statistic. Fam Med. 2005;37(5):360–3.
13. Hall-Lord ML, Larsson BW. Registered nurses' and student nurses' assessment of pain and distress related to specific patient and nurse characteristics. Nurse Educ Today. 2006;26(5):377–87.
14. Holm K, Cohen F, Dudas S, Medema PG, Allen BL. Effect of personal pain experience on pain assessment. Image—the. J Nurs Scholarsh. 1989;21(2):72–5.
15. Gregersen M, Melin AS, Nygaard IS, Nielsen CH, Beedholm-Ebsen M. Reliability of the Danish Abbey pain scale in severely demented and non-communicative older patients. Int J Palliat Nurs. 2016;22(10):482–8.
16. Takai Y, Yamamoto-Mitani N, Chiba Y, Nishikawa Y, Hayashi K, Sugai Y. Abbey pain scale: development and validation of the Japanese version. Geriatr Gerontol Int. 2010;10(2):145–53.

17

ECMO use and mortality in adult patients with cardiogenic shock

Rayan El Sibai[1], Rana Bachir[1] and Mazen El Sayed[1,2*]

Abstract

Background: Extracorporeal membrane oxygenation (ECMO) is increasingly used in resuscitation of critically ill patients with documented improved survival. Few studies describe ECMO use in cardiogenic shock. This study examines ECMO use and identifies variables associated with mortality in patients treated for cardiogenic shock in US hospitals.

Methods: A retrospective observational study of the US Nationwide Emergency Department Sample (NEDS) database of 2013 was conducted. Weighted visits for cardiogenic shock (discharge diagnosis) with ECMO use were included. Collected data was analyzed and variables associated with mortality were identified.

Results: A total of 922 weighted patients with cardiogenic shock and ECMO were included. Mean age was 50.8 years. They were more commonly males (66.3%; $n = 658$). Slightly over half (51.0%, $n = 506$) survived to hospital discharge. Mean charges per patient were $589,610.5. Mean length of stay was 21.8 days.
Increased mortality was associated with presence of respiratory diseases (OR = 3.83), genitourinary diseases (OR = 4.97), undergoing an echocardiogram (OR = 4.63), and presenting during seasons other than Fall. Lower mortality was noted in patients with injury and poisoning (OR = 0.47), in those who underwent certain vascular procedures (OR = 0.49) and those with increasing length of stay (OR = 0.90).

Conclusion: Mortality in patients with cardiogenic shock remains high despite ECMO use. Season of admission (other than Fall) and presence of specific comorbidities (Respiratory and genitourinary diseases) are associated with increased mortality in this population. Familiarity with these variables can help identify patients at higher risk of death and can help improve outcomes further in cardiogenic shock.

Keywords: Extracorporeal circulation, Extracorporeal membrane oxygenation, Shock, cardiogenic, Emergency service, hospital, Resuscitation, Critical illness

Background

Mechanical cardiopulmonary assistance, which is often utilized as an integral part of certain invasive cardiac surgeries, is increasingly used in resuscitation of patients in intensive care settings and emergency departments [1–12]. Prolonged cardiopulmonary assistance is called extracorporeal membrane oxygenation (ECMO) or extracorporeal life support (ECLS) and is a sophisticated and resource-intensive intervention for critically ill patients with cardiac or respiratory dysfunction [11, 12]. ECMO and ECLS are often used interchangeably [13].

There are two types of ECMO – veno-venous (VV) and veno-arterial (VA) ECMO – depending on differences in vascular access. During VV ECMO, blood is extracted from the vena cava or right atrium and returned oxygenated to the right atrium. During VA ECMO, blood is extracted from the right atrium and returned oxygenated to the arterial system, most commonly the iliac artery. VA ECMO provides hemodynamic support in addition to respiratory support [11].

Although ECMO use is more commonly described in the pediatric population, ECMO use in adults for cardiac and respiratory indications more recently

* Correspondence: melsayed@aub.edu.lb
[1]Department of Emergency Medicine, American University of Beirut Medical Center, P.O. Box - 11-0236, Riad El Solh, Beirut 1107 2020, Lebanon
[2]Emergency Medical Services and Prehospital Care Program, American University of Beirut Medical Center, Beirut, Lebanon

became the largest contributing group in the Extracorporeal Life Support Organization Registry, which was established to improve quality and outcome of ECMO use [4, 12]. ECMO is used for various cardiac or pulmonary diseases including: post-cardiotomy, myocarditis, acute coronary syndrome or refractory cardiac arrest, as a bridge to heart/lung transplant, cardiogenic shock, respiratory failure, trauma/drowning as well as other conditions [14]. In 2015, cardiogenic shock was found to be the most common diagnosis associated with ECLS use in adults with VA ECMO, occurring in 60.7% of such patients [4]. Cardiogenic shock is a clinical condition of inadequate tissue perfusion due to cardiac dysfunction that is associated with persistent hypotension and end organ damage. Cardiogenic shock often results from myocardial infarction but can also result from other cardiac diseases such as myocarditis, pericarditis, and cardiomyopathy [15].

ECMO use improves survival in patients with cardiac disease with survival rates ranging from 20 to 50% [1–10]. ECMO also increases 30-day survival rates when used to bridge patients in cardiogenic shock to coronary intervention procedures [16]. Additionally, ECMO improves outcomes in patients with cardiac arrests – mainly survival without neurologic deficit – when added to cardiopulmonary resuscitation (CPR) [3, 17].

Contraindications for VA ECMO in cardiac failure do exist and include the following: ethical considerations and patient's will, no bridging goal, severe aortic regurgitation, aortic dissection, severe peripheral artery disease (iliac), left ventricular thrombus (relative contraindication) [18]. Despite several observational and registry studies on ECMO use, few studies describe the extent of ECMO use in patients with cardiogenic shock. This study examines cardiogenic shock presentations that involved ECMO use and identifies variables associated with mortality in this U.S. hospital population sample.

Methods

Data and materials

NEDS is a product of Healthcare Cost and Utilization Project (HCUP) under the auspices of the Agency for Healthcare Research and Quality (AHRQ) [19]. It is the largest U.S. all-payer ED database, combining medical and non-clinical data from both national and state sources. Data from this stratified sample is accrued from 945 hospital-owned EDs located across 30 States and the District of Columbia, reflecting approximately 20% of all hospital-based EDs located in the United States. The following stratification variables were used to weight data per HCUP specifications: U.S. Census region, urban-rural location, ownership, and teaching status of the hospital as well as trauma center designation [20]. This stratified sample of patients is statistically weighted using the above stratification variables to approximate and examine national estimates. Weighting of sample compensates for different probabilities of selection as part of the dataset sample. As per requirements for publishing HCUP data and to safeguard patients' privacy, data on any variable with size less than or equal to 10 are excluded.

Study design and population

This retrospective study used the 2013 public release dataset of the US Nationwide Emergency Department Sample (NEDS) database. The 2013 NEDS dataset contains information on weighted 134,869,015 ED visits. Patients were included in this study if they met the following criteria: Adult patients (age 18 or older) who presented with cardiogenic shock and underwent ECMO procedure and died in the ED or were admitted to the same hospital during the selected visit.

Data definitions

The NEDS data elements include: demographic patient information; mechanism, intent, and severity of injury; admission and discharge status; payment source; healthcare expenses and general hospital characteristics. The AHRQ Clinical Classifications Software (CCS) was used to select all patients with cardiogenic shock. CCS is a tool for grouping patient diagnoses and procedures into a convenient number of clinically meaningful categories similar and equivalent to than the International Classification of Diseases (ICD) coding system.

The following CSS codes are specific for cardiogenic shock: CCS 97, CCS 100, CCS 101, CCS 103, CCS 106, CCS 107, CCS 108 [12]. A list of Equivalent ICD-9 CM codes and variable classification is included (See attachment, Additional File 1 which illustrates code and variable classifications). Additionally, the ICD-9 CM procedure code 39.65 was used to gather all patients who underwent ECMO procedure.

Chronic diseases and procedures with frequencies less than 10% were removed from the analysis and were not displayed results. Injury severity score (ISS) is considered as the gold standard trauma severity score to predict morbidity, increased hospital stay and mortality in trauma patients. An ISS score greater than 15 is historically used as a cutoff value for severe trauma injury [21]. This study used a more conservative cut off value for ISS of >8 since very few patients had an ISS score greater than 15. Previous studies have also shown that increasing injury severity (ISS of >8) is associated with increased hospital stay and ICU admission [22].

AHRQ provides a database and a software tool, called the Chronic Condition Indicator (CCI), that allows for the identification of chronic diseases using ICD-9 CM coding. CCI was utilized in this study for the purposes of investigating presence of chronic conditions according to body system categories affected. According to CCI, the definition of a chronic disease is "a medical condition which lasts for twelve months or longer with either one of the following criteria being met: (1) the medical condition restricts self-care, independent living, and social interaction; (2) the medical condition results in the need of ongoing medical intervention."

Additionally, NEDS categorizes ICD-9 CM procedure codes into four broad categories labeled as either major or minor and therapeutic or diagnostic. An ICD-9 CM procedure is classified as "minor if the procedure is a non-operating room procedure and major if the procedure is a valid operating room procedure by the Diagnosis Related Group (DRG) grouper" (an ICD-9 CM grouping system). CCS procedure codes were also used to examine most common procedures other than ECMO.

Statistical analysis

IBM-SPSS 24 was used to carry out descriptive analysis on the socio-demographic, clinical and hospital characteristics. Mean with associated 95% confidence intervals (CI) was used for continuous variables, while frequencies, percentages and 95% CI were used for categorical variables.

The standard statistical methods that treat the data as being emerged from a simple random sampling data were inappropriate for the NEDS survey design and would yield biased estimates, overly-narrow confidence levels and misleading significance tests due to the type I error generated from the biased results. The Rao-Scott chi-square test, a modified version of the Pearson's chi-square test, as well as a general linear model (GLM) for complex sampling (CS) were used to assess the significance of the statistical association of the independent categorical and continuous variables respectively between the two groups (those who survived and those who did not). Logistic regression was conducted to identify significant associations with mortality in ECMO patients with cardiogenic shock. Variables that were significantly different between the two groups when compared by outcome (mortality) were included in the multivariate analysis.

All estimates (means, percentages, odds ratio and confidence intervals) were drawn by complex sampling methods, particularly, CSTABULATE, CSDESCRIPTIVES, CSGLM and CSLOGISTIC to adjust for the NEDS survey design and to ensure the results are accurate. CSTABULATE is a complex sample procedure that produces analysis for categorical variables. CSDESCRIPTIVES and CSGLM are two different complex sample procedures that allow for analysis of continuous variables at the univariate and bivariate levels respectively. Lastly, the Complex Samples Logistic Regression procedure, CSLOGISTIC, performs logistic regression for samples drawn by complex sampling methods.

Complex sampling design of the study resulted in decimal places among sample frequencies. To avoid rounding errors and for the sake of clarity, variables were restored to discrete format by discarding decimals. In addition, a maximal value for total sample frequency was capped at 992 patients. Analysis was verified using *HCUPnet*, a free on-line query system based on data from HCUP [23]. Lastly, a p-value of < 0.05 was used to indicate statistical significance.

Results

A total of 8,605,807 weighted adult visits were admitted to the emergency department with cardiogenic shock. Of those, 992 weighted adult patient visits included an ECMO procedure yielding a rate of 0.1 per 1000 ED visits for cardiogenic shock.

The mean age of the study population was 50.8 years (95%CI 48.8–52.7). Patients were more commonly males (66.3%; 95%CI 60.3–71.8). Visits were equally distributed across all four seasons and were mainly during the weekday (Monday through Friday) (70.6%, $n = 700$). Over half of visits were to large metropolitan hospitals (fringe 39.4%, $n = 389$ and central 29.1%, $n = 287$). Private insurance (47.8%, $n = 472$) as well as Medicare and Medicaid (43.6%, $n = 430$) were the most common primary expected payer types. (Table 1).

All patients had diseases of the circulatory system, and most patients had diseases of the respiratory system (82.7%, $n = 820$) as well as endocrine, nutritional, and metabolic diseases/immunity disorders (80.1%, $n = 795$) (Table 2). Few patients had injury diagnosis reported on record (14.2%, $n = 141$). The most frequent injury reported was suffocation injury (1.9%, $n = 19$) followed by falling injury (1.5%, $n = 15$). Only 5.3% ($n = 52$) had increased injury severity defined by an ISS of 9 or greater. The mean for total charges (both ED and inpatient services) was $589,610.5 (95% CI 512,270.0 – 666,950.9). The mean hospital length of stay was 21.8 days (95% CI 19.0–24.6).

In addition to ECMO, patients with cardiogenic shock underwent different types of procedures (Table 3). By procedure class, all patients had major therapeutic procedures on record since ECMO procedure is categorized as major therapeutic. Most patients (89.1%, $n = 884$) also had minor therapeutic procedures. The most common procedure other than ECMO was respiratory intubation and mechanical ventilation (56.7%, $n = 562$).

For Patients who underwent ECMO, there were significant differences between those who survived to

Table 1 Characteristics of Study Population

Continuous Variables	Range	Median (IQR)	Mean (95% CI)
Age (years)	18–90	54 (23)	50.8 (48.8–52.7)
Categorical Variables		*Count (N = 992)*	*Percent (95% CI)*
Gender (male)		658	66.3 (60.3–71.8)
Median household income[a]			
$1 - $37,999		126	13.2 (9.8–17.6)
$38,000 - $47,999		238	25.1 (19.9–31.0)
$48,000 - $63,999		238	25.0 (20.2–30.7)
$64,000 or more		348	36.7 (31.1–42.6)
Season of admission			
Winter		223	23.2 (18.3–29.0)
Spring		244	25.4 (20.5–31.0)
Summer		259	27.0 (21.8–33.0)
Autumn		234	24.3 (19.5–29.9)
Admission day			
Monday - Friday		700	70.6 (64.7–75.8)
Saturday - Sunday		292	29.4 (24.2–35.3)
Patient location[b]			
Large central metropolitan		287	29.1 (24.4–34.3)
Large fringe metropolitan		389	39.4 (34.5–44.5)
Medium metropolitan		147	14.9 (11.5–19.0)
Small metropolitan		66	6.6 (4.1–10.7)
Micropolitan		51	5.1 (3.2–8.1)
Not metropolitan or micropolitan		48	4.9 (3.0–7.9)
Primary expected payer			
Private insurance		472	47.8 (41.6–54.1)
Medicare & Medicaid		430	43.6 (37.3–50.1)
Self-pay		60	6.1 (3.8–9.7)
Other		25	2.5 (1.1–5.5)

[a]According to national quartile for patient ZIP code derived from ZIP Code-demographic data obtained from Claritas
[b]According to National Center for Health Statistics (NCHS) Urban-rural code

hospital discharge and those who did not. Table 4 lists only the statistically significant variables between the two groups and which included age, season of admission, presence of certain chronic conditions and certain procedures, whether injury was reported, total charges, and length of stay (LOS). Those who survived were slightly younger than those who did not (49.5 vs 52.1, years respectively $p = 0.009$) and had significantly higher total hospital charges for services as well as total length of stay.

Table 5 shows the variables associated with mortality in ECMO patients. Having diseases of either the respiratory system (OR = 3.83, 95%CI 1.76–8.31) or genitourinary system (OR = 4.97, 95%CI 2.39–10.33) as well as undergoing an echocardiogram (OR = 4.63, 95%CI 1.300–16.504) were significantly associated with increased mortality. Higher mortality was also associated with visits during all seasons when compared to autumn.

Conversely, having a chronic disease of injury and poisoning (OR = 0.382, 95%CI 0.191–0.765), undergoing other operating room procedures on vessels other than head and neck (OR = 0.49, 95%CI 0.24–1.00), as well as increasing total charges (OR = 0.993 95%CI 0.988–0.999) were associated with decreased mortality.

Discussion

ECMO use is increasing in adult patients with cardiogenic shock, but few studies that describe ECMO use or associations with mortality in this population are available. This study is the first to use the largest US ED database, NEDS, to describe socio-demographic, clinical, and hospital characteristics for patients with cardiogenic shock who underwent ECMO.

This study also described patterns of ECMO use and outcomes of patients with cardiogenic shock. ECMO was used in 0.1 per 1000 ED/hospital visits with cardiogenic shock in 2013. Survival to hospital discharge was 51%. This finding is consistent with survival rates from previous studies that range from 20 to 50% [1–10].

The mean age of patients who presented to US EDs with cardiogenic shock and who underwent ECMO was 50.8 years (95%CI 48.4–52.7). Previous studies have shown similar characteristics [12, 24]. Maxwell et al. examined national ECMO use between the years 1998 to 2009 and found an overall mean age of 53.9 ± 0.4 years and a mean age of 48.9 ± 0.8 years among those with cardiogenic shock specifically [12]. Schmidt et al., on the other hand, analyzed ECMO use only for refractory cardiogenic shock between the years of 2003 and 2013 and found a mean age of 54 years (range 39–64) [24].

ECMO use as expected was mostly in large metropolitan hospitals. ECMO is considered a complex procedure and is fraught with complications such as stroke, neurologic complications, lower extremity ischemia, fasciotomy or compartment syndrome, amputation, acute kidney injury, renal replacement therapy, significant infection, major or significant bleeding and re-thoracotomy for bleeding or tamponade [14, 18]. Thus, it is usually reserved for when conventional treatments have failed and is usually undertaken in larger specialized centers.

Seasonal variation in mortality among patients presenting with cardiogenic shock and undergoing ECMO procedure was also identified in this study. The association of seasonal patterns on both hospital admission and mortality has been previously examined and described among patients with cardiovascular disease. Previous studies have reported increased adverse effects (hospital admission and mortality) during colder months

Table 2 Chronic Conditions, Injuries, and Outcomes of Sample Patients

Categorical Variables			Count (*N* = 992)	Percent (95% CI)
Chronic conditions body system indicator				
Circulatory system			992	100
Respiratory system			820	82.7 (77.5–86.9)
Endocrine/nutritional/metabolic/immunity			795	80.1 (74.7–84.6)
Symptoms, signs, and ill-defined conditions			779	78.5 (73.1–83.1)
Genitourinary system			724	72.9 (67.1–78.1)
Blood and blood-forming organs			636	64.1 (58.0–69.7)
Injury and poisoning			617	62.2 (56.3–67.7)
Digestive system			414	41.8 (35.8–47.9)
Infectious and parasitic disease			393	39.7 (33.7–45.9)
Health status/contact with health services factors			383	38.6 (33.1–44.4)
Nervous system and sense organs			313	31.5 (26.1–37.5)
Mental disorders			186	18.8 (14.3–24.2)
Injury diagnosis reported on record				
No injury diagnoses reported			851	85.8 (80.8–89.7)
Injury is reported			141	14.2 (10.3–19.2)
Injuries Specified by the NEDS Database				
Injury by suffocation			19	1.9 (0.8–4.4)
Injury by falling			15	1.5 (0.5–4.1)
More than one injury diagnosis				
One or no injury diagnosis reported			938	94.5 (90.9–96.7)
More than one injury diagnosis			54	5.5 (3.3–9.1)
Unintentional injury indicated				
Intention not specified			924	93.1 (89.2–95.6)
Unintentional injury			68	6.9 (4.4–10.8)
Injury severity score[a]				90.3 (85.9–93.5)
No injury severity score			896	4.4 (2.4–7.8)
1–8			44	5.3 (3.0–9.0)
9–75			52	
Disposition of patient				
Admitted to same hospital			992	100
Survival to discharge			506	51.0 (44.8–57.1)
Died in the ED/hospital			486	49.0 (42.9–55.2)
Continuous Variables	Frequency	Range	Median (IQR)	Mean (95% CI)
Total charges[b] (USD$)	988	3773–4,292,990	409,138 (468,598)	589,610.5 (512,270.0 – 666,950.9)
Length of stay (days)	992	0–131	16 (24)	21.8 (19.0–24.7)

[a]Assigned by ICPIC Stata program
[b]Total charges are for accumulated ED and Inpatient services

(up to 10–20% increased mortality) [25–27]. Similarly, our study shows that the winter season was associated with the highest mortality (OR: 8.85; 95%CI: 3.39–23.11). Reasons for these seasonal variations though not directly identified in our study are multiple and complex, involving both physiologic and behavioral causes. Previously identified causes include sudden cold acclimatization, change in dietary patters, change in physical activity, changes in mental health, vitamin D deficiency, increased air pollution, and increased incidence of infectious disease [26].

This study also identified variables associated with mortality in patients with cardiogenic shock requiring ECMO. In addition to previously described associated

Table 3 Extracorporeal Membrane Oxygenation Among Cardiogenic Shock: Procedures

Procedure class for inpatient	Count ($N = 992$)	Percent (95% CI)
Minor diagnostic	534	53.8 (47.8–59.7)
Minor therapeutic	884	89.1 (84.6–92.4)
Major diagnostic	62	6.2 (3.8–10.1)
Major therapeutic	992	100
Specific procedures using CCS codes	Count ($N = 992$)	Percent (95% CI)
Circulator system procedures		
Extracorporeal circulation auxiliary to open heart procedures[a]	992	100
Other operating room heart procedures[b]	510	51.4 (45.3–57.5)
Diagnostic cardiac catheterization; coronary arteriography	231	23.3 (18.6–28.9)
Conversion of cardiac rhythm	183	18.4 (14.4–23.3)
Heart valve procedures	179	18.1 (13.9–23.1)
Coronary artery bypass graft (CABG)	150	15.1 (11.5–19.6)
Other non-operating room therapeutic cardiovascular procedures	123	12.4 (9.0–16.9)
Percutaneous transluminal coronary angioplasty (PTCA)	113	11.4 (8.1–15.8)
Echocardiogram	107	10.8 (7.6–15.3)
Swan-Ganz catheterization for monitoring	102	10.2 (7.2–14.4)
Blood transfusion	220	22.2 (17.9–27.2)
Respiratory system procedures		
Respiratory intubation and mechanical ventilation	562	56.7 (50.5–62.7)
Other operating room procedures on respiratory system and mediastinum	182	18.4 (14.0–23.7)
Diagnostic bronchoscopy and biopsy of bronchus	135	13.6 (10.0–18.3)
Tracheostomy; temporary and permanent	111	11.2 (7.8–15.9)
Other procedures		
Other operating room procedures[b]	365	36.8 (31.1–42.9)
Other vascular catheterization; not heart	330	33.3 (27.8–39.3)
Other therapeutic procedures[c]	207	20.9 (16.5–26.1)

[a]This CCS procedure code also includes ICD-9 procedure code 39.65 for ECMO procedures
[b]Examples include operations on valves and septa of the heart, heart vessels, and the heart and pericardium
[c]Specifically procedures on vessels other than head/neck
[d]Nervous, ophthalmic, gastrointestinal procedures not otherwise specified

clinical variables, the study examined different socio-economic and system level factors that might be affecting mortality in this population. Patients with specific chronic conditions such as diseases of the respiratory system or the genitourinary system were more likely to die. This was expected given that patients with multiple organ dysfunction syndrome require ventilator support or dialysis and are more likely to die. These findings are similar to previous studies where pre-ECMO predictive survival score (SAVE-score) in patients with refractory cardiogenic shock identified chronic renal failure as risk factor associated with mortality [24].

The study also examined the costs and impact associated with ECMO use. The mean total charges for cardiogenic shock visits with ECMO procedure was $589,610.5 (95%CI $512,270.0 – $666,950.9) per admission. This mean is more than 10 times the national mean cost of patients with cardiogenic shock post ST-Elevation Myocardial Infarction in 2010 ($45,625) [28]. The mean length of stay for the study population was 21.8 days (95%CI 19.0–24.7). Both the mean cost and mean length of stay are higher than what Maxwell et al. previously reported on resource use trends in ECMO between 1998 and 2009 where the mean total hospital charges was $344,009 ± $30,707 per admission and the mean length of stay was 18.3 ± 1.3 days [12]. Resources utilization with ECMO seem to be increasing without an associated increase in survival benefit. Future research is therefore needed to document trends in survival and the impact of ECMO use on outcomes of patients suffering from cardiogenic shock and from other conditions. ECMO is just one of several mechanical assist

Table 4 Comparison of Study Groups Stratified by Outcome (Mortality)

	Survival to Discharge (*N* = 506)		Mortality (*N* = 486)		
Categorical Variables[a]	Count	Percent (95% CI)	Count	Percent (95% CI)	*p*-value
Season of admission					
Winter	85	17.4 (11.7–25.2)	138	29.2 (21.8–37.8)	0.006
Spring	104	21.3 (15.0–29.1)	140	29.7 (22.2–38.5)	
Summer	140	28.7 (21.3–37.5)	119	25.2 (18.2–34.0)	
Autumn	159	32.6 (25.6–40.3)	75	15.9 (10.3–23.7)	
Chronic conditions	506	100	487	100	
Respiratory system	389	76.9 (69.1–83.2)	431	88.6 (81.4–93.3)	0.014
Injury and poisoning	375	74.2 (65.9–81.0)	242	49.7 (41.1–58.3)	< 0.001
Genitourinary system	305	60.4 (51.7–68.4)	419	86.0 (79.6–90.7)	< 0.001
Digestive system	178	35.3 (27.5–43.9)	236	48.5 (39.8–57.3)	0.034
Nervous system & sense organs	127	25.1 (18.4–33.4)	186	38.2 (30.1–46.9)	0.025
Injury diagnosis					
No injury diagnoses	392	77.7 (69.3–84.3)	459	94.3 (88.7–97.2)	< 0.001
Injury is reported	113	22.3 (15.7–30.7)	28	5.7 (2.8–11.3)	
Procedures					
Other operating room procedures[b]	225	44.5 (36.0–53.3)	140	28.8 (21.4–37.6)	0.012
Tracheostomy[c]	82	16.1 (10.5–23.9)	30	6.1 (3.0–12.1)	0.015
Echocardiogram	36	7.1 (3.8–12.9)	71	14.7 (9.5–22.0)	0.05
Continuous Variables[d]	Count	Mean (95% CI)	Count	Mean (95% CI)	*p*-value
Age (years)	506	49.5 (46.8–52.1)	487	52.1 (49.3–54.9)	0.009
Total charges[e] (USD)	501	695,089.0 (560,971.1-829,206.8)	487	480,927.5 (398,015.8-563,839.2)	< 0.001
Length of stay (days)	506	28.8 (24.4–33.1)	487	14.6 (11.5–17.6)	< 0.001

[a]The *p*-values for the categorical variables were calculated using the Rao-Scott chi-square test of the complex sample procedure
[b]Specifically procedures on vessels other than head and neck
[c]Temporary and permanent
[d]The *p*-values for the continuous variables were calculated using the general linear model of the complex sample procedure
[e]Total charges are for accumulated ED and Inpatient services

devices used in cardiogenic shock. Other devices include intra-aortic balloon pumps (IABP) and LV assist devices (LVADs). ECMO however, is the only intervention that compensates for both the right and left heart function as well as lung function. As such, ECMO decreases requirements for catecholamine, vasodilator, and mechanical ventilation in the treatment of cardiogenic shock and reduces the complications that are usually associated with these treatment modalities [18, 29]. ECMO use therefore holds promise for use in selected cardiogenic shock patients and further prospective studies are recommended.

The limitations of this study are directly related to structural features of the NEDS database. First, ICD-9 CM codes do not differentiate between VA or VV ECMO. This may be resolved with future use of ICD-10 CM codes. Second, information on the duration of ECMO use or timing of initiation is not available and costs are allocated to the whole hospital admission and not to a specific resource. Other limitations are related to the retrospective nature of the study. The quality and quantity of the data depends on the knowledge and experience of the coder, the completeness and accuracy of the patient record, and the state requirements. The study findings portray however trends in ECMO use for cardiogenic shock from a large sample from US based hospitals and can be generalized to other hospitals from similar settings.

Conclusion

Mortality in adult patients with cardiogenic shock remains high despite ECMO use. Season of admission (other than Fall) and presence of specific comorbidities (Respiratory and genitourinary diseases) are associated with increased mortality in this population. Familiarity with patients' characteristics and variables associated with mortality after ECMO use is important to improve outcomes further in cardiogenic

Table 5 Mortality with ECMO use in Cardiogenic Shock[a]

	Odds Ratio	95% CI	*p*-value
CCI[b] - Nervous system and sense organs diseases	1.22	0.64–2.32	0.541
CCI - Respiratory system diseases	3.83	1.76–8.31	0.001
CCI - Digestive system diseases	1.72	0.82–3.61	0.150
CCI - Genitourinary system diseases	4.97	2.39–10.33	< 0.001
CCI - Injury and poisoning	0.47	0.24–0.94	0.032
Injury diagnosis reported	0.45	0.15–1.36	0.156
Tracheostomy; temporary and permanent	0.46	0.14–1.48	0.190
Other operating room procedures[c]	0.49	0.24–1.00	0.048
Echocardiogram	4.63	1.30–16.50	0.018
Season of admission (Autumn)			
Winter	8.85	3.39–23.11	< 0.001
Spring	5.44	2.16–13.73	< 0.001
Summer	4.02	1.54–10.46	0.005
Age (1 year)	1.01	1.00–1.04	0.239
Length of Stay (1 day)	0.94	0.90–0.98	0.003
Total charges[d] (per $10,000)	1.01	1.00–1.02	0.069

[a]Variables included in the model are: significant chronic conditions and procedures found at the bivariate level, injury diagnosis, season of admission, age, and total charges
[b]CCI denotes body system categories affected by chronic conditions
[c]Specifically procedures on vessels other than head and neck
[d]Total charges are for accumulated ED and Inpatient services

shock. With rising costs and resources utilization, future research should focus on the impact of ECMO use on survival and on outcomes of patients with critical illnesses including but not limited to cardiogenic shock.

Abbreviations

AHRQ: Agency for Healthcare Research and Quality; CCS: Clinical Classifications Software; CI: confidence intervals; CPR: Cardiopulmonary Resuscitation; ECLS: extracorporeal life support; ECMO: Extracorporeal membrane oxygenation; ED: emergency department; ELSORIR: Extracorporeal Life Support Organization Registry International Report; HCUP: Healthcare Cost and Utilization Project; IABP: include intra-aortic balloon pumps; ICD: International Classification of Diseases; IRB: Institutional Review Board; LOS: length of stay; LVADs: LV assist devices; NEDS: Nationwide Emergency Department Sample; VA: veno-arterial; VV: veno-venous

Funding

There are no sources of funding for the research reported.

Authors' contributions

ME provided substantial involvement in the conception, design, and execution of the manuscript as well as reviewing and revising the manuscript for its credible content. RE provided substantial involvement in the design, and execution of the manuscript as well as drafting and revising the manuscript. RB provided substantial involvement in design and reviewing the manuscript as well as analysis of data. All authors read and approved the final manuscript.

Competing interests

The authors declare that they have no competing interests.

References

1. Massetti M, Tasle M, Le Page O, Deredec R, Babatasi G, Buklas D, Thuaudet S, Charbonneau P, Hamon M, Grollier G, et al. Back from irreversibility: extracorporeal life support for prolonged cardiac arrest. Ann Thorac Surg. 2005;79(1):178–83. discussion 183-174
2. Kelly RB, Porter PA, Meier AH, Myers JL, Thomas NJ. Duration of cardiopulmonary resuscitation before extracorporeal rescue: how long is not long enough? ASAIO J (Am Soc for Artif Inter Organs : 1992). 2005;51(5): 665–7.
3. Shin TG, Choi JH, Jo IJ, Sim MS, Song HG, Jeong YK, Song YB, Hahn JY, Choi SH, Gwon HC, et al. Extracorporeal cardiopulmonary resuscitation in patients with inhospital cardiac arrest: a comparison with conventional cardiopulmonary resuscitation. Crit Care Med. 2011;39(1):1–7.
4. Thiagarajan RR, Barbaro RP, Rycus PT, McMullan DM, Conrad SA, Fortenberry JD, Paden ML. Extracorporeal life support organization registry international report 2016. ASAIO J (Am Soc for Artif Inter Organs : 1992). 2017;63(1):60–7.
5. Younger JG, Schreiner RJ, Swaniker F, Hirschl RB, Chapman RA, Bartlett RH. Extracorporeal resuscitation of cardiac arrest. Acad Emerg Med Off J Soc Acad Emerg Med. 1999;6(7):700–7.
6. Combes A, Leprince P, Luyt CE, Bonnet N, Trouillet JL, Leger P, Pavie A, Chastre J. Outcomes and long-term quality-of-life of patients supported by extracorporeal membrane oxygenation for refractory cardiogenic shock. Crit Care Med. 2008;36(5):1404–11.
7. Smedira NG, Blackstone EH. Postcardiotomy mechanical support: risk factors and outcomes. Ann Thorac Surg. 2001;71(3 Suppl):S60–6. discussion S82–65
8. Bednarczyk JM, White CW, Ducas RA, Golian M, Nepomuceno R, Hiebert B, Bueddefeld D, Manji RA, Singal RK, Hussain F, et al. Resuscitative extracorporeal membrane oxygenation for in hospital cardiac arrest: a Canadian observational experience. Resuscitation. 2014;85(12):1713–9.
9. Pagani FD, Aaronson KD, Swaniker F, Bartlett RH. The use of extracorporeal life support in adult patients with primary cardiac failure as a bridge to implantable left ventricular assist device. Ann Thorac Surg. 2001;71(3 Suppl): S77–81. discussion S82–75
10. Kagawa E, Dote K, Kato M, Sasaki S, Nakano Y, Kajikawa M, Higashi A, Itakura K, Sera A, Inoue I, et al. Should we emergently revascularize occluded coronaries for cardiac arrest?: rapid-response extracorporeal membrane

oxygenation and intra-arrest percutaneous coronary intervention. Circulation. 2012;126(13):1605–13.

11. Squiers JJ, Lima B, DiMaio JM. Contemporary extracorporeal membrane oxygenation therapy in adults: fundamental principles and systematic review of the evidence. J Thorac Cardiovasc Surg. 2016;152(1):20–32.
12. Maxwell BG, Powers AJ, Sheikh AY, Lee PHU, Lobato RL, Wong JK. Resource use trends in extracorporeal membrane oxygenation in adults: an analysis of the Nationwide inpatient sample 1998-2009. J Thorac Cardiovasc Surg. 2014;148(2):416–21. e411
13. Lazzeri C, Bernardo P, Sori A, Innocenti L, Stefano P, Peris A, Gensini GF, Valente S. Venous-arterial extracorporeal membrane oxygenation for refractory cardiac arrest: a clinical challenge. Europ Heart J Acute Cardiovasc Care. 2013;2(2):118–26.
14. Cheng R, Hachamovitch R, Kittleson M, Patel J, Arabia F, Moriguchi J, Esmailian F, Azarbal B. Complications of extracorporeal membrane oxygenation for treatment of cardiogenic shock and cardiac arrest: a meta-analysis of 1,866 adult patients. Ann Thorac Surg. 2014;97(2):610–6.
15. Reyentovich A, Barghash MH, Hochman JS. Management of refractory cardiogenic shock. Nat Rev Cardiol. 2016;13(8):481–92.
16. Sheu J. Early extracorporeal membrane oxygenator-assisted primary percutaneous coronary intervention improved 30-day clinical outcomes in patients with ST-segment elevation myocardial infarction complicated with profound cardiogenic shock. Crit Care Med. 2010;38(9):1810–7.
17. Chen YS, Lin JW, Yu HY, Ko WJ, Jerng JS, Chang WT, Chen WJ, Huang SC, Chi NH, Wang CH, et al. Cardiopulmonary resuscitation with assisted extracorporeal life-support versus conventional cardiopulmonary resuscitation in adults with in-hospital cardiac arrest: an observational study and propensity analysis. Lancet. 2008;372(9638):554–61.
18. Napp LC, Kühn C, Bauersachs J. ECMO in cardiac arrest and cardiogenic shock. Herz. 2017;42(1):27–44.
19. HCUP Nationwide Emergency Department Sample (NEDS). In.: Healthcare Cost and Utilization Project (HCUP); 2013.
20. Barrett M, Lopez-Gonzalez L, Coffey R, Levit K. Population Denominator Data for Use with the HCUP Databases (Updated with 2013 Population Data). 2014. HCUP Methods Series Report # 2014-02 ONLINE. August 18, 2014. U.S. Agency for Healthcare Research and Quality. Available: http://www.hcup-us.ahrq.gov/reports/methods/methods.jsp. Accessed 10 Oct 2017.
21. Sasser SM, Hunt RC, Faul M, Sugerman D, Pearson WS, Dulski T, Wald MM, Jurkovich GJ, Newgard CD, Lerner EB. Guidelines for field triage of injured patients: recommendations of the National Expert Panel on field triage, 2011. MMWR Recommendations and reports. Morb Mortal Wkly Rep Recomm Rep / Ctr Dis Control. 2012;61(Rr-1):1–20.
22. Palmer C. Major trauma and the injury severity score - where should we set the bar? Ann Proc / Assoc for the Adv of Automotive Med. 2007;51:13–29.
23. HCUPnet [https://hcupnet.ahrq.gov/#setup].
24. Schmidt M, Burrell A, Roberts L, Bailey M, Sheldrake J, Rycus PT, Hodgson C, Scheinkestel C, Cooper DJ, Thiagarajan RR, et al. Predicting survival after ECMO for refractory cardiogenic shock: the survival after veno-arterial-ECMO (SAVE)-score. Eur Heart J. 2015;36(33):2246–56.
25. Spencer FA, Goldberg RJ, Becker RC, Gore JM. Seasonal distribution of acute myocardial infarction in the second National Registry of myocardial infarction. J Am Coll Cardiol. 1998;31(6):1226–33.
26. Stewart S, Keates AK, Redfern A, McMurray JJ. Seasonal variations in cardiovascular disease. Nat Rev Cardiol. 2017;14(11):654.
27. Turin TC, Kita Y, Rumana N, Nakamura Y, Takashima N, Miura K, Ueshima H. Increased risk of acute myocardial infarction during colder periods is independent of the conventional cardiovascular risk factors: Takashima AMI Registry, Japan. CVD Prev Cont. 2011;**6**(3):109–11.
28. Kolte D, Khera S, Aronow WS, Mujib M, Palaniswamy C, Sule S, Jain D, Gotsis W, Ahmed A, Frishman WH, et al. Trends in incidence, management, and outcomes of cardiogenic shock complicating ST-elevation myocardial infarction in the United States. J Am Heart Assoc. 2014;3(1):e000590.
29. Shock C. Current concepts and improving outcomes. Hochman. Harmony R Reynolds and Judith S sl. Circulation. 2008;117(**5**):686–97.

Prior CT imaging history for patients who undergo whole-body CT for acute traumatic injury and are discharged home from the emergency department

Mary Matthews[1], Peter Richman[1*], Scott Krall[1], Kimberly Leeson[1], K Tom Xu[2], Albert L Gest[1] and Osbert Blow[3]

Abstract

Background: Recurrent CT imaging is believed to significantly increase lifetime malignancy risk. We previously reported that high acuity, admitted trauma patients who received a whole-body CT in the emergency department (ED) had a history of prior CT imaging in 14% of cases. The primary objective of this study was to determine the CT imaging history for trauma patients who received a whole-body CT but were ultimately deemed safe for discharge directly home from the ED.

Methods: This was a retrospective cohort study conducted at an academic ED. All trauma patients who were discharged directly home from the ED after whole-body CT were analyzed. The decision to utilize whole-body CT was at the discretion of the caring physician during the study period. Clinical data for the most recent trauma visit was recorded in a structured fashion on a standardized data collection instrument utilizing the hospital system electronic medical record (EMR). Subsequently, study investigators reviewed a shared, electronic radiological archive for the 6-hospital system to evaluate prior CT exposure for each patient.

Results: 165 patients were in the study group. The mean age of the study group was 39+/− 16 years old, 40% were female and 64% were Hispanic. The most common mechanism of injury in our study group was motor vehicle crash (MVC) (66%). In our study group, 25% had at least one prior CT. The most common prior studies performed were: CT abdomen/pelvis (13%), CT head (9.1%), CT face (6.7%), and CT chest (1.8%). Within a multivariate logistic regression model we found that the large majority of patient characteristics and mechanisms of injury were not associated with a positive prior CT imaging history.

Conclusion: We found a positive history for prior CT for 25% of trauma patients who received whole-body CT scan but were discharged from the ED to home.

Keywords: Acute traumatic injury, Discharge from ED, CT scans

Background

CT imaging has the capacity to detect a variety of different pathologies encountered in the emergency department (ED). Rosen described that CT is beneficial to the emergency medicine physician by increasing the certainty of diagnosis within a short period of time and significantly decreasing the need for surgical exploration [1]. In light of these benefits, CT use in the ED increased from 2 million studies (1980) to 72 million (2007) [2]. More recently, Levin reported that CT use in the ED tripled from 2002 to 2012, rising from 57.2 scans to 147.9 scans per 1,000 patient encounters [3].

One area, in particular, for which there has been significant expansion in CT utilization is the evaluation of trauma patients. From 1998 to 2007 there was a national 3-fold increase in the use of CT scans in the ED for injury-related conditions [4]. Such an increase is undoubtedly due to the potential for such imaging to

* Correspondence: PRichmanMDMBA@gmail.com
[1]Department of Emergency Medicine, CHRISTUS HEALTH/Texas A&M Residency in Emergency Medicine, Corpus Christi, TX 78404, USA
Full list of author information is available at the end of the article

reduce the risk of missed injury. CT scanning has been shown to increase diagnostic accuracy for blunt trauma patients compared to conventional radiological imaging. Several investigators have reported that whole-body (brain, c-spine, trunk) CT frequently identifies unexpected findings and can lead to a change of treatment as high as 33% of patients [5–7].

When considering the increased use of CT imaging, clinicians must weigh the risks inherent to this modality. A single whole-body CT provides significantly more radiation exposure than a conventional x-ray, and at a dose in excess of which is felt to be safe within a one-year period, by the International Symposium on the System of Radiological Protection. (20 mSv) [8]. Reviews of published analyses suggest whole-body CTs could directly result in cancers as often as 1 in 380 and cause 12.5 additional cancer deaths in 10,000 patients [9]. Furthermore, CT scans in children will result in significantly increased lifetime radiation risk over adult CT, both because of the increased dose per milliampere-second, and the increased lifetime risk per unit dose [10]. With increased CT use, it is prudent to assess whether patients understand the risks associated with this modality. Investigators recently reported that patients were more confident when CT imaging was part of their medical evaluation, but, unfortunately, they had a poor understanding of the concomitant radiation exposure/risk and underestimated their previous imaging experience [11].

A recent study published at our center in 2015 revealed that 14% of trauma patients that received whole-body CT and were admitted to the hospital had prior CT imaging before their traumatic injury [12]. This study was limited in that it focused on a patient population that represents the subset of trauma patients with more significant injuries such that whole-body CT was likely unavoidable. On the other hand, there is a segment of trauma patients with significant mechanisms for which there may be some risk of injury but clinical suspicion may be more moderate or even low. These patients represent an opportunity for shared decision-making where clinicians may discuss the balance between clinical concerns for serious injury vs. the risk of imaging. We believe physicians will find it helpful in that context to understand the prior imaging exposure for this cohort of trauma patients. For that purpose, we conducted a retrospective cohort study to examine the imaging history for trauma patients who underwent a whole-body CT but were ultimately considered safe from discharge from the ED.

Methods

Study design

This was a multicenter, retrospective cohort study to assess the prior imaging history for patients with significant trauma mechanisms and clinical suspicion for important traumatic injuries that were ultimately deemed to be safe for discharge from the ED to home following whole-body CT. Data from all trauma patients who were discharged directly home from the ED after whole-body CT from 3/25/2016 to 10/25/2016 were analyzed.

Setting

The study was conducted at Christus Spohn Memorial Hospital (site of patient enrollment) and electronic records were reviewed from Memorial Hospital along with five other Christus Spohn hospital sites. Christus Spohn Memorial is a major teaching affiliate of Texas A&M College of Medicine, a level-two trauma center, and serves an inner city population. The annual ED census is 45,000 patients. The six affiliated hospitals comprise 192,073 annual ED visits, which, based on administrative data available locally, constitutes approximately 70% of all ED visits within our twelve-county region of southern Texas. The study was approved by the Spohn Institutional Review Board prior to initiation of data collection.

Population

The study included all adult ED patients, age > 17 years, from 3/25/16–10/25/16 for whom there was clinical suspicion for important traumatic injuries but were ultimately deemed by the emergency physician to be safe for discharge home following whole-body CT (i.e. patients discharged home from the ED). Patients were excluded if they were pregnant, prisoners, admitted to the hospital from the ED, or had less than a full whole-body CT to evaluate their traumatic injuries. Inclusive electronic radiological logs were reviewed on a weekly basis by study authors to include any patients that were not identified at point of care.

Study protocol

Evaluation of trauma patients and the decision to utilize whole-body CT was at the discretion of the caring physician during the study period. Clinical data for the current visit were recorded in a structured fashion on a standardized data collection instrument utilizing data from the hospital system EMR with all study data points determined a priori. In a similar structured fashion, study investigators reviewed a shared, electronic radiological archive for the 6-hospital system to evaluate prior CT exposure for each patient.

Statistical analysis

Data were entered into Excel 2013 for Windows (Microsoft Corporation, Redmund, WA), and, then, transported into STATA 11 software (StataCorp LLC, College Station, TX) for statistical analysis. Continuous data are presented as means +/− standard deviations and were analyzed by t-tests. Categorical data are presented as frequency of occurrence and were analyzed by chi-square. We calculated odds ratios with 95% CIs.

Our primary outcome parameter was the percentage of patients who were discharged from the hospital from the ED following whole-body CT and determined to have had a prior history of CT(s) before their traumatic event. Prior CT was defined as CT imaging of any protocol/body area identified on a dedicated page within our system-wide EMR. Data was available for review from this system from 2009 to the present time.

As bivariate analyses often mask confounding of other independent variables, we utilized multivariate logistic regression to delineate the effect of each independent variable. The dependent variable was whether patients had any CT(s) performed previously, The independent variables were sex, age, race/ethnicity and mechanism of injury. In view of our methodology for data collection that involved chart review, we were limited to analyzing patient characteristic variables available in the EMR. Physician and examination characteristics were not included within the model.

Results

Over the seven-month period, 165 patients were discharged home from the ED after receiving whole-body CT scan. The mean age of the study group was 39 (SD +/− 16) years old, 40% were female (66/165), and 64% (106/165) were Hispanic. The most common mechanism of injury in our study group was MVC (66%; 109/165). Other mechanisms included fall (6.7%; 11/165), stab head (11%; 18/165), and other (16%; 27/165).

Within the study group, one-fourth (25%; 41/165, 95% CI = 19–32%) had at least one prior CT. The prior studies performed in order of frequency were: CT abdomen/pelvis 13% (21/165), CT head 9.1% (15/165), CT face 6.7% (11/165), CT cervical spine 5.5% (9/165), CT limb 4.2% (7/165), CT thoracic spine 3%(5/165), CT lumbar spine 3%(5/165), CT neck 1.8% (3/165), and CT chest 1.8% (3/165).

With respect to aggregate exposure to chest and/or abdominal CT, studies with typically higher doses of radiation, we found 11 patients (6.7%) had at least one previous study prior to enrollment in our study, five (3%) had two previous studies, and one patient (0.6%) has 13 previous CT studies.

A multivariate model which included patient characteristics and mechanism injury found that age 41–64 years (p = .025, OR = 2.6; 95% CI 1.12–6.14) and "other" trauma mechanisms (non-fall, non-stab wound to head, non-MVC; ($p < 0.001$; OR 7.40; 95% CI 2.6–21) were associated with positive prior CT history We did not find that other patient characteristics were associated with a prior CT history, including age > 64 years ($p = 0.098$; OR; 95% CI 0.78–20) female gender ($p = 0.84$; OR 0.92; 95% CI 0.39–2.1), Hispanic race ($p = 0.82$; OR 0.90; 95% CI 0.37–2.2), non-white/non--Hispanic race ($p = 0.73$; OR 0.73; 95% CI 0.14–3.78), fall mechanism ($p = 0.86$; OR 1.2; 95% CI 0.22–6.1), and stab wound head ($p = 0.068$; OR3.2; 0.92–11).

A similar multivariate model found that age 41–64 years (p = .03, OR = 1.0; 95% CI 1.0–1.1) was associated with positive prior CT abdomen and/or chest history. We did not find that other patient characteristics were associated with such an imaging history, including age > 64 years ($p = 0.054$; OR 6.1; 95% CI 0.96–39), female gender ($p = 0.88$; OR 0.92; 95% CI 0.32–2.6), Hispanic race ($p = 0.39$; OR 1.7; 95% CI 0.50–6), non-white/non-Hispanic race ($p = 0.38$; OR 2.4; 95% CI 0.33–18), stab wound head ($p = 0.15$; OR 2.8; 95% CI 0.43–6.5), and other non-MVC, no stab wound head mechanisms ($p = 0.46$;; OR 1.7; 95% CI 0.43–6.5).

Discussion

We found that 25% of patients within our cohort who received a whole-body CT but then were deemed low risk for discharge had a prior history of CT imaging. Of note, 6% of the study group had more than one prior CT in our health system. We believe our results provide a context for clinicians to understand the risk of prior imaging beyond their reliance on patient recall and single hospital records. As much as physicians might desire a complete imaging history, for a variety of reasons the available information may be limited. Many patients have had CTs in unrelated hospitals and private imaging centers. Furthermore, the accuracy of patient recall is poorly understood to date. While we cannot account for imaging performed in private centers and in distant locations, our 6-hospital system provides a significant proportion of the care for patients within a 12-county area, thus, providing a better window to evaluate previous exposure for our patients compared with most centers.

Our study fits within the context of the growing body of literature on CT utilization in the setting of trauma and efforts to limit radiation exposure to those most likely to have medically important injuries. In recent years, a significant proportion of patients who come to the ED after a high-energy traumatic event undergo whole-body CT Scan for evaluation of suspected injuries [11]. In view of the associated radiation risks, investigators have worked to identify patient characteristics that reduce the likelihood that CT will identify unexpected injuries [13–15]. Linder et al. conducted a two-center retrospective cohort study of 523 alert trauma patients for which 139 were classified as low risk [15]. The authors did not identify any significant injuries in this segment of the study group.

Similarly, Gupta et al. conducted a prospective, observational study of 600 patients with blunt trauma who underwent whole-body CT and 101 who underwent limited scanning respectively after evaluation by the senior most emergency physician and the treating trauma surgeon [13]. The authors note that one or both of these physicians was willing to omit 35% of the individual scans performed and a critical action only occurred for 3 of these patients. The results of this study provide a framework upon which clinicians may discuss their clinical impression versus the risk of missed injury with a patient for the purposes of shared decision-making. Moreover, addressing the need for CT imaging (or lack thereof) with the trauma team may reduce CT ordering since the consulting physicians have been shown to be the driving factor for CTs deemed unnecessary by emergency physicians [16].

At the same time, in order to adequately assess the delicate balance between imaging exposure vs. risk of injury for patients, physicians need to have as complete as possible picture of a patient's prior imaging history. Griffey et al. surveyed 155 emergency physicians to characterize their attitudes and practices with respect to CT utilization [17]. The investigators reported that 87% of the physician respondents indicated that they would utilize information regarding prior imaging history as a component of their discussions with patients regarding imaging options. We believe our report provides clinicians with some context of the prior imaging exposure for a cohort that represents the subset of trauma patients most likely to benefit from such shared decision making discussions.

Limitations and future directions

Our study has several limitations that warrant discussion. Undoubtedly, our results underestimate the actual number of patients who had prior imaging and those who had more than one prior CT. We were able to review previous imaging records only within our hospital system, from 2009 to present, so CTs performed before that time would not be included. Further, we cannot account for scans performed in non-system facilities.

In addition, the retrospective design of our study allows for the possibility that bias may have been introduced both with respect to patients included, how they were managed, and their ultimate disposition. We do believe it is likely that all eligible patients were captured by our methods as we reviewed an inclusive electronic radiological database for all whole-body CTs ordered during the study period. Patients were only eligible for inclusion if at the discretion of their treating emergency physician a whole body CT was ordered and, ultimately, the patient was deemed safe for discharge directly from the ED. We are anecdotally not aware of physicians within our department specifically using standardized algorithms for selective CT in the setting of trauma. However, practice patterns for imaging as well as disposition surely vary between practitioners and, thus, this likely introduced some heterogeneity in the study group compared with the structure that a prospective protocol for imaging would alternatively provide.

Another limitation to our retrospective design is the possibility of bias and/or error in the data abstraction from the EMR and radiological databases. We did not perform an assessment of interobserver agreement for a sample of charts to assess the reliability of the chart review method. However, in view of the fact that the majority of data collected for the purpose of this study were objective (e.g. presence and type of prior CTs in the hospital system are provided in a vertical list by dates), we are confident that errors in the structured abstraction were likely minimal.

The characteristics of our study group may also raise concerns for external validity. Our local population is largely indigent and predominately Hispanic. It is unclear if patients from different socioeconomic and ethnic groups would be more or less at risk to have had prior imaging. Another source of potential concern for the generalizability of our results is with respect to our definition of low risk patients. We defined low risk patients as those discharged after ED evaluation. Future studies could improve upon our methods by utilizing low risk criteria identified previously [13].

Conclusions

We found a positive history for prior CT for 25% of trauma patients who received whole-body CT scan but were discharged from the ED to home. Our results should encourage clinicians to evaluate prior CT imaging history and consider shared decision making/use of selective CT algorithms in case for which pretest assessment for risk of serious injury is relatively low.

Abbreviations

CT: Cat Scan; ED: Emergency Department; EMR: Electronic Medical Record

Acknowledgements

This study was performed at CHRISTUS Spohn Memorial Hospital. We wish to thank the Office of Research & Academics, CHRISTUS Health for their administrative support throughout the project.

Authors' contributions

MM—Was the primary investigator and contributed in all facets of the study including study conception/design, data collection, data analysis, and was the lead author for all drafts of the manuscript. SK—contributed to study conception/design, data analysis, and edited all drafts of the manuscript KL-- contributed to study conception/design, data analysis, and edited all drafts of the manuscript KTX-- contributed to study conception/design, was the primary data analyst, and edited all drafts of the manuscript. AG-- contributed to study conception/design, data analysis, and edited all drafts of the manuscript. PR— contributed to study conception/design, data analysis, and manuscript writing and editing of all drafts/revisions. OB – contributed to study conception/design, data analysis, and edited several drafts of the manuscript. All authors read and approved the final manuscript.

Competing interests
The authors declare that they have no competing interests.

Author details
[1]Department of Emergency Medicine, CHRISTUS HEALTH/Texas A&M Residency in Emergency Medicine, Corpus Christi, TX 78404, USA. [2]Department of Emergency Medicine Texas Tech College of Medicine, Lubbock, TX, USA. [3]Department of Acute Care Surgery, Trauma & Surgical Critical Care, CHRISTUS Spohn Hospital, Corpus Christi, TX, USA.

References
1. Rosen MP, Sands DZ, Longmaid HE 3rd, Reynolds KF, Wagner M. Raptopoulos. Impact of abdominal CT on the management of patients presenting to the emergency department with acute abdominal pain. AJR Am J Roentgenol. 2000;174:1391–6.
2. Brenner DJ, Hall EJ. Computed tomography--an increasing source of radiation exposure. NEJM. 2007;357:2277–84.
3. Levin D, Rao V, Parker L, Frangos M. Continued growth in emergency department imaging is bucking the overall trends, 2002-2012. J Am Coll Radiol. 2014;11:1044–7.
4. Korley F, Pham J, Kirsch T. Use of advanced radiology during visits to US emergency departments for injury-related conditions, 1998-2007. JAMA. 2010;304(13):1465–71.
5. Self ML, Blake AM. The benefit of routine thoracic, abdominal, and pelvic computed tomography to evaluate trauma patients with closed head injuries. Am J Surg. 2003;186(6):609–13.
6. Deunk J, Dekker HM, Brink M, van Vugt R, Edwards MJ, van Vugt AB. The value of indicated computed tomography scan of the chest and abdomen in addition to the conventional radiologic work-up for blunt trauma patients. J Trauma. 2007;63(4):757–63.
7. Deunk J, Brink M, Dekker HM, Kool DR, van Kuijk C, Blickman JG, van Vugt AB, Edwards MJ. Routine versus selective computed tomography of the abdomen, pelvis, and lumbar spine in blunt trauma: a prospective evaluation. J Trauma. 2009;66(4):1108–17.
8. ICRP. The 2007 Recommendations of the international commission on radiological protection. ICRP publication 103. Ann ICRP. 2007;37(2–4).
9. Tien HC, Tremblay LN, Rizoli SB. Radiation exposure from diagnostic imaging in severely injured trauma patients. J Trauma. 2007;62(1):151–6.
10. Brenner D, Elliston C. Estimated risks of radiation-induced fatal cancer from pediatric CT. AJR Am J Roentgenol. 2001;176(2):289–96.
11. Repplinger MD, Li AJ, Svenson JE, Ehlenbach WJ, Westergaard RP, Reeder SB, Jacobs EA. Emergency department Patients' perceptions of radiation from medical imaging. WMJ. 2016;115(1):22–8.
12. Kenter J, Blow O, Krall SP, Gest A, Smith C, Richman PB. Prior CT imaging history for patients who undergo PAN CT for acute traumatic injury. PeerJ. 2015;3:e963. https://doi.org/10.7717/peerj.963
13. Gupta M, Schriger DL. Selective use of computed tomography compared with routine whole body imaging in patients with blunt trauma. Ann Emerg Med. 2011;58(5):407–16.
14. Linder F, Mani K, Juhlin C, Eklof H. Routine whole body CT of high energy trauma patients leads to excessive radiation exposure. Scand J Trauma Resusc Emerg Med. 2016;24:7.
15. Davies RM, Scrimshire AB, Sweetman L, Anderton MJ, Holt EM. A decision tool for whole-body CT in major trauma that safely reduces unnecessary scanning and associated radiation risks: an initial exploratory analysis. Injury. 2016;47(1):43–9.
16. Broder JS, Bhat R, Boyd JP, Ogloblin IA, Limkakeng A, Hocker MB, Drake WG, Miller T, Harringa JB, Repplinger MD. Who explicitly requests the ordering of computed tomography for emergency department patients? A multicenter prospective study. Emerg Radiol. 2016;23(3):221–7.
17. Griffey RT, Jeffe DB, Bailey T. Emergency physicians' attitudes and preferences regarding computed tomography, radiation exposure, and imaging decision support. Acad Emerg Med. 2014;21(7):768–77.

19

Burnout and safety outcomes - a cross-sectional nationwide survey of EMS-workers in Germany

Natalie Baier[1*], Karsten Roth[1,2], Susanne Felgner[1] and Cornelia Henschke[1]

Abstract

Background: The association between burnout and patient safety has been analyzed in many studies for nurses, physicians, and residents. However, studies concerning prehospital emergency medical services (EMS) workers are limited, although they are particularly under risk for emotional stress. This study aims to descriptively analyze the overall degree of burnout among EMS-workers, and potential adverse events that might harm patients as well as the relationship between burnout and perceived safety outcomes for EMS-workers in Germany.

Methods: EMS-workers were recruited via German EMS-journals, social media and a professional association to participate in an online survey. The questionnaire includes the 'Maslach Burnout Inventory' (MBI), the 'Emergency Medical Services Safety Inventory' (EMS-SI), and items about job satisfaction and the individual person. Data was descriptively analyzed by calculating frequencies, means, percentages and Pearson correlation coefficients. The association between burnout and patient safety was analyzed using linear and logistic regression models.

Results: A total of $n = 1101$ questionnaires were considered for data analysis. The vast majority of participants were male, younger than 40 years old, and full-time employees with an EMS-experience of 12 years on average. Between 19.9 and 40% of the participants showed a high degree of burnout in one of the burnout dimensions. Safety compromising behavior was the outcome measure with the highest percentage of participants reporting a negative outcome measure. The dimensions emotional exhaustion and depersonalization were positively associated with the safety outcomes injury and safety compromising behavior. Additionally, experiences, job satisfaction and the intention to leave the current job were significantly associated with the outcome measures.

Conclusion: This is the first study that examines the association between the degree of burnout and patient safety for EMS-workers. The results suggest that an expansion of psychological support for EMS-workers should be considered. Further research should concentrate on the complex relations between working conditions, burnout and patient safety.

Keywords: EMS, Prehospital, Burnout, Safety outcomes

Background

Psychological burden of health care professionals is an intensively discussed topic, especially in the context of potential negative consequences for patients. It is in the nature of these professions that they have a high risk for psychological diseases as they are exposed to situations with high emotional stress levels. Persistent emotional stress might lead to the burnout syndrome [1], first mentioned by Herbert Freudenberger for helping professions which sacrifice themselves for others resulting in a burnout [2, 3]. Maslach and Jackson [1] conceptualized the burnout syndrome by three dimensions: emotional exhaustion, depersonalization and personal accomplishment [1] which are the basis of the Maslach Burnout Inventory, the most commonly used self-assessment instrument to evaluate the degree of burnout [4]. Based on this conceptualization, there are different results for the prevalence of burnout with regard to the considered medical profession. Prevalence for emotional exhaustion ranges from 27% (nurses [5]) and 47% (physicians from

* Correspondence: natalie.baier@tu-berlin.de
[1]Institute of Health Care Management, Berlin Centre of Health Economics Research (BerlinHECOR), Technische Universität Berlin, Straße des 17. Juni 135 (H80), 10623 Berlin, Germany
Full list of author information is available at the end of the article

all specialty disciplines [6]) to 57% (residents [7]) of the study participants and for depersonalization from 10% (nurses [5]) and 35% (physicians from all specialty disciplines [6, 8]) to 50% (residents [7]) of the study participants.

Following Leiter [9], employees that experience burnout (emotional exhaustion) a more likely to move away from people associated with their jobs including the patients. Based on an imbalance between investment of work resources and return of investment, employees or health care providers will be more reserved regarding future investments and may develop negative attitudes towards their patients [10]. This conservation of resources can have a negative impact on the patient safety. The association between burnout and patient safety has been examined in many studies focusing on physicians and nurses [11–13]. A systematic review by Hall et al. [11] found a significant association between burnout and patient safety for 24 studies ($n = 30$). However, EMS-workers (providing care out-of-hospital) are only examined in a few studies although they are particularly under risk for emotional stress as they often provide care in public environments with a high potential of traumatizing effects. National and international studies of EMS-workers focused on the correlation between burnout and organizational working conditions [14], coping strategies [15], job related stress factors [16, 17] and/or the exposure to critical incidents as a child victim or particularly severe injuries [18]. Only one study by Hammer et al. [19] focused on patient safety measured by judgement errors in patient care and its association with wellbeing measures as job satisfaction and somatic distress for paramedics in the US.

However, the relation between burnout and patient safety has not been analyzed for EMS-workers so far. Although, research on this association is imperative in light of workforce shortages e.g. due to high rates of sick leave and an increasing number of cases that cause growing concerns regarding the prehospital emergency care in Germany and other developed countries [20–22]. This study aims to fill this research gap by (1) evaluating the frequency of self-perceived negative safety outcomes and the prevalence of burnout among EMS-workers and (2) analyzing the association between the degree of burnout and patient safety for EMS-workers in Germany.

Method

Recruitment of participants and data collection

EMS-workers were recruited via call for joining the survey at social media channels including specialized groups at Facebook and Twitter, German EMS-journals ('Rettungsdienst' and 'retten!'), and the professional association for non-medical EMS-workers ('Deutscher Berufsverband Rettungsdienst e.V.'). The main reason for this recruitment was to avoid employer-biased responses, which might have occurred when recruiting EMS-workers via their employers. Three reminders were used in social media after one, two, and four months. EMS-workers in this study are defined as trained professionals in prehospital emergency medical care according to their level of qualification excluding emergency physicians. Their tasks cover medical care on-site and in ambulances as well as the transport of patients to hospitals.

With the aim of testing the comprehensibility of the instructions and the appropriateness concerning the order of questions in the questionnaire, a pilot survey including 10 EMS-workers was conducted. As a result, some minor changes regarding the order of questions were implemented before starting the large-scale survey. Data collection was performed from June to December 2015 using the online survey tool SoSciSurvey, which records data according to the German privacy policy. The study makes use of a cross-sectional design by conducting a nationwide survey to EMS-workers.

Instrument

The final survey consists of the Maslach Burnout Inventory - Human Services Survey (MBI-HSS), the EMS-Safety Inventory (EMS-SI), accompanied by the EMS-Safety Attitudes Questionnaire (EMS-SAQ) as well as items of job satisfaction adapted from the nurse survey within the project Nurse forecasting in Europe (RN4Cast) [23], and items to collect individual data of the respondents, e.g. socioeconomic characteristics. Most items of the RN4Cast study (inclusion of questions regarding satisfaction) and all items of the EMS-SAQ are not considered in this study as they are not focused in this study or were collected for a planned comparative study with nurses. The MBI – HSS uses a total of 22 items grouped in three dimensions to examine the degree of burnout [24]. Each statement is rated according to the frequency of occurrence adapting a seven-point Likert scale [1]. The subscale emotional exhaustion (EE) assesses feelings according to an emotional overextension, the exhaustion in someone's work or the contact with other people. The subscale depersonalization (DP) measures the callousness and impersonal response towards people receiving service, care, treatment, or instruction. The subscale personal accomplishment (PA) assesses feelings of being competent and successful in working with people [1, 24]. Specific sum scores of the items per dimension indicate the degree of burnout, ranging from 'high' to 'low'. Based on the manual of Maslach et al. [24] respondents are assigned to a high degree of burnout with a sum score ≥ 27 in the subscale EE, ≥ 13 in DP and ≤ 31 in PA [24]. In line with current studies [6, 25, 26], high scores for emotional exhaustion and depersonalization were additionally considered.

The EMS-SI has been used for identifying and rating safety outcomes in EMS. This self-reporting instrument is seen as an alternative to incomplete and inaccurate data of electronic patient care reports [27, 28]. It includes 44 items within three safety outcome measures: 'provider injury', 'error or adverse events', and 'safety-compromising behaviors' as these issues bear the risk of harming providers and patients [29]. Two nominal, seven-option, categorical scales were used (A – 35 items, B – 19 items) for extracting answers which have to be referred to the previous three months of working [27].

The demographic section includes years of working in EMS, current EMS-area, highest apprenticeship, employment relationship and federal state of participants' workplace. In addition, the respondents were asked about their age when reaching the highest level of EMS-education, satisfaction with occupational choice (6-point Likert scale), and the operating ranges.

As the MBI was translated into German language by the study group of the project RN4CAST, no further adaption was necessary. The EMS-SAQ and EMS-SI used for the first time in the German context were translated using the back translation method [30]. The original and translated EMS-SAQ and EMS-SI as well as details regarding the items of each instrument, used scales and corresponding dimensions/categories are available in the Additional file 1.

Analysis of the data

Data screening process

The target population were EMS-workers actively working in their position at the time of the survey period. Before starting the survey, participants had to approve a data privacy statement including (1) details about the content and duration of the survey, (2) indications that participation may evoke negative experiences, and (3) information on the possibility to interrupt the survey at any time. The last point includes the possibility to withdraw participants' data. In this context, participants received an e-mail address assuring that their data can be deleted anytime. Therefore, they had to enter an eight-digit code. Missing approvals of the data privacy statement and the eight-digit code led to the exclusion of participants. For those participants who opened the survey link, the following criteria resulted in an exclusion of the questionnaires: (1) multiple records, and (2) questionnaires, where less than 50% of the items are completed. Implausible answers as typing errors for single questions ($n = 10$) were handled like missing data and substituted applying unconditional mean imputation [24].

Statistical analysis

The MBI, EMS-SI and the participants' characteristics were descriptively analyzed on the respondent-level using the manuals of the different instruments. Percentages and frequencies were calculated for the MBI and the EMS-SI. Frequencies, percentages, means, their corresponding standard deviations (SD) and min/max were examined for the participant characteristics. The Fisher exact test was used to compare the dimensions of the MBI between EMS workers who reported negative safety outcomes and EMS workers who did not report negative safety outcomes. Additionally, the association between the EMS-SI und the MBI was analyzed using the Pearson correlation coefficient. Linear and logistic regression models were used to evaluate the association between the dimension of burnout and the three safety outcomes. The dimension personal accomplishment was not included in the linear regression models as several studies have questioned the validity of this dimension [31, 32]. For the regression analysis all results with a p-value < 0.1 were considered significant, for the Pearson correlation coefficient and for the Fisher exact test all result with a p-value < 0.01. Analyses were performed using the statistical software package Stata 12.

Results

Participants' characteristics

Based on the data screening process described in the method section, 1101 questionnaires could be considered for the data analysis.

The majority of all participants were male (86.2%) and younger than 40 years old (73.2%). On average, the participants had an experience in EMS-work of 12 years. Experiences in their current EMS-area comprised 9 years. The questions regarding the level of the participants' EMS-qualification include the German terms of occupational profiles (See Additional file 2 for detailed description on EMS-qualification). The majority of the respondents (85.3%) had the qualification level of a paramedic and worked in a full-time position (89.6%). Half of the respondents (53.7%) were satisfied with their current job, 24% of the respondents with their wages and 33% with their professional status. No intention to leave their current job due to dissatisfaction was reported by 45% of the respondents. Nearly half of the respondents (46.2%) would recommend their current EMS area as a good place to work. Participants' demographic and occupational characteristics are outlined in Table 1.

Descriptive results regarding the degree of burnout and safety outcomes

Based on the cut-off point presented in the method section the answers of the participants regarding the three dimensions of the MBI were categorized in high degree and low degree of burnout. High degrees could be shown for 25.3% ($n = 290$) of the participants in EE, for 40.2% ($n = 443$) of the participants in DP and 19.9% ($n = 219$) in PA. A high degree for EE and DP could be shown for 18.5% ($n = 204$) of the study participants. Figure 1 shows, furthermore, that the percentage of participants with a high degree of EE and

Table 1 Characteristics of the study participants

Participants; $n = 1101$ (%) or (SD/min – max)	
Gender	
Male	949 (86.2)
Female	152 (13.8)
Age in years	
≤ 29	439 (39.9)
30–39	367 (33.3)
40–49	205 (18.6)
≥ 50	90 (8.2)
Experience in EMS in years	
Mean	12.34 (9.11/0.5–42)
Experience in current EMS-area in years	
Mean	9.01 (8.22/0–42)
Level of EMS-qualification*	
Paramedic 'Notfallsanitäter'	121 (11.0)
Paramedic 'Rettungsassistent'	818 (74.3)
EMT-I 'Rettungssanitäter'	115 (10.4)
EMT-B 'Rettungshelfer'	4 (0.4)
Other	43 (3.9)
Employment relationship	
Full-time	986 (89.6)
Part-time	94 (8.5)
Voluntary	21 (1.9)
Satisfaction	
Satisfaction in the current job	591 (53.7)
Satisfaction with wages	266 (24.2)
Satisfaction with the professional status	371 (33.7)
Intention to leave/Recommendation	
No intention to leave the current job within the next year as a result of job dissatisfaction	500 (45.4)
Recommendation of the current EMS-area as a good place to work	509 (46.2)

Caption: *B* basic, *EMS* emergency medical services, *EMT* emergency medical technician, *I* intermediate
* A more detailed description on EMS-qualification can be found in the Additional file 1: Appendix B

DP is greater for those who reported injuries or errors and adverse events. This is especially the case for the dimension DP where a high degree could be shown for 50% (reported injuries) and 44% (reported errors and adverse events) of the participants.

Comparisons were conducted for the domains injury and errors and adverse events. As nearly all respondents (99.4%) reported at least one factor of the domain safety comprising behavior a comparison between reported and not reported safety comprising behavior was impossible. Table 2 shows the frequency and the percentage (in brackets) of the negative safety outcomes as well as the greatest contributing factors for the domains error and adverse events and safety compromising behavior. Approximately one third of the participants (36.2%) reported that they experienced an injury in the last three months, 73.7% positively responded to one of the items measuring error or adverse events. Greatest contributing factors in the measure safety comprising behavior included speed limits and the check of the ambulance. For the measure error and adverse events factors are more diverse ranking from not printing and properly interpreting an EKG strip to not checking the glucose level in a patient with altered mental status.

Table 3 shows the Pearson correlation coefficients for the dimensions of the MBI and the domains of EMS-SI. All correlation coefficients are significant except the one between personal accomplishment and injury. Following Cohen [33] regarding the effect size of the Pearson correlation coefficient, a moderate and positive correlation can be shown between the measure safety comprising behavior and the dimensions EE and DP of the MBI.

Regression results

The results of the regression models for the three safety outcomes are summarized in Table 4. For the safety outcomes injury and error and adverse events a logistic regression was conducted, consequently the odds ratios are presented. For the safety outcome safety compromising behavior a linear regression was used as a differentiation between those who reported safety compromising behavior and those who did not was not possible. Therefore, the regression coefficients are displayed in Table 4. The association between burnout and safety outcomes is assessed by the dimensions emotional exhaustion and depersonalization. We observed a positive and significant association between both dimensions and the three safety outcomes besides between emotional exhaustion and error and adverse events. Age is negatively associated with the safety outcomes (except the age category 40–49 for the safety outcomes injury). A positive association between experience in EMS and the safety outcomes injury and safety compromising behavior is observed. Satisfaction with the current job is negatively associated with the safety outcome safety compromising behavior, satisfaction with the professional status with the safety outcome safety compromising behavior and error and adverse events. We observed a negative association between no intention to leave the current job within the next year and all safety outcomes. Additionally, a negative effect between the safety compromising behavior and the recommendation of the EMS area as a good place to work is observed.

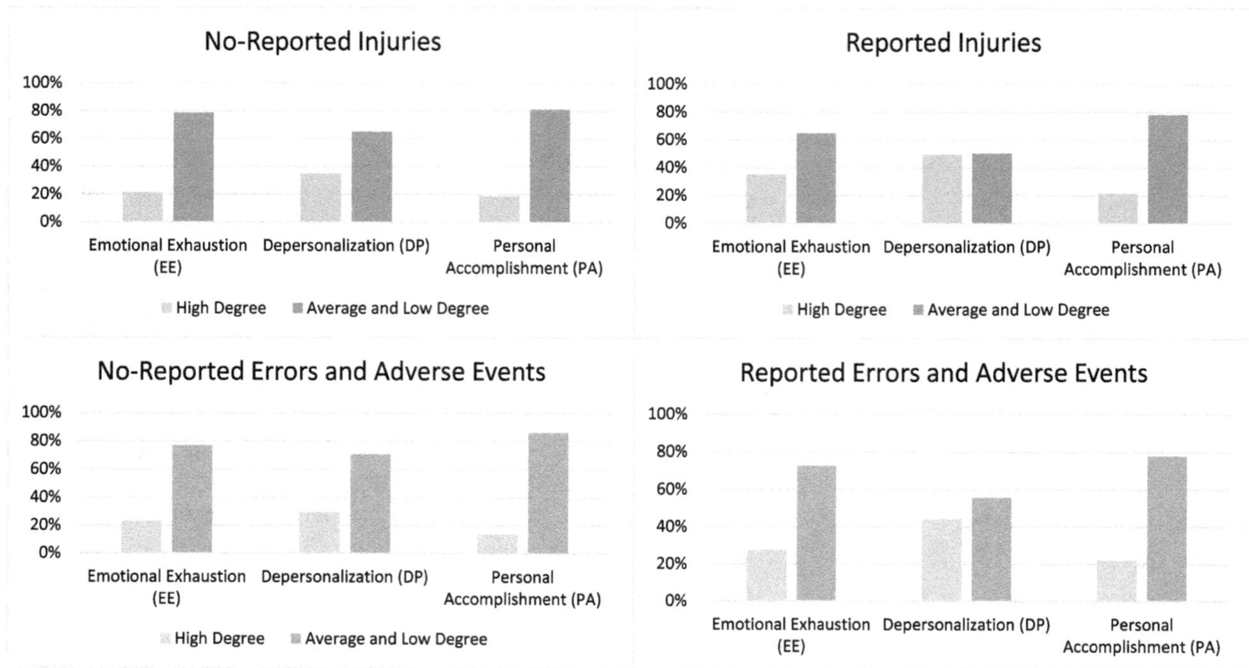

Fig. 1 Degree of burnout for reported and not reported negative safety outcomes

Discussion

Burnout among health care workers is seen as an important issue in patient care. Several studies have analyzed the risk factors and potential consequences of the burnout syndrome for EMS-workers. Especially in the context of health threatening diseases medical errors and failure may lead to fatal consequences [34]. Burnout of health care professionals may pose a risk to patients' safety and health outcomes. Therefore, this study focuses on investigating the association between burnout and safety outcomes by combining tools measuring the degree of burnout and adverse events (safety outcomes) for EMS-workers.

We got the result that between 19.9 and 40% of the participants showed a high degree of burnout in one of the burnout dimensions with the highest percentages of participants in the dimension depersonalization. Compared with the prevalence of burnout for nurses and surgeons presented in the introduction our results for depersonalization were in the higher range. A potential reason might be that with 86% the majority of our participants were male and men are more affected by depersonalization than women [35]. Our results are furthermore not fully in line with the results of the presented burnout studies for EMS-workers. The only German study [14] examining the degree of burnout using the MBI, got the result that the dimension with the highest percentage of participants with a high degree of burnout was personal accomplishment. However, the number of 98 considered questionnaires was considerably low and the analysis was limited to two regions in Germany. Alexander and Klein [18] could show for ambulance personnel in the UK that personal accomplishment is the dimension with the highest percentage of a high degree of burnout. In contrast Essex and Scott [15] showed the highest percentage of a high degree of burnout for the dimension depersonalization. They reported significantly higher scores than other studies (92% high level for EE, 99.3% high level for DP, and 76.1% high level for PA). A potential reason might be the combination of full or part-time job and EMS volunteering which may result in a double burden.

Regarding safety outcomes, the comparison of our results of the EMS-SI with the results by Weaver et al. [27] shows that a greater percentage of participants reported negative safety outcomes in all domains. A potential reason for difference might be various regional settings. Furthermore, the regression results show that burnout is significantly associated with the safety outcomes injury, error and adverse events, and safety-compromising behavior. This is especially in line with studies investigating the association of self-reported medical errors and self-reported burnout of healthcare staff [36–39]. One of those studies could furthermore show a mediating role of burnout for patient outcomes and job turnover indicating that the working environment supports psychological well-being and ensures patients safety [38].

Table 2 Number of negative safety outcomes measured by the EMS-SI

Safety outcome measures	N(%) N = 1101
Injury	
Yes	398 (36,2)
No	703 (63,9)
Error and adverse events	
Yes	811 (73,7)
No	290 (26,3)
Greatest contributing factors	
Did not print and properly interpret a 6 in. EKG strip	357 (44,0)
Made patient with chest pain ambulate instead of using stretcher	322 (39,7)
Did not administer necessary treatment for specific condition/malady	257 (31,7)
Did not establish an IV after two attempts	190 (23,4)
Did not check glucose level in a patient with altered mental status	135 (16,6)
Safety Comprising Behavior	
Yes	1094 (99,4)
No	7 (0,6)
Greatest contributing factors	
Greatly exceeded speed limit while responding lights and sirens	876 (80,0)
Exceeded speed limit while routinely driving	790 (72,2)
Did not complete pre-shift check of equipment and medications	760 (69,5)
Did not restock the ambulance before a call or shift	742 (67,8)
Overly stressed during a shift	728 (66,5)

Our survey shows that 46% of the EMS-workers are dissatisfied with their current job and 54% intend to leave their job within the next year. Compared to a study of Linda Aiken and colleagues [40], who investigated these items for nursing professionals, our results exceed the findings for nurses surveyed in Germany, 11 other European countries and the US (except for the item job satisfaction in Greece). Furthermore, they could show a significant association between satisfaction and intention to leave and the quality of care. Results of Patterson and colleagues who investigated job satisfaction of EMT-Basics and EMT-Paramedics showed that satisfaction varies across several important personal and organizational factors. They recommend a longitudinal study design to explore fully the importance of these factors in predicting job satisfaction [41].

In summary, job satisfaction, the intention to leave the current position and burnout in the EMS-workers workforce are critical issues as they pose safety risks for patients as well as EMS-workers. Given the increasing numbers of cases in prehospital emergency care, EMS managers should be aware of factors that affect the items such as the intention to leave a job. Therefore, identifying predictors of job satisfaction, intention to leave and burnout is an essential issue to ensure prehospital emergency care and improve its safety outcomes.

Table 3 Pearson correlation coefficients for the MBI and the EMS-SI

MBI	Emotional Exhaustion	Depersonalisation	Personal Accomplishment
EMS-SI			
Injury	0.2109*	0.1895*	− 0.0409
Error and Adverse Events	0.1605*	0.2679*	− 0.1562*
Safety Comprimising Behavior	0.4355*	0.4052*	− 0.1717*

* $p < 0.01$

Limitations

Several limitations need to be mentioned. Online surveys might lead to a selection bias, as people without internet access are not able to participate. Studies have shown that variables such as "high age group" and "female" are associated with less internet use [42]. Another limitation is that the calculation of a response rate is not possible. The study population is all EMS-workers in Germany. Since no standardized data on the number of EMS-workers on federal state level and information on the number of voluntary EMS-workers for Germany is available, a clear numerical number for the study population could not defined. However, the characteristics of our study population regarding gender and EMS-qualification is similar to nationwide data (77% are male and 71% have the EMS-qualification paramedic) [43, 44]. A further methodological limitation of the study findings might be the use of self-report measures for burnout and safety outcomes. Study participants with high burnout levels may over-report adverse events due to their negative emotional state [45]. Fahrenkopf and colleagues [46] used objective and subjective measures of error. They could show that burned out residents and non-burned out residents showed similar rates of error when using objective measurement. However, burned out residents reported a higher mean number of errors. Without taking into account the degree of burnout, prior studies have shown non-reporting rates of 4–19% for adverse events [47–49]. Reasons for underreporting might be a poor safety culture resulting in an unwillingness to report adverse events or that EMS-workers might not realize that an adverse event occurred. Finally,

Table 4 Results of the regressions analysis

	Injury		Error and Adverse Events		Safety-Compromising Behavior	
	Odds Ratio	95% CI	Odds Ratio	95% CI	Coefficient	95% CI
Burnout						
Emotional Exhaustion	1.48225**	1.07–2.05	1.04878	.72–1.54	.892386***	.40–1.39
Depersonalization	1.53438***	1.16–2.03	1.57450***	1.13–2.19	1.20405***	.78–1.62
Age						
30–39	.721825*	.49–1.06	.570877***	.38–.87	−.908149***	−1.43 - -.38
40–49	.746867	.40–1.39	.371898***	.19–.71	−1.71182***	−2.59 - -.84
> =50	.342833**	.13–0.92	.296491**	.11–.80	−3.57810***	−4.91 - -2.25
Gender	1.05635	.72–1.54	.827610	.54–1.26	−.3577269	−.89–.17
Experience in EMS	1.04295**	1.01–1.08	1.00161	.97–1.03	.0453481**	.001–.09
Full-time	1.33335	.86–2.07	1.39728	.89–2.20	.2312638	−.41–.88
Satisfaction						
Satisfaction current job	1.15952	.85–1.59	1.24126	.88–1.76	−.4735402**	−.93 - -.01
Satisfaction professional status	.826897	.62–1.10	.666836***	.49–.91	−.833566***	−1.21 - -.45
Satisfaction Wages	1.01309	.73–1.40	1.22432	.86–1.74	−.2322153	−.66–.19
Intention to leave/Recommendation						
No intention to leave	.659769**	.47–0.92	.549649***	.38–.79	−.777390***	−1.24 - -.31
Recommendation	1.07947	.78–1.50	1.40473*	.97–2.02	−.656998***	−1.11 - -.20
Level of EMS-qualification						
Paramedic 'Notfallsanitaeter'	.562515	.27–1.18	1.12939	.51–2.51	−.1906393	−1.35 - .97
Paramedic 'Rettungsassistent'	.653700	.35–1.23	1.24601	.62–2.50	−.100563	−1.10 - .90
EMT I 'Rettungssanitaeter'	.738753	.36–1.51	1.15101	.52–2.55	−.6527509	−1.77 - .46
Constant	.399562**	.16–.98	3.24927**	1.22–8.63	9.20007***	7.77–10.63

*** $p < 0.01$, ** $p < 0.05$, * $p < 0.1$

the cross-sectional study design prohibits determination of causality. Whether a high degree of burnout preceded negative safety oucomes cannot be analyzed.

Conclusion

This first large German study analyzing burnout and safety outcomes could show that the share of EMS-workers with a high degree of burnout in one dimension varies between 20 and 40%. A high percentage of the surveyed EMS-workers reported at least one negative safety outcome in the three measures of the EMS-SI. It could be shown that burnout is significantly associated with safety outcomes. An expansion of the psychological support of EMS-workers in Germany seems to be necessary. Setting-based prevention could be a beneficial approach e.g. by enhancing the information flow between the EMS-workers and their management. Further analysis is needed to understand the nature and complex relations between various factors for example by using a structural equation model. Those further investigations have the potential to identify predictors for negative safety outcomes as well as determinants of burnout. Policymakers and managers of EMS should take care of the burnout prevalence and safety outcomes when qualifying EMS-workers and planning their working environments.

Abbreviations

DP: Depersonalization; EE: Emotional exhaustion; EKG: Electrocardiogram; EMS: Emergency medical services; EMS-SAQ: Emergency medical services-Safety Attitudes Questionnaire; EMS-SI: Emergency medical services-Safety Inventory; EMT: Emergency medical technician; MBI: Maslach Burnout Inventory; MBI-HSS: Maslach Burnout Inventory-Human Services Survey; PA: Personal Accomplishment; RN4CAST: Nurse forecasting in Europe; SD: Standard deviation

Funding

The project was funded as part of the Berlin Centre for Health Economics Research by the German Federal Ministry of Education and Research, Bonn, Germany (grant no. 01EH1202A).

Authors' contributions

KR, CH, and NB had the main responsibility for the conception of the study.

NB had the main role in the conception of the manuscript. The preparation of the data was mainly performed by KR, CH and SF. Descriptive statistics were performed by SF and NB. Regression analysis was performed by NB. NB, SF and CH had the main role in manuscript preparation. All listed authors were responsible for reading, commenting upon, and approving the final manuscript.

Competing interests
The authors declare that they have no competing interest.

Author details
[1]Institute of Health Care Management, Berlin Centre of Health Economics Research (BerlinHECOR), Technische Universität Berlin, Straße des 17. Juni 135 (H80), 10623 Berlin, Germany. [2]ASB Köln e.V, Sülzburgstraße 146, 050937 Köln, Germany.

References
1. Maslach C, Jackson SE. The measurement of experienced burnout. J Organ Behav. 1981;2:99–113. https://doi.org/10.1002/job.4030020205.
2. Freudenberger HJ. The issues of staff burnout in therapeutic communities. J Psychoactive Drugs. 1986;18:247–51. https://doi.org/10.1080/02791072.1986.10472354.
3. Institute for Quality and Efficiency in Health Care. Depression: What is burnout? 2017. https://www.ncbi.nlm.nih.gov/pubmedhealth/PMH0072470/. Accessed 13 Apr 2018.
4. Schaufeli WB, van Dierendonck D. A cautionary note about the cross-national and clinical validity of cut-off points for the Maslach burnout inventory. Psychol Rep. 1995;76:1083–90.
5. Dall'Ora C, Griffiths P, Ball J, Simon M, Aiken LH. Association of 12 h shifts and nurses' job satisfaction, burnout and intention to leave: findings from a cross-sectional study of 12 European countries. BMJ Open. 2015;5:e008331. https://doi.org/10.1136/bmjopen-2015-008331.
6. Shanafelt TD, Hasan O, Dyrbye LN, Sinsky C, Satele D, Sloan J, West CP. Changes in burnout and satisfaction with work-life balance in physicians and the general US working population between 2011 and 2014. Mayo Clin Proc. 2015;90:1600–13. https://doi.org/10.1016/j.mayocp.2015.08.023.
7. Elmore LC, Jeffe DB, Jin L, Awad MM, Turnbull IR. National Survey of burnout among US general surgery residents. J Am Coll Surg. 2016;223:440–51. https://doi.org/10.1016/j.jamcollsurg.2016.05.014.
8. Shanafelt TD, Oreskovich MR, Dyrbye LN, Satele DV, Hanks JB, Sloan JA, Balch CM. Avoiding burnout: the personal health habits and wellness practices of US surgeons. Ann Surg. 2012;255:625–33. https://doi.org/10.1097/SLA.0b013e31824b2fa0.
9. Leiter MP. Burnout as a developmental process: consideration o models. In: Schaufeli W, Maslach C, Marek T, editors. Professional burnout: Recent developments in theory and research. Philadelphia, Pa., London: Taylor & Francis; 1993. p. 237–50.
10. Bakker AB, Schaufeli W, Sixma HJ, Bosveld W, van Dierendonck D. Patient demands, lack of reciprocity, and burnout: a five-year longitudinal study among general practitioners. J Organ Behav. 2000:425–41.
11. Hall LH, Johnson J, Watt I, Tsipa A, O'Connor DB. Healthcare staff wellbeing, burnout, and patient safety: a systematic review. PLoS One. 2016;11:e0159015. https://doi.org/10.1371/journal.pone.0159015.
12. Dewa CS, Loong D, Bonato S, Trojanowski L. The relationship between physician burnout and quality of healthcare in terms of safety and acceptability: a systematic review. BMJ Open. 2017;7:e015141. https://doi.org/10.1136/bmjopen-2016-015141.
13. Dewa CS, Loong D, Bonato S, Trojanowski L, Rea M. The relationship between resident burnout and safety-related and acceptability-related quality of healthcare: a systematic literature review. BMC Med Educ. 2017;17:195. https://doi.org/10.1186/s12909-017-1040-y.
14. Hering T, Beerlage I. Arbeitsbedingungen, Belastungen und Burnout im Rettungsdienst. Notfall Rettungsmed. 2004;7:415–24. https://doi.org/10.1007/s10049-004-0681-7.
15. Essex B, Scott LB. Chronic stress and associated coping strategies among volunteer EMS personnel. Prehosp Emerg Care. 2008;12:69–75. https://doi.org/10.1080/10903120701707955.
16. Boudreaux E, Mandry C, Brantley PJ. Stress, job satisfaction, coping, and psychological distress among emergency medical technicians. Prehosp Disaster Med. 1997;12:242–9.
17. Sterud T, Hem E, Lau B, Ekeberg O. A comparison of general and ambulance specific stressors: predictors of job satisfaction and health problems in a nationwide one-year follow-up study of Norwegian ambulance personnel. J Occup Med Toxicol. 2011;6:10. https://doi.org/10.1186/1745-6673-6-10.
18. Alexander DA, Klein S. Ambulance personnel and critical incidents: impact of accident and emergency work on mental health and emotional well-being. Br J Psychiatry. 2001;178:76–81. https://doi.org/10.1192/bjp.178.1.76.
19. Hammer JS, Mathews JJ, Lyons JS, Johnson NJ. Occupational stress within the paramedic profession: an initial report of stress levels compared to hospital employees. Ann Emerg Med. 1986;15:536–9. https://doi.org/10.1016/S0196-0644(86)80988-X.
20. Senatsverwaltung für Inneres und Sport. Aktuelle Personalengpässe im Berliner Rettungsdienst. 2018. https://kleineanfragen.de/berlin/18/13653-aktuelle-personalengpaesse-im-berliner-rettungsdienst/viewer. Accessed 18 Jun 2018.
21. Chapman S, Lindler V, Kaiser JA. The emergency medical services workforce agenda for the future. 2011. https://www.ems.gov/pdf/2011/EMS_Workforce_Agenda_052011.pdf. Accessed 18 Jun 2018.
22. National Audit Office. NHS Ambulance Services. 2017. https://www.nao.org.uk/wp-content/uploads/2017/01/NHS-Ambulance-Services.pdf. Accessed 18 June 2018.
23. Sermeus W, Aiken LH, van den Heede K, Rafferty AM, Griffiths P, Moreno-Casbas MT, et al. Nurse forecasting in Europe (RN4CAST): rationale, design and methodology. BMC Nurs. 2011;10:6. https://doi.org/10.1186/1472-6955-10-6.
24. Maslach C, Jackson SE, Leiter MP. Maslach burnout inventory manual: third edition. Palo Alto, California: Consulting Psychologists Press, Inc.; 1996.
25. Halbesleben JRB, Wakefield BJ, Wakefield DS, Cooper LB. Nurse burnout and patient safety outcomes: nurse safety perception versus reporting behavior. West J Nurs Res. 2008;30:560–77. https://doi.org/10.1177/0193945907311322.
26. Thomas NK. Resident burnout. JAMA. 2004;292:2880–9. https://doi.org/10.1001/jama.292.23.2880.
27. Weaver MD, Wang HE, Fairbanks RJ, Patterson D. The association between EMS workplace safety culture and safety outcomes. Prehosp Emerg Care. 2012;16:43–52. https://doi.org/10.3109/10903127.2011.614048.
28. Zohar D. Safety climate in industrial organizations: theoretical and applied implications. J Appl Psychol. 1980;65:96–102. https://doi.org/10.1037/0021-9010.65.1.96.
29. Patterson PD, Weaver MD, Frank RC, Warner CW, Martin-Gill C, Guyette FX, et al. Association between poor sleep, fatigue, and safety outcomes in emergency medical services providers. Prehosp Emerg Care. 2012;16:86–97. https://doi.org/10.3109/10903127.2011.616261.
30. Maneesriwongul W, Dixon JK. Instrument translation process: a methods review. J Adv Nurs. 2004;48:175–86. https://doi.org/10.1111/j.1365-2648.2004.03185.x.
31. Green DE, Walkey FH, Taylor AJW. The three-factor structure of the Maslach burnout inventory: a multicultural, multinational confirmatory study. J Soc. Behav. Personal. 1991;6:453–73.
32. Demerouti E, Bakker AB, Nachreiner F, Schaufeli WB. The job demands-resources model of burnout. J Appl Psychol. 2001;86:499–512. https://doi.org/10.1037/0021-9010.86.3.499.
33. Cohen J. Statistical power analysis for the behavioral sciences. In: Hillsdale NJ, editor. . 2nd ed: L. Erlbaum Associates; 1988.
34. Kerby JD, Cusick MV. Prehospital emergency trauma care and management. Surg Clin North Am. 2012;92:823–41, vii. https://doi.org/10.1016/j.suc.2012.04.009.
35. Maslach C, Schaufeli WB, Leiter MP. Job burnout. Annu Rev Psychol. 2001;52:397–422. https://doi.org/10.1146/annurev.psych.52.1.397.
36. Chen K, Yang C, Lien C, Chiou H, Lin M, Chang H, Chiu W. Burnout, job satisfaction, and medical malpractice among physicians. Int J Med Sci. 2013;10:1471–8. https://doi.org/10.7150/ijms.6743
37. Block L, Wu AW, Feldman L, Yeh H, Desai SV. Residency schedule, burnout and patient care among first-year residents. Postgrad Med J. 2013;89:495–500. https://doi.org/10.1136/postgradmedj-2012-131743.
38. Spence Laschinger HK, Leiter MP. The impact of nursing work environments on patient safety outcomes: the mediating role of burnout/engagement. J Nurs Adm. 2006;36:259–67.

39. Shanafelt TD, Balch CM, Bechamps G, Russell T, Dyrbye L, Satele D, et al. Burnout and medical errors among American surgeons. Ann Surg. 2010;251: 995–1000. https://doi.org/10.1097/SLA.0b013e3181bfdab3.
40. Aiken LH, Sermeus W, van den Heede K, Sloane DM, Busse R, McKee M, et al. Patient safety, satisfaction, and quality of hospital care: cross sectional surveys of nurses and patients in 12 countries in Europe and the United States. BMJ. 2012;344:e1717. https://doi.org/10.1136/bmj.e1717.
41. Patterson PD, Moore CG, Sanddal ND, Wingrove G, LaCroix B. Characterizing job satisfaction and intent to leave among nationally registered emergency medical technicians: an analysis of the 2005 LEADS survey. J Allied Health. 2009;38:e84–91.
42. Statistisches Bundesamt. IT-Nutzung. 2015. https://www.destatis.de/DE/ZahlenFakten/GesellschaftStaat/EinkommenKonsumLebensbedingungen/ITNutzung/ITNutzung.html. Accessed 26 Oct 2017.
43. Die Bundesregierung. Neue Ausbildung zum Notfallsanitäter. 2013. https://www.bundesregierung.de/ContentArchiv/DE/Archiv17/Artikel/2013/11/2013-11-29-notfallsanitaeter.html. Accessed 14 Jun 2018.
44. Statistisches Bundesamt. Gesundheit. 2017. https://www.destatis.de/DE/Publikationen/Thematisch/Gesundheit/Gesundheitspersonal/PersonalPDF_2120731.pdf%3F__blob%3DpublicationFile. Accessed 14 June 2018.
45. Jong MA, de Nieuwenhuijsen K, Sluiter JK. Common mental disorders related to incidents and behaviour in physicians. Occup Med (Lond). 2016; 66:506–13. https://doi.org/10.1093/occmed/kqw030.
46. Fahrenkopf AM, Sectish TC, Barger LK, Sharek PJ, Lewin D, Chiang VW, et al. Rates of medication errors among depressed and burnt out residents: prospective cohort study. BMJ. 2008;336:488–91. https://doi.org/10.1136/bmj.39469.763218.BE.
47. Fairbanks RJ, Crittenden CN, O'Gara KG, Wilson MA, Pennington EC, Chin NP, Shah MN. Emergency medical services provider perceptions of the nature of adverse events and near-misses in out-of-hospital care: an ethnographic view. Acad Emerg Med. 2008;15:633–40. https://doi.org/10.1111/j.1553-2712.2008.00147.x.
48. Hobgood C, Bowen JB, Brice JH, Overby B, Tamayo-Sarver JH. Do EMS personnel identify, report, and disclose medical errors? Prehosp Emerg Care. 2006;10:21–7. https://doi.org/10.1080/10903120500366011.
49. Vilke GM, Tornabene SV, Stepanski B, Shipp HE, Ray LU, Metz MA, et al. Paramedic self-reported medication errors. Prehosp Emerg Care. 2007;11:80–4. https://doi.org/10.1080/10903120601021358.

20

Seasonal prevalence of hyponatremia in the emergency department: impact of age

Naohiko Imai*, Kiyomi Osako, Nagayuki Kaneshiro and Yugo Shibagaki

Abstract

Background: Hyponatremia is one of the most commonly encountered electrolyte disorders in emergency department (ED). Seasonal fluctuations of the prevalence of hyponatremia has been reported. We investigated the impact of age on the seasonal prevalence of hyponatremia in the emergency department in Japan.

Methods: Total of 8377 patients presented to the ED between January 2015 and December 2016 were reviewed. The adult group aged between 18 and 64 years old consisted of 3656 patients and the elderly group aged over 65 years consisted of 4721 patients. Information collected included age, sex, serum sodium, and serum creatinine. Hyponatremia was defined as a serum sodium leve1 < 135 mEq/L and severe hyponatremia was defined as a serum sodium level < 125 mEq/L.

Results: Prevalence of hyponatremia was significantly higher in the elderly group than in the adult group (17.0% vs. 5. 7%, $p < 0.001$). Similarly, the prevalence of severe hyponatremia was significantly higher in the elderly group than in the adult group (1.9% vs. 0.3%, $p < 0.001$). Prevalence of hyponatremia and severe hyponatremia was significantly higher in the elderly group than in the adult group in all seasons. In the elderly group, there was a significant correlation between weather high temperature during summer and prevalence of hyponatremia ($r = 0.510$, $p = 0.011$).

Conclusion: There was a major impact of age on the seasonal prevalence of hyponatremia and severe hyponatremia. Strategies to prevent hyponatremia and severe hyponatremia should be taken especially in the elderly patients during summer.

Keywords: Hyponatremia, Severe hyponatremia, Emergency department, Prevalence

Background

Hyponatremia is one of the most commonly encountered electrolyte disorders in the emergency departments [1, 2]. Hyponatremia is known for its high morbidity and mortality and age is a strong independent risk factor of hyponatremia [3–7]. Only a few studies have investigated the impact of age on the seasonal prevalence of hyponatremia in patients admitted to emergency departments [7, 8]. Considering the aging population in Japan, the increased susceptibility of the elderly to develop hyponatremia is particularly important. The impact of age on the seasonal fluctuations on the prevalence of hyponatremia has not been reported in Japan. Thus, we investigated the impact of age on the seasonal prevalence of hyponatremia in the emergency department in Japan.

* Correspondence: naohiko.imai@gmail.com
Division of Nephrology and Hypertension, Department of Internal Medicine, St. Marianna University School of Medicine, 2-16-1 Sugao, Miyamae-ku, Kawasaki, Kanagawa, Japan

Methods

All adult patients (18 years old or older) who had their serum sodium levels measured at the emergency department between January 2015 and December 2016 were included. Hyponatremia was defined as serum sodium levels of less < 135 mEq/L. Severe hyponatremia was defined as serum sodium level < 125 mEq/L. Information collected included age, sex, serum sodium, and serum creatinine. We used the meteorological parameters provided by the Japan Meteorological Agency. The seasons are defined as follows: spring: March–May; summer: June–August; fall: September–November; winter: December–February. The study was approved by the Institutional Review Boards at our institution.

Table 1 Patients characteristic

	All	Adult	Elderly
N	8377	3656	4721
Male (N)	4152	1882	2270
Age (years)	63.3 ± 22.2	41.3 ± 13.6	80.3 ± 8.3
Serum creatinine	1.03 ± 1.0	0.87 ± 0.9	1.11 ± 1.1
eGFR (mL/min/1.7m^2)	67.5 ± 27.0	81.5 ± 23.5	56.7 ± 27.4

Statistical analyses

Data analysis was performed using SPSS, Version 21.0 (IBM Corp, Armonk, NY). Student t test or analyses of variance were used to compare means for continuous variables. Chi-square tests were used to test statistical differences for categorical variables. A p-value of < 0.05 was considered statistically significant.

Results

Patients characteristics

From January 2015 to December 2016 a total of 8377 adult patients had their serum sodium measured at the emergency department. The key characteristics of the patients are summarized (Table 1). The mean age of the patients was 63.3 ± 22.2 years and 49.6% of patients were male. Patients were divided into adult group aged from 18 to 64 years and elderly group aged 65 years and over. The mean age of the adult group ($N = 3656$) was 41.3 ± 13.6 years and 51.5% of patients were male. The mean age of the elderly group ($N = 4721$) was 80.3 ± 8.3 years and 48.1% of patients were male.

Prevalence of hyponatremia and severe hyponatremia

Prevalence of hyponatremia was significantly higher in the elderly group than in the adult group (17.0% vs. 5.7%, $p < 0.001$). Similarly, the prevalence of severe hyponatremia was significantly higher in the elderly group than in the adult group (1.9% vs. 0.3%, $p < 0.001$).

Seasonal prevalence of hyponatremia and severe hyponatremia

The prevalence of hyponatremia was significantly higher in the elderly group than in the adult group in all seasons (Fig. 1). Similarly, the prevalence of severe hyponatremia was significantly higher in the elderly group than in the adult group in all seasons (Fig. 2). In the adult group, the prevalence of hyponatremia and sever hyponatremia didn't differ between the seasons (Table 2). On the other hand, in the elderly group, although the prevalence of severe hyponatremia didn't differ between the seasons, the prevalence of hyponatremia was significantly higher in summer ($p < 0.001$ vs. spring and winter) (Table 3).

Monthly weather temperature and prevalence of hyponatremia

The monthly weather temperature during the 2-year period is summarized (Table 4). In the adult group, the monthly weather temperature didn't show any correlation with monthly prevalence of hyponatremia ($r = 0.094$, $p = 0.661$). On the other hand, in the elderly group, the monthly weather temperature showed a linear

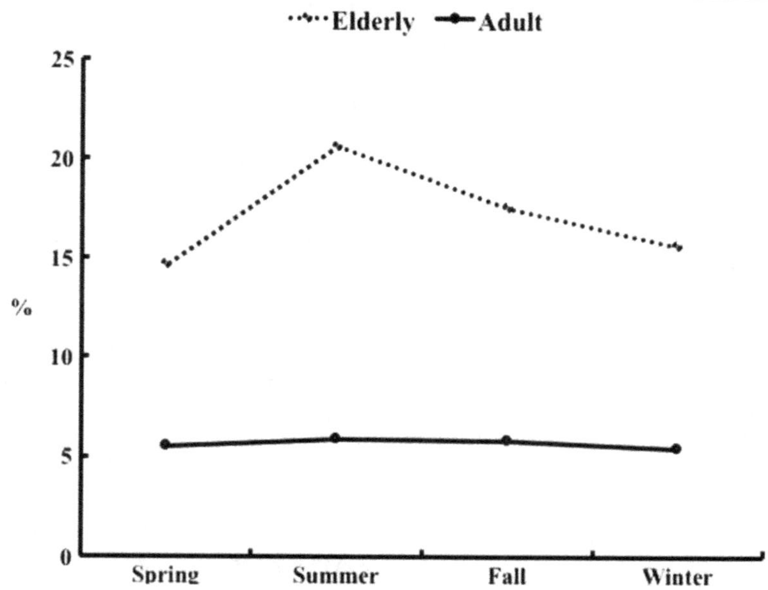

Fig. 1 Seasonal prevalence of hyponatremia in adult group and elderly group

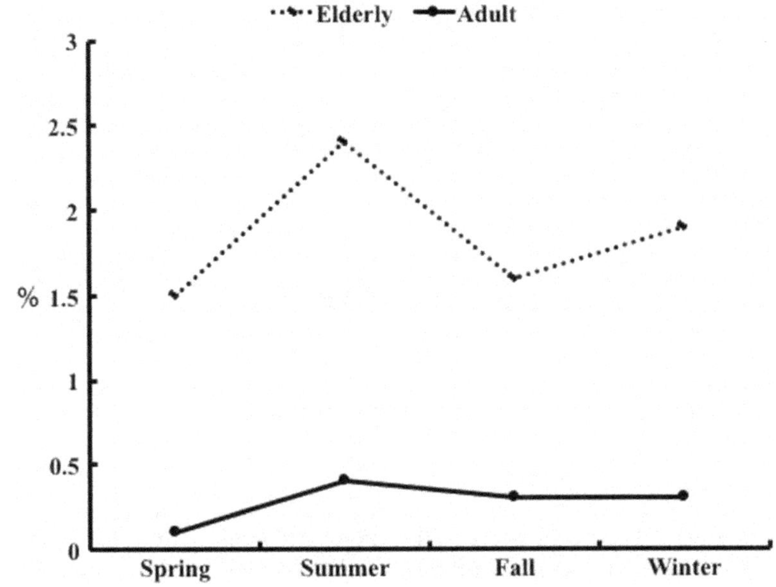

Fig. 2 Seasonal prevalence of severe hyponatremia in adult group and elderly group

correlation with monthly prevalence of hyponatremia ($r = 0.510$, $p = 0.011$) (Fig. 3).

Discussion

The prevalence of hyponatremia including severe hyponatremia was significantly higher in elderly group compared to adult group during the two-year period. Also, the seasonal prevalence of hyponatremia including severe hyponatremia was significantly higher in elderly group compared to adult group during the two-year period.

The prevalence of hyponatremia observed in emergency departments varies between studies. The 5.7% prevalence of hyponatremia in the adult group observed in our study was close to the previous report [7, 9]. Similarly, the 0.3% prevalence of severe hyponatremia in the adult group observed in our study was also close to the previous report [10]. On the other hand, the 17.0% prevalence of hyponatremia in the elderly group was higher than the previous report [7].

The prevalence of hyponatremia is strongly affected by age and is higher in elderly patients [3, 7, 8]. Various risk factors including a decline in renal function, excessive water intake, reduced salt intake, and medications could all contribute to developing hyponatremia in the elderly patients [7, 11, 12]. Although we could not assess in this study, diuretics, especially thiazides, is a known risk factors for developing hyponatremia [13, 14]. The risk associated potassium-sparing diuretics are also reported [10, 15]. It is important that physician taking care of elderly patients is fully aware of the fact that elderly patients are susceptible to develop hyponatremia because the increased morbidity and mortality associated with hyponatremia can't be ignored [11, 15, 16].

The prevalence of hyponatremia is also strongly affected by the high weather temperature and is higher during the summer [7, 8, 10]. An increased prevalence of hyponatremia during heat periods has been reported too [11]. In our study, the prevalence of hyponatremia in the elderly group was highest during the summer. Water intake and loss are approximately 40% higher in the summer than in the winter [17]. Also, it is reported that salt appetite is not

Table 2 Seasonal prevalence of hyponatremia and serve hyponatremia: Adult

	Spring	Summer	Fall	Winter
Hyponatremia (%)	5.5	5.9	5.8	5.4
Sever hyponatremia (%)	0.1	0.4	0.3	0.3

Table 3 Seasonal prevalence of hyponatremia and sever hyponatremia: Elderly

	Spring	Summer	Fall	Winter
Hyponatremia (%)	14.6	20.6*	17.2	15.6
Sever hyponatremia (%)	1.5	2.4	1.6	1.9

*$p < 0.01$ vs Spring and Winter

Table 4 Mean monthly weather temperature during the 2 year period

	Jan	Feb	Mar	Apr	May	Jun	Jul	Aug	Sep	Oct	Nov	Dec
2015	4.6	5.0	9.5	14.0	20.5	21.6	26.1	26.2	22.1	17.7	13.1	8.3
2016	4.8	6.3	9.5	14.9	19.8	22.0	25.1	26.8	24	18.1	10.7	7.7

increased in summer heat [18]. These findings could have caused the high prevalence of hyponatremia during the summer in the elderly. The strong correlation between the prevalence of hyponatremia in the elderly group and the monthly weather temperature was confirmed in our study [7]. This correlation was not observed in the adult group.

This study is not without limitations. First, this is a single center study and there is a possibility of selection bias in the patients enrolled. Secondary, serum sodium was not corrected for plasma glucose levels, when elevated. Thus, patients with pseudohyponatremia are not completely ruled out. Third, several potential confounders such as reason for visit, medications which could induce hyponatremia, history of hyponatremia, and past medical history were not collected.

Conclusions

In conclusion, we observed a major impact of age on the seasonal prevalence of hyponatremia. Elderly patients had significantly higher seasonal prevalence of hyponatremia and severe hyponatremia compared to adult patients. Strategies to prevent hyponatremia and severe hyponatremia should be taken especially in the elderly patients.

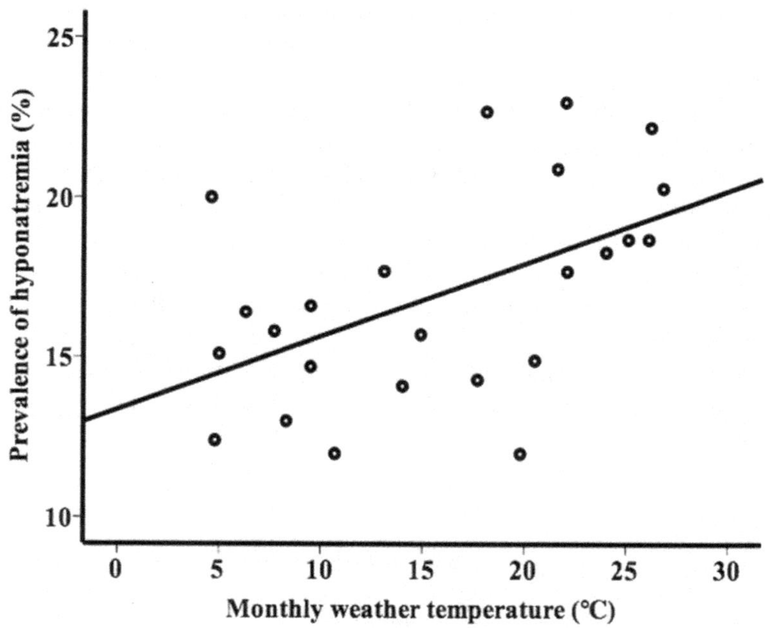

Fig. 3 Relationship between prevalence of hyponatremia and monthly weather temperature in elderly group ($r = 0.510$, $p = 0.011$)

Abbreviation
ED: Emergency department

Authors' contributions
NI, KO, NK, and YS designed the study. NI performed data collection and data analysis, and wrote the manuscript. KO, NK, and YS interpreted the data and critically reviewed the manuscript. YS revised the intellectual content of the manuscript. All authors read and approved the final manuscript.

Competing interests
The authors declare that they have no competing interests.

References
1. Giordano M, Ciarambino T, Castellino P, Malatino L, Di Somma S, Biolo G, et al. Diseases associated with electrolyte imbalance in the ED: age-related differences. Am J Emerg Med. 2016;34(10):1923–6.
2. Funk G-C, Lindner G, Druml W, Metnitz B, Schwarz C, Bauer P, et al. Incidence and prognosis of dysnatremias present on ICU admission. Intensive Care Med. 2009;36(2):304–11.
3. Hawkins RC. Age and gender as risk factors for hyponatremia and hypernatremia. Clin Chim Acta. 2003;337(1–2):169–72.
4. Renneboog B, Musch W, Vandemergel X, Manto MU, Decaux G. Mild chronic hyponatremia is associated with falls, unsteadiness, and attention deficits. Am J Med. 2006;119(1):71.e1–8.
5. Sajadieh A, Binici Z, Mouridsen MR, Nielsen OW, Hansen JF, Haugaard SB. Mild hyponatremia carries a poor prognosis in community subjects. Am J Med. 2009;122(7):679–86.
6. Waikar SS, Mount DB, Curhan GC. Mortality after hospitalization with mild, moderate, and severe hyponatremia. Am J Med. 2009;122(9):857–65.
7. Giordano M, Ciarambino T, Castellino P, Malatino L, Cataliotti A, Rinaldi L, et al. Seasonal variations of hyponatremia in the emergency department: age-related changes. Am J Emerg Med. 2017;35(5):749–52.
8. Giordano M, Ciarambino T, Adinolf LE. Severe hyponatremia in the elderly: the seasonalvariability in the emergency department. Italian Journal of Emergency Medicine. 2018;1:1–14.
9. Lee CT, Guo HR, Chen JB. Hyponatremia in the emergency department. Am J Emerg Med. 2000;18(3):264–8.
10. Huwyler T, Stirnemann J, Vuilleumier N, Marti C, Dugas S, Poletti PA, et al. Profound hyponatraemia in the emergency department: seasonality and risk factors. Swiss Med Wkly. 2016;146:w14385.
11. Pfortmueller CA, Funk G-C, Leichtle AB, Fiedler GM, Schwarz C, Exadaktylos AK, et al. Electrolyte disorders and in-hospital mortality during prolonged heat periods: a cross-sectional analysis. PLoS One. 2014;9(3):e92150.
12. Hoorn EJ, Lindemans J, Zietse R. Acute and concomitant deterioration of hyponatremia and renal dysfunction associated with heart and liver failure. Clin Nephrol. 2006;65(4):248–55.
13. Rodenburg EM, Hoorn EJ, Ruiter R, Lous JJ, Hofman A, Uitterlinden AG, et al. Thiazide-associated hyponatremia: a population-based study. Am J Kidney Dis. 2013;62(1):67–72.
14. Spital A. Diuretic-induced hyponatremia. Am J Nephrol. 1999;19(4):447–52.
15. Liamis G, Rodenburg EM, Hofman A, Zietse R, Stricker BH, Hoorn EJ. Electrolyte disorders in community subjects: prevalence and risk factors. Am J Med. 2013; 126(3):256–63.
16. Assen A, Abouem D, Vandergheynst F, Nguyen T, Taccone FS, Melot C. Hyponatremia at the emergency department: a case-control study. Minerva Anestesiol. 2014;80(4):419–28.
17. Malisova O, Bountziouka V, Panagiotakos DB, Zampelas A, Kapsokefalou M. Evaluation of seasonality on total water intake, water loss and water balance in the general population in Greece. J Hum Nutr Diet. 2013;26(Suppl 1):90–6.
18. Leshem M. Salt appetite is not increased in summer heat. Appetite. 2017; 108:28–31.

Emergency response time and pre-hospital trauma survival rate of the national ambulance service, Greater Accra

Mohammed-Najeeb Mahama[1], Ernest Kenu[2*], Delia Akosua Bandoh[2] and Ahmed Nuhu Zakariah[1]

Abstract

Background: Every year, about 1.2 million people die through road traffic crashes worldwide. Majority of these deaths occur in Africa where most of their emergency medical services are underdeveloped. In 2004, Ghana established the National Ambulance Council to provide timely and efficient pre-hospital emergency medical care to the sick and injured. Pre-hospital emergency medical service is essential for accident victims since it has the potential of saving lives. The study sought to determine the relationship between pre-hospital trauma survival rate and response time to emergencies and factors associated to pre-hospital trauma survival in Accra, Ghana.

Methods: The study was a cross sectional study which reviewed pre-hospital care forms of trauma patients from the fourteen ambulance stations in the Greater Accra region from January to December 2014. Data were extracted from these forms and the response time estimated. Conscious patients who were alert were categorized as responsive under the AVPU scale. The proportion of patients who survived pre-hospital trauma and the time pre-hospital trauma cases were responded to was estimated. Multiple logistic regression analysis was conducted to determine which variables were associated with survival.

Results: A total of 652 pre-hospital care forms were reviewed. About 87% survived pre-hospital trauma. The average response time to patients was (16.9 ± 0.7) minutes and the median transportation time of the patient was 82 min. Level of consciousness of a patient and response time of patients transported was found to be significantly associated with pre-hospital trauma survival.

Conclusion: There was a high trauma patient survival rate among victims attended to by an NAS. The average response time in Greater Accra region in the 14 ambulance stations is 16.9 min which is not different from the 17 min recorded in 2013 by NAS. Factors that were associated with pre-hospital survival were alertness in the level of consciousness and response time less than 17 min.

Keywords: Pre-hospital trauma, Ambulance, Survival, Response time

* Correspondence: ernest_kenu@yahoo.com
[2]Ghana Field Epidemiology and Laboratory Training Program, Department of Epidemiology, School of Public Health, University of Ghana, Accra, Ghana
Full list of author information is available at the end of the article

Background

Each year about 1.2 million people die through road traffic crashes in the world [1]. Many of these deaths could have being prevented if there was adequate pre-hospital medical care worldwide. Africa bears majority of the deaths and yet with the most underdeveloped emergency medical service (EMS) [2]. The Ghana national road safety 2012 report indicates that 2249 people lost their lives whiles about 14,000 were injured by Road Traffic Crash (RTC) [3]. The Greater Accra region has become infamous for topping the list of cities in Ghana for trauma disaster.

Trauma refers to bodily injury resulting from the application of an external physical force [4]. It ranges from motor vehicle crashes, to burns and blunt assault and is the leading cause of death between the 15 to 45-years age group [5]. Most trauma cases occur in out -of -hospital settings. Road traffic Crash (RTC) is the leading cause of deaths in trauma cases and has unfortunately earned the name "the neglected disease of modern society" since much attention has not been given to it [6].

Pre-hospital Emergency Medical Service (EMS) is the first level of treatment given to patient suffering life threatening conditions by emergency medical technicians (EMTs) and paramedics before they are handed over to the hospital. EMS seeks to reduce response time. That is the time between an emergency call made to an ambulance station and the time a dispatched ambulance gets to the scene for assistance. A shorter response time is known to greatly improve survival [7].

The occurrence of the May 9th Accra sports stadium disaster in 2001 which led to the loss of about 127 lives, provided the leverage for the establishment of the national ambulance service (NAS) in Ghana. The core mandate of the service is to provide timely and efficient emergency medical care to the sick and injured and to transport them to an appropriate facility. The target set for response time in Ghana is eight (8) minutes [8]. Though the total number of ambulance has increased from 24 to 124, the response time target of 8-min has not been achieved. The country's current response time is 17 min [8].

It has been well documented that shorter response time has the potential of saving lives [9]. However, designing EMS systems to meet these response time targets requires substantial investment which include ambulances, personnel and other resources across the region in other to reduce response time. Work done by Fischer and colleagues in 2000, explains that meeting the set response time target would require substantial cost. [10, 11]. Even though the response time target has not been met. No recent assessment has been made on how Ghana's response time affects its pre-hospital trauma survival. This study determined the National Ambulance Service's pre-hospital trauma survival rate, its response time to emergencies attended to the in Greater Accra and factors associated to pre-hospital trauma survival.

Methods

Study design

This was a record review of pre-hospital trauma patients' data for the period January to December 2014. Pre-hospital care forms (PCR forms) of trauma patients responded to by the fourteen (14) Ambulance Stations in the Greater Accra Region [Ridge hospital, Accra Airport, Weija, Tema, Accra City, Ashaiman, Teshie, Atomic, Dodowa, Pantang hospital, Mamprobi, La General hospital, Accra Sports Stadium, and Ada Ambulance Stations] were reviewed and data extracted.

Study area

The Greater Accra Region occupies a total land surface of 1.4% of the total land area of Ghana. Its capital is Accra, which is also the capital of the Republic of Ghana. This region is the second most populated region in the country after the Ashanti Region. Greater Accra Region has a population of 4,010,054, accounting for 15.4% of Ghana's total population.

The NAS has fourteen ambulance stations (Accra Airport, Accra city (Makola), Amasaman, Ashaiman, Atomic, Dodowa, La General, LEKMA, Accra Sports Stadium, Ridge, Tema, and Weija) which offers service to 62.5% of the region and record an average of 1358 cases annually. The region was chosen because it has 14 ambulance stations and heavy traffic making it difficult for movement of ambulances to the scene of emergencies.

We reviewed records of all trauma cases in the Greater Accra region transported to various health care facilities by the 14 ambulance stations in 2014. These records were obtained from a PCR forms registry provided by NAS. The study focused on trauma which was defined in the context of road traffic crashes. Trauma was limited to road traffic crashes patients who have been conveyed to various hospitals by the national ambulance service.

Inclusion criteria

Records of patients who sustained pre-hospital trauma and were directly attended to by the National Ambulance Service as well those who were picked by private or commercial vehicles to clinics and subsequently transported to an appropriate hospital by NAS in the Greater Accra Region were included in the study.

Exclusion criteria

Data from patients with ineligible or missing records that were difficult to decipher were excluded and all pre-hospital trauma (stable) cases that were transported for diagnostic purposes such as X-ray and CT scan in the region were as well excluded. All the cases that the time of transfer from site of injury to the hospital could not be ascertained were not included in the study.

Data collection

This data was extracted from the records of operations department of the NAS where Pre-hospital care forms filled by EMTs for each patient they transported are kept. Research assistants were trained to help in the extraction of the data. Stations were also visited to confirm and clarify inconsistent data. This was done by going through their occurrence books at the stations.

Data extracted from the forms were:

- Patient characteristics: age, sex, type of injury
- Time the emergency call was made to the station
- Time the ambulance departed to scene,
- Time the ambulance arrived at scene time,
- Time the ambulance departed the scene to the health facility
- Time the ambulance arrived at the health facility
- The time the patient was handed over to the health facility.

Data processing and analysis

Data extracted was entered into Microsoft Excel 2010 to estimate the following variables: Response time, transportation time and time spent on scene.

Response time was estimated as the duration between the time a call was made for the emergency and time of arrival of the ambulance at the scene of the emergency.

Transportation time was estimated as the duration between when the call was made to the station and the time the patient was handed over to the facility.

On-scene time was estimated as the duration of time the ambulance spent at the scene of the emergency before transporting the patient to the health facility. That is time of arrival at scene of emergency to time of departure.

Case handling time was estimated as time the patient is taken from the scene to the time the patient is handed over to the facility.

EMTs on the field sort patients according to their degree of injuries and transport those with life threating conditions but salvageable injuries first as it is done in triaging. However, this process is not color coded or recorded on their PCR forms.

Conscious patients that were alert were categorized as responsive under the AVPU scale.

Analysis was done using the Stata Version 13. Response time in minutes was categorized as < 4 vs. ≥4, < 8 vs. ≥8 and < 17 vs. ≥17 min respectively. The proportion of patients who survived pre-hospital trauma as well as the proportion of pre-hospital trauma cases that was responded to within eight minutes was estimated. In line with Eisenerg and colleagues findings of response time between 4 and 8 min increasing the rate of survival for cardiac patients, we determined the four (4) to eight (8) minutes response times [12].

Bivariate analysis was conducted to determine which variables were associated with survival. Chi-squared test of proportions was used to determine the relationship between independent variables (response time categories, on-scene time (< 10 vs. ≥10 min), transportation time (< 60 vs. ≥ 60 min), level of consciousness, type of injuries and age) and dependent variable (pre-hospital trauma survival). Level of significant association was determined at 95% confidence interval and p-value of less than 0.05. A multiple logistic regression was conducted to test the association between pre-hospital trauma survival and the significant dependent variables while adjusting for age, and sex.

Ethical considerations

The study protocol was reviewed and approved by the Ghana Health Service Ethical Review Committee of the Research and Development Division of the Ghana Health Services GHS-ERC: 59/12/15. In addition, permission was obtained from the National Ambulance Service to use their data for the conduct of the study. Patient identifiers such as name and address were not extracted. To assure confidentiality, the forms were kept in locked cabinets and the data entered kept in password protected files on the researcher's personal computer.

Results

Description of data

The 14 ambulance stations of the National Ambulance Service from January to December 2014 transported a total of 20,236 patients. Of these 652 were trauma cases that had all been involved in road traffic crashes.

Description of patient characteristics

About 70% (435/652) of the trauma cases transported were male. The mean age was (33.0 ± 18.6) years. Almost 66% (415/652) of them were within the age group 15 to 44 years.

The mean response time was (16.9 ± 0.7) minutes, with a range of (1–151) minutes. The median time spent on the scene in managing patients was 17 min with a range of (1–150) minutes. The median transportation time for patients was 82 min with a range of (5–552) minutes.

Response time and patient characteristics

A total of 8 patients did not survive pre-hospital trauma, only one (12.5%) had a response time of < 8 min.

However, no significant difference was found between the patients' characteristics and response times of eight minutes. (Table 1).

Pre-hospital trauma survival and patient characteristics

Response time and level of consciousness were found to be associated with pre-hospital survival ($p < 0.05$). Other patient characteristics observed such as transportation time and type of injury were not found to be associated with survival. The other response time categories were not significantly associated with survival (Table 2).

Patients that were conscious had higher odds of pre-hospital survival compared to unconscious patients Table 3. We observed that a response time less than 17 min was associated with survival [aOR = 0.08, 95%CI (0.009–0.59)].

Table 1 Characteristics for trauma patients attended to NAS in Greater Accra region, 2014 based on the 8 Minute Response Time Criterion

Variable	Number of trauma patients for each response time N (%)		*P*-value
	< 8 min	> 8 min	
Sex	239	413	0.311
Female	69 (33.8)	135 (66.2)	
Male	170 (38.0)	278 (62.0)	
Age			0.121
> 15	37 (43.6)	48 (56.5)	
15 to 44 years	157 (37.9)	258 (62.2)	
45 to 59 years	18 (26.5)	50 (73.5)	
> 60 years	20 (31.3)	44 (68.8)	
Not stated	7 (35.0)	13 (65.0)	
Body parts injured	221	390	0.887
Head	60 (36.8)	103 (63.2)	
Limbs	77 (38.0)	126 (62.1)	
Multiple trauma	22 (33.3)	44 (62.7)	
Body trunk	16 (30.8)	36 (69.2)	
No obvious injuries	35 (34.7)	66 (65.3)	
Neck injuries	11 (42.3)	15 (57.7)	
Not stated	19 (46.4)	22 (53.6)	
Level of consciousness	200	356	0.211
Alert	179 (37.5)	299 (62.6)	
Verbal	4 (25.0)	12 (75.0)	
Pain	9 (36.0)	16 (64.0)	
Unresponsive	8 (21.6)	29 (78.4)	
Not stated	35 (36.5)	61 (63.5)	
Survival	239	413	0.269
Dead	1 (12.5)	7 (87.5)	
Alive	238 (37.0)	406 (63.3)	

Table 2 Bivariate analysis between trauma survival and independent variables of pre-hospital trauma cases attended to in Greater Accra, 2014

Variables	Pre-hospital trauma Survival		*P*-values
	Died	Alive	
Level of consciousness			< 0.0001**
Responsive	3 (0.6)	516 (99.5)	
Unresponsive	5 (13.5)	32 (86.5)	
Response time			0.209
Based on 4 min			
< 4 min	0 (0.0)	155 (100)	
> 4 min	8 (1.6)	489 (98.4)	
Based on 8 min			0.269
< 8 min	1 (0.4)	238 (99.6)	
> 8 min	7 (1.7)	406 (98.3)	
Based on 17 min			0.003*
< 17 min	1 (0.3)	422 (99.8)	
> 17 min	7 (3.1)	222 (97.0)	
Types of injuries			1.00
Obvious	7 (1.8)	502 (98.7)	
Not obvious	1 (1.0)	100 (99.0)	
Time spent on scene[a]			0.183
< 10 min	0 (0.0)	197 (100)	
> 10 min	5 (1.2)	415 (98.8)	
Transportation time[a]			1.00
< 60 min	3 (0.9)	371 (99.2)	
> 60 min	2 (0.8)	235 (99.2)	
Age groups			0.175
> 15	1 (1.2)	84 (98.8)	
15 to 44	3 (0.7)	412 (99.3)	
45 to 59	2 (2.9)	67 (97.1)	
> 60	2 (3.1)	62 (96.9)	

[a]missing data
* - p<0.05, ** - p<0.001

Discussion

Our study sought to determine the pre-hospital trauma survival rate and response time to emergencies and its associated factors in the Greater Accra region, Ghana. Our findings revealed that, 98.8% of the cases attended to and transported to various facilities in the Greater Accra Region by NAS survived pre-hospital trauma. According to WHO, timely pre-hospital care can save lives [13]. EMTs at the scene of an emergency perform Basic Life Support skills such as controlling bleeding, oxygen administration and splinting which can lead to high patient survival. Lack of Pre-hospital care can lead to death from airway compromise, respiratory failure or uncontrolled bleeding. The common practice of commercial and private vehicles carrying trauma patients from

Table 3 Logistic Regression Analyses to Model Emergency Response Time as a Predictor for pre-hospital trauma Survival

Variables	Pre-hospital trauma survival		Crude odds ratio (95% Confidence Interval)	Adjusted odds Ratio (95% Confidence Interval)
	Died	Alive		
Level of consciousness				
Responsive	3 (0.6)	516 (99.5)	Ref	Ref
Unresponsive	5 (13.5)	32 (86.5)	26.8 (6.1–117.5)**	37.87 (6.0–239.2)**
Response time based on 17 min				
< 17 min	1 (0.3)	422 (99.8)	0 .08 (0.092–0.61)*	0.08 (0.009–0.59)*
> 17 min	7 (3.1)	222 (97.0)	Ref	Ref
Types of injuries				
Obvious	7 (1.8)	502 (98.7)	1.4 (0.18–63.4)	1.8 (0.16–19.7)
No obvious	1 (1.0)	100 (99.0)	Ref	Ref
Sex				
Male	3 (0.7)	445 (99.3)	0.33 (0.05–2.0)	4.6 (0.69–30.8)
Female	5 (2.0)	200 (98.0)	Ref	
Age	8 (1.3)	625 (98.7)	0.95 (0.92–0.98)	0.78 (0.30–2.03)

* - p<0.05, ** - p<0.001

accident scene to hospitals have resulted in the death of some patients. This is because these vehicle were not designed for that purpose and also the drivers lack the needed skills required at the accident scene.

Our study also found the average emergency response time for the region to be 16.9 min. This finding is very similar to the national average of 17 min recorded in NAS, 2013 annual report [14]. In Ghana, response time calculations are still based on estimating the mean response time. However, in many countries, emergency response time is estimated by calculating the proportion of ambulances that were able to respond to cases within 8 min. This is referred as fractal response time. In line with that, a suggested target response time of 8 min for at least 90% of emergency responses has become the guideline for many EMS providers worldwide [7]. This is to prevent extreme values from skewing the mean response time in their direction.

In line with fractile response time, England as at April 2015, had more than 75.6% life threatening cases responded to within 8 min [15]. These higher response times recorded are possibly due the fact that Accra is a city in developing country with a lot of traffic. Driving an ambulance through the traffic-laden city involves a lot of maneuvering. In addition, there are no dedicated emergency lanes for ambulances. These factors eventually increases the response time to emergency. Also, many road users do not obey traffic road regulations or are ignorant of them. These reasons could be contributory factors to the delay in the emergency response time. In order to achieve this national response time target, these situations need to be addressed to improve timely response to medical emergencies.

The median transportation time estimated was 82 min with a range 5 to 552 min. This means that after an incident occurs, it takes an ambulance approximately 82 min to get the case to the hospital. In trauma management, it is believed that the first one-hour after trauma incident is crucial to the patient getting to the emergency department in the hospital in order to improve patient outcome. This principle is usually termed as the golden hour guideline. The NAS is therefore not able to meet the golden hour guideline in trauma cases. Thus morbidity and mortality are likely to increase significantly since the injured person does not receive definitive care within 60 min of injury [16]. In our test of association, transportation time was however not significantly associated with pre-hospital trauma survival ($p > 0.05$). This is similar to a study conducted in Germany in 2012 which also found no significant association between survival advantage for trauma patients with shorter pre-hospital transportation times [17]. Another study in Pakistan assessing the trauma outcomes as a result of hospital transfers and delays in transport time also did not find a significant difference in mortality between patients who were presented within 60 min and those presented after 60 min of response times [18]. Shorter transportation times are therefore essential for the survival of trauma patients. From our study, this was however not found to be significantly associated with survival of trauma patients.

The median time spent on scene managing trauma patients was 17 min with minimum of 1 to maximum of 180 min. The platinum ten-minute guideline recommends that patients should be managed for a maximum of 10 min in trauma situations. Spending more than ten-minutes on the scene can lead to splinting patient to death. It is necessary to initiate transport and continue with treatment on the way to the hospital. The first 10 min is crucial in the management of patients. When the platinum 10 min is violated, it decreases the chances of survival [19]. However, from our study, 10 min spent on scene was not found to be associated with trauma survival ($p > 0.05$).

Our results further suggest that, the level of consciousness is significantly associated with pre-hospital trauma survival. The odds of surviving a pre-hospital trauma increased when a patient was conscious and alert. This confrims the findings of a study in Germany that concluded that patients with Glasgow Coma score of 3 (unresponsive patients) had a poor outcome and even with treatment only 5% of them had good recovery [20].

Response time of 8-min standard was not also significantly associated with trauma survival in our study ($p > 0.05$). We rather observed 17-min response time to be associated with trauma survival ($p < 0.05$). Since Ghana's current response time is 17 min, reducing the 17-min response time has the potential of improving pre-hospital survival. Blanchard and colleagues found that after controlling for several important confounders, such as severity of injury, age and sex, the response time standard of within 8 min was not associated with improved survival which supports our findings [6].

Limitations of the study

Ideally, response time would have been appropriately estimated as the time the accident occurred to the time the ambulance arrived at the scene. However, it was not possible to determine the exact response time, since the EMT was not present at the time of the accidents. We therefore estimated response time as the time between the call being made for the ambulance to the time the ambulance arrived at the scene. Also, distances corresponding to various transport times were not recorded on the PCR forms, which made it virtually impossible for us to factor in an important possible predictor like distance in the study. However, the location of the emergencies was indicated on the form and gave a fair idea of distance.

Conclusion

There is a high trauma patient's survival rate among victims of accident attended to by the Ghana National Ambulance Service. The average response time in Greater Accra region in the 14 ambulance stations is 16.9 min which is not different from the 17 min recorded in 2013 by NAS. Factors that were associated with pre-hospital survival were alertness in the level of consciousness and response time less than 17 min. NAS should put in measures to reduce the response time and also put in structures to measure fractal response time. Public education on how to reach an ambulance, what should be done when there is an emergency are some of the efforts that have been made to reduce the response time.

Abbreviations

CPR: Cardiopulmonary Resuscitation; EMS: Emergency Medical Service; EMT: Emergency Medical Technician; NAS: National Ambulance Service; PCR: Pre-hospital Care forms; RTC: Road Traffic Crashes; WHO: World Health Organization

Acknowledgements

We would like to acknowledge Christana Aching Boatema, Michael Kwesi Badu, Puala Beeri and Dr. Joseph Atia Akamah for their assistance with data extraction and in other areas of the project.

Funding

The first author funded the project.

Authors' contributions

M-NM and EK conceptualized the idea. M-NM collected data, did the analysis and wrote the draft manuscript. DB reviewed the manuscript and edited come out with the final manuscript. ANZ and EK reviewed the completed manuscript and made intellectual inputs. All authors read and approved the final manuscript.

Competing interest

The authors declare that they have no competing interests.

Author details

[1]National Ambulance Service, Accra, Ghana. [2]Ghana Field Epidemiology and Laboratory Training Program, Department of Epidemiology, School of Public Health, University of Ghana, Accra, Ghana.

References

1. Bigdeli M, Khorasani-zavareh D, Mohammadi R. Pre-hospital care time intervals among victims of road traffic injuries in Iran . A cross-sectional study. BMC Public Health. 2010;10:406. https://doi.org/10.1186/1471-10-406.
2. Mould-Millman N, Sasser SM, Wallis LA. Prehospital Research in Sub-Saharan Africa: Establishing Research Tenets; 2013. p. 1304–9. https://doi.org/10.1111/acem.12269
3. National Road Safety Commission. National Road Saftey Commission Report. Accra Ghana: NRSC; 2012.
4. Hamilton H, Hamilton H, Hodge SD, Hodge SD. Trauma, Emergency Medicine, And The Golden Hour. Pract Litig. 2011;1609:25–38.
5. Ogunmola JO, Oladosu YO, Drolamoyegun MA, Drayodele L. Mortality Pattern in Adult Accident and Emergency Department of a Tertiary Health Centre situated in a Rural Area of Developing Country. IOSR J Den Med Sci. 2013;5(2):12–5.
6. Blanchard IE, Doig CJ, Hagel BE, Anton AR, Zygun DA, Kortbeek JB, et al. Emergency medical services response time and mortality in an Urban setting. Prehosp Emerg Care. 2012;16(1):142–51 https://doi.org/10.3109/10903127.2011.614046.
7. The National Highway Traffic Safety Adminstration, National EMS Scope Of Practice Model. (2007).Washington Available: https://www.ems.gov/education/EMSScope.pdf. Accessed 15 June 2015.
8. National Ambulance Service. Annual Report, NAS 2014. Ghana: Accra; 2014.
9. Gonzalez RP, Cummings DM, Phelan H, Mulekar MS, Rodning CB. Does increased emergency medical services prehospital time affect patient mortality in rural motor vehicle crash ? A statewide analysis. AJS. 2009;197(1):30–4 https://doi.org/10.1016/j.amjsurg.2007.11.018.
10. Fischer AJ, O'Halloran PO, Littlejohns P, Kennedy A, Buston G. Ambulance Economics. J Public Health Med. 2000;22(3):pp413–21.
11. Stein C, Wallis L, Adetunji O. Meeting national response time targets for priority 1 incidents in an urban emergency medical services system in South Africa: More ambulances won't help. S Afr Med J. 2015;105(10):840–4. https://doi.org/10.7196/SAMJnew.8087.

12. Eisenberg M, Bergner L, Hallstrom A. Cardiac resuscitation in the community. Importance of rapid provision and implications for program planning. JAMA. 1979;241(18):1905–7.
13. WHO. World report on road traffic injury prevention: summary. Geneva: WHO Library Cataloguing-in-Publication Data; 2004.
14. Ghana National Ambulance Service. National Ambulance Service Anual Report. Accra: Ghana National Ambulance Service; 2013.
15. Turner N. Emergency Ambulance Services In England. (2015). NHS Support Fedaration Available from: http://www.nhsforsale.info/uploads/images/ambulance_report_low_res_july27.pdf. Accessed 10 Sept 2016.
16. Rogers FB, Rittenhouse K. The Golden Hour in Trauma: Dogma or Medical Folklore? J Lancaster Gen Hosp. 2014;9(1):11–3.
17. Kleber C, Giesecke MT, Tsokos M, Haas NP, Schaser KD, Stefan P, et al. Overall distribution of trauma-related deaths in Berlin 2010: advancement of stagnation. World J Surg. 2012;36(9):2125–30.
18. Khan A, Zafar H, Naeem SN, Raza SA. Transfer delay and in-hospital mortality of trauma patients in Pakistan. Int J Surg. 2010;8(2):155–8. https://doi.org/10.1016/j.ijsu.2009.10.012.
19. Bukowski MCW. The PLATINUM 10 2nd BCT, 101st Airborne Improves Medidical Training to Help Save Lives. Infantry Pressional Forum. 2006;2006:11–5.
20. Nijboer JM, van der Naalt J, ten Duis HJ. Patients beyond salvation? Various categories of trauma patients with a minimal Glasgow coma score. Injury. 2010;41(1):52–7. https://doi.org/10.1016/j.injury.2009.05.030.

22

Emergency and disaster management training; knowledge and attitude of Yemeni health professionals

Waheeb Nasr Naser[1*] and Huda Ba Saleem[2]

Abstract

Background: Medical professionals together with other first responder teams are the first to attend an emergency or disaster. Knowledge and training in emergency and disaster preparedness are important in responding effectively. This study aims to assess the current knowledge, attitude and training in emergency and disaster preparedness among Yemeni health professionals.

Method: A descriptive, cross-sectional, non-probability based study was conducted in Yemen using self-reported on-line and paper surveys in 2017. A total of 531 health professionals responded. The Chi-Square test was used to identify any significant difference in the knowledge and attitude of the professional categories. The p-value of <0.05 was used as a statistical significant.

Results: The overall knowledge status of Yemeni health professionals was insufficient with regards to emergency and disaster preparedness. Of all respondents, 32.0% had good knowledge, 53.5% had fair and 14.5% exhibited poor knowledge. The educational level was a key factor in the knowledge gap amongst respondents. Regardless of the period of experience, postgraduate staff were more knowledgeable than graduates. Physicians were better in knowledge than other subgroups of health specialties. Health administrators seemed insufficiently qualified in emergency and disaster planning. Medical teachers performed better in responding to knowledge test than managers. However, the majority of study respondents appeared in the 'positive attitudes' level to emergency and disaster preparedness. 41.0% of all respondents had received no courses in disaster preparedness. The trained staff used NGOs, and online-related programs more frequently for learning disaster planning (15.7%, and 13.6%) respectively. In contrast, formal resources such as MoPHP, health facility, medical schooling programs were used by (10.2%, 9.6, and 7.3%) of respondents, respectively. 58.9% of respondents had not participated in any exercise in emergency and disaster preparedness. Of all respondents, triage and mass causality response exercises were attended by only (13.5%, and 9.7%) respectively.

Conclusion: The absence of teaching programs is a major issue in the lack of knowledge of health professionals regarding disaster preparedness. Thus, emergency and disaster preparedness has to be included in the primary medical school curricula and continuing medical education programs of the health facilities. Long-term formal training such as undergraduate and postgraduate programs is necessary. Operational simulations enrolled key personnel of multi-agencies focus on an organizational training rather than individual based training are recommended.

Keywords: Training, Knowledge, Attitude, Emergencies, Disaster management, Health professionals, Yemen

* Correspondence: waheeb_nasr@yahoo.com
[1]King Khalid Hospital Najran, King Abdul-Aziz Road, Najran, Kingdom of Saudi Arabia
Full list of author information is available at the end of the article

Background

A disaster is a situation or event which overwhelms local capacity, necessitating a request to a national or international level for external assistance [1]. Global reports show that disasters are usually associated with a serious physical, mental, environmental and economic crisis to the affected vulnerable population [2–5]. Yemen is a disaster-prone country, with flooding being the main natural disaster [6]. Over the past several decades, due to poverty, social unrest, and civil conflicts, Yemen has experienced many human impact related emergencies. Recently, the huge complex humanitarian crisis caused by the ongoing war has left thousands killed or injured in this country [7].

Additionally, Yemen's population has faced the world's worst cholera outbreak [8, 9]. According to WHO, the country has been hit by two epidemic waves since October 2016 to the end of February 2018. The reported cumulative number of cholera cases is 1,097,735 including 2,392 related deaths with a case fatality rate of 0.22% [9]. In 2017, an Inter-Agency Standing Committee (IASC) in collaboration with the European Commission based on the physical exposure, vulnerability and the socio-economic status of the country ranked Yemen with a Risk Index 7.6 of 10. (INFORM) a measure of risk management to disaster and humanitarian crisis [10].

At the time of response to disasters and emergencies, the priority is to help, support and treat the victims; to save lives. Therefore, disaster relief and assistance are mainly carried out by rescue or emergency medical teams [11]. Moreover, when an emergency event such as fire occurs for instance; within the health facility, medical professionals will be on the frontline. Thus, they must be knowledgeable in disaster management and able to respond effectively to any disaster and emergency crisis. Education and training are necessary for health professionals to gain knowledge and develop the skills that make an effective response to disaster and emergency possible [12]. However, the lack of training programs in disaster preparedness was one of the main issues contributing to the negative outcomes of two regional studies on Yemen assessing hospital disaster preparedness [13, 14].

To the best of our knowledge, there has never been a national study carried out in Yemen evaluating the knowledge, attitude and training of health professional's towards disaster management. Therefore, the main aim of this study is to assess the above issues.

Other specific objectives of the study are as follows:

1. To find out the training courses in emergency and disaster medicine attended by Yemeni health professionals.
2. To ascertain common hazards that might cause disasters or emergencies on the local and national level.
3. To highlight the necessary educational and training programs that might help policymakers to improve emergency and disaster management.

Methods

Study design

This is a descriptive and cross-sectional study carried out in May through June 2017 using a self-reported survey of both web and paper form questionnaires.

Study setting

The setting of this study is the Republic of Yemen. Five main governorates were purposefully selected for an on-site visit to collect the data using a paper survey. These include the capital Sana'a, Aden, Hadramout, Shabwa and Lahj governorates. The authors assumed that if any training programs and more knowledgeable staff could be found they would be in the main cities; Sana'a and Aden, where most of the teaching institutions and university hospitals are sited. Hence, over 50% of papers were distributed in those two cities. The on-site visits targeted both governmental and private hospitals as well as ambulance rescue points.

In order to expand the sample, and bearing in mind time limitations, funding and safety concerns related to the ongoing war, authors used an online survey to collect additional data from other governorates where possible. Moreover, the circulated online survey helped to reach to a wide range of eligible participants from other non-visited facilities or agencies such as primary health care centres, health authorities and non-governmental organizations (NGOs).

Study population

The targeted subjects were the health professionals who provide health care to the Yemeni people at the time of the study under the auspices of the Ministry of Public Health and Population (MoPHP) of Yemen. The enrolled subjects were categorized based on educational level, professional career, specialty, type of facility, the period of experience and workplace and used as independent variables.

Sample

A non-probability purposive sampling technique was used in selecting the samples. The total number of the targeted population was assumed unknown. Therefore, we used the Daniel formula to estimate the minimum sample size for the study [15, 16]. Where (p) a value of expected proportion considered as 50%, (z) the confidence interval of 95%, (d) an error of deviation of 5 % and the calculated minimum sample size was 384.

$$n = \frac{z^2\, p(1-p)}{d^2}$$

Study Tool

Two types of self-reported questionnaires were used; a paper survey and an online survey of google drive. Authors developed the tool after an extensive search of relevant literature of similar studies [17–22]. To our knowledge, disaster medicine and training are still not included in the programs of MoPHP of Yemen. Furthermore, studies reported that neither an incident command centre nor an emergency plan has yet been implemented in Yemen's health facilities. [13, 14]. Therefore, the questionnaires were designed to outline the basic principles of disaster management stages such as mitigation, preparedness and response.

The questionnaire consists of 28 items of both structured and open-ended questions, and divides into six sections as follows; 1) an introduction: describes the purpose of the study and illustrates how to answer the questions. 2) Knowledge test: includes 11 items of correct and incorrect questions. 3) Attitude test: includes six items of 3 points Likert scale questions (agree, disagree and not sure). 4) Training and practice: consists of three items of multiple choice questions. 5) Anticipated disasters: consists of two items of multiple chooses questions. 6) Demographic data: consists of six categories: an educational level, professional career, specialty, facility, the period of experience and workplace. The majority of Yemeni staff use the Arabic language; hence, the tool was made both in English and Arabic to simplify an item's meanings. Furthermore, to test the tool validity before use, a pilot study was conducted on 50-health personnel. It was excluded from the main data. The authors used the feedback from the pilot study respondents to revise the questionnaire content.

Data collection

Before the start, data collectors were trained in how to clarify respondent's enquiries about the questions content. In addition to a list of emails and mobile numbers that were assembled from the contact list in some hospitals, the authors used WhatsApp, Facebook messenger, and groups to distribute the online survey to other professional colleagues and texted mobile messages to those not using these applications. The online survey link sent through email, mobile numbers and social media groups of the health personnel was left open for two months.

Within the web survey timeline, the paper survey was distributed to the health facilities of the selected cities as enumerated above. All non-medical profession and non-health administrative staff, as well as the piloting respondents, were excluded from this evaluation. Furthermore, 27 of the online survey respondents were found to be non-health professionals and were therefore removed from the study sample. A total of 531 eligible responses were gathered within the timeline of the study; 300 responses to the paper survey, and 231 to a web survey.

Data analysis

The data collected from both survey types was compiled and then introduced into an Excel spreadsheet for coding. It was then transferred to the SPSS version 23 for analysis. Based on a similar study [19], the data was analyzed to get the final scores of the staff knowledge and attitude. In the knowledge test, the participants could get one score for each correctly answered question and zero for an incorrect answer. The maximum score was 11. Respondents with total correct scores of 9 or higher were graded "good," those with scores between 5 and 8 were graded "fair" and those with scores of 4 or less were graded as having "poor" knowledge. In the attitude test; each question with an 'agree' response was scored 5 marks and both 'disagree' and 'not sure' were scored 0, with the maximum score of 30. The final respondent's attitude was said to be positive if the respondent scored ≥15, and negative when a participant scored <15. Chi-square was used to compare the difference of knowledge and attitude status between the independent categorical variables. A p value of < 0.05 was used as a statistical significant cut off point. Other sections were analyzed by obtaining the frequencies and percentages.

Ethical issues

An official written consent to carry out the study was obtained from the Research and Ethical Committee of the Faculty of Medicine and the Health Sciences University of Aden. To avoid having different approaches of informed consent because we have an online and in place participants, Research Committee agreed on having verbal consent. Therefore, during the visits, verbal permission to question the staff was granted by the facility's administrators. Although the participation was voluntary, verbal consent was obtained from the respondents who were ensured the study was for educational purposes and the findings would be treated as facts.

Results

Demographic characteristic of the respondents

A total of 531 health professionals responded to the questionnaire. Of all respondents, 66.7% were graduates and 33.3% post-graduates. In respect to their position or career in the facility, around two-thirds were practitioners, 9.8% medical teachers and 16.0% managers. Of all respondents, only 6.4% were health administrators and the others were physicians and non-physician medical staff (mostly nurses) (50%, 44.6%) respectively. Around three-quarters of respondents were practicing in the public facilities and another was in private or non-profit facilities. One-half of all respondents had less than 5 years' experience, while the remaining had from 5-10 years or more than 10 years (33%, 17.5%) respectively. Of all cities enrolled in the current study, 26.6% of respondents were in Aden, 25.2% Sana'a and the remaining were from other governorates (Table 1).

Anticipated national and facility disasters

Violence due to either armed conflicts and/or terrorism was the major hazard concerning 41.3 % of subjects that might lead to mass casualty incidents, followed by pandemic, flood, earthquake (36.6%, 10.7, and 8.5%) respectively. While 2.2% of respondents were expecting other threats such as transportation accidents, drought and famine; 0.7% cited no risk Fig. 1a. A shortage of medical supplies is the main threat that might cause a hospital emergency crisis. It was ticked by 41.26% of respondents. Communication failure, fire, structural collapse was 21.4%, 19.9, and 10.2% respectively. 3.4% of respondents expected other potential hazards, such as chemical spillage or security threats, and 3.9% said no risks Fig. 1b.

Table 1 The demographic characteristics of respondents

Variable	Frequency	Percentage
Educational level		
Post graduate	177	33.3
Graduate	354	66.7
Professional Career		
Medical teacher	52	9.8
Practitioner	394	74.2
Manager	85	16.0
Specialty		
Physician	260	49.0
Non-physician medical staff[a]	237	44.6
Health administrator	34	6.4
Facility		
Governmental facility	403	75.9
Non-governmental facility	128	24.1
Experience		
Less than 5 years	263	49.5
5-10 y	175	33.0
More than 10 y	93	17.5
Workplace		
Sana'a	134	25.2
Aden	141	26.6
Hadramout	60	11.3
Taiz	34	6.4
Lahj	41	7.7
Abyan	32	6.0
Shabwa	44	8.3
Other	45	8.5

[a]Non-physician medical staff such as nurses, paramedics, technicians, pharmacists

Training in disaster medicine

Media was the frequent informative source for disasters and emergencies in more than one-third of the study population (35.9%). The facility, schooling lessons, MoPHP and NGO related programs were indicated by 15.2%, 14.7, 14%, and 12.4% respectively. Self-reading was the source of information for 3.9% of participants. A negligible number had no source (3.5%).

Of the study sample, 41.0% had not been taught disaster planning. Amongst those who had been taught, NGOs were the main learning source (15.7%) followed by online programs (13.6%). MoPHP, health facility related programs and schooling lessons accounted for 10.2%, 9.6, and 7.3% respectively. Additionally, 2.5% of participants used others ways of learning such as such self-study Fig. 2a. More than half of enrolled health professionals (58.9%) had not received any training courses in emergency and disaster preparedness. The remainder had received courses in triage, mass causality responses, fire responses and evacuation drills (13.5, 9.7, 7.6, 7.3%) respectively. Other courses such as first aid and infection control workshops were cited by 2.9% Fig. 2b.

Disaster knowledge

Table 2 depicts the correct answer rates to the 11 knowledge questions (Q1-Q11). Overall, about one-third of participants (32.0%) had good knowledge, while the others had fair or poor knowledge in disaster management (53.5%, and 14.5%) respectively Fig. 3a. Moreover, there was a significant difference ($p < 0.05$) in knowledge level between graduates and postgraduates. Postgraduates responded better to almost all knowledge test questions. As far as professional experience was concerned, there was no significant difference in the individual's knowledge level related to their level of experience Table 3.

With regards to professional specialties, there was a significant difference in eight items of the knowledge test ($p < 0.05$). Physicians represented better than health administrators while non-physician medical staff did not get any higher score than other specialty subgroups. Regarding professional career, there was no significant difference in knowledge status amongst the career subgroups except the medical teachers responded correctly to Q2, Q3, Q9 with ($p = < 0.05$). The other

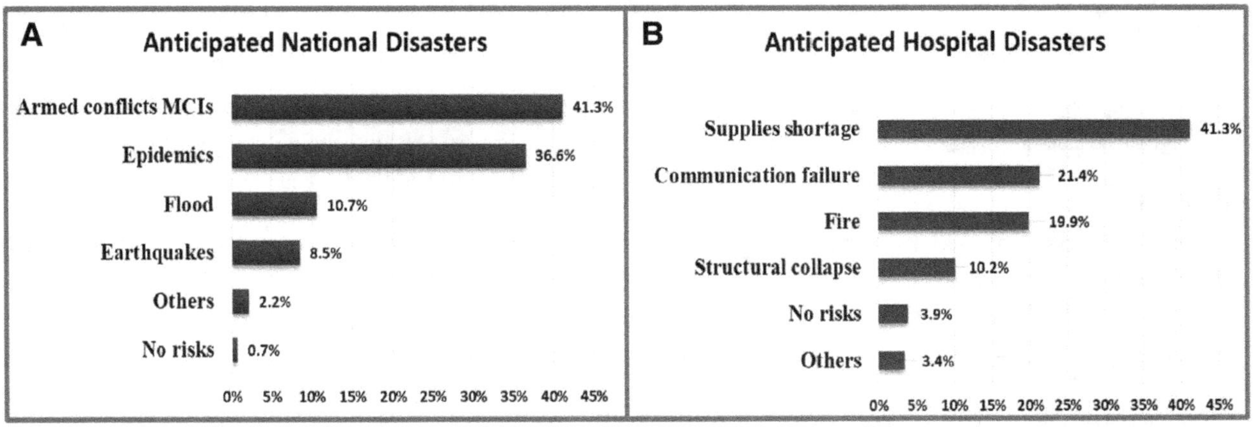

Fig. 1 The frequency of emergencies or disasters expected by the respondents. **a** National or local emergencies or disasters. **b** Hospital emergencies or disasters

questions had no significant difference between the career subgroups Table 4.

Attitude to disaster

Table 2 shows the agreed upon responses of study participants to the attitudes test (Q12-Q17). The study concluded that the respondent's attitude toward disaster management was generally positive. Of study participants, 84.9% agreed to the teaching of disaster management in the country (Q12). They want to have an emergency plan, to know their roles during the response to emergency events, as well as wanting to train on disaster planning Fig. 3b.

The findings also elicited that the level of attitude regarding disaster planning among the health professions was statistically different. Postgraduates agreed with most attitude questions compared to graduates ($p < 0.05$). The length of experience seemed to have no effect on the professional attitude towards disaster management. However, those who had worked a long time appeared slightly more eager for training and the implementation of an emergency plan in their workplaces Table 5.

Health administrators were interested in implementing simulation-training programs in their facilities. They considered that hands-on or field exercises and workshops were an appropriate method in disaster training rather than lectures and presentations ($p< 0.05$). Physicians preferred to know their role during disaster and emergency responses in their workplaces ($p < 0.05$). Among the careers, medical teachers appeared higher in attitude to disaster management, in terms of risk analysis, planning and committee supervision ($p < 0.05$). Leaders or managers were higher in attitude to hospital and field hands-on training Table 6.

Discussion

The present study aimed to ascertain the current knowledge, attitude and training attributes among Yemeni health professionals in relation to disaster management. The findings indicate that the overall knowledge level of the health professionals was insufficient and needed

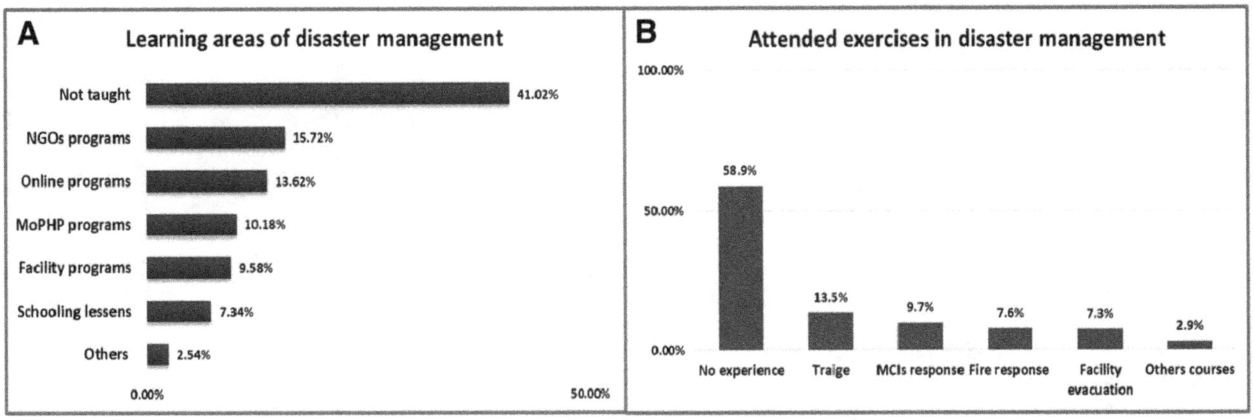

Fig. 2 Emergency and disaster management. **a** The learning sources used by respondents. **b** The exercises or workshops attended by respondents

Table 2 Knowledge and attitude of health professionals regarding emergency and disaster preparedness

Knowledge items	YES		NO
Have you heard about disaster?	501 (94.4)		30 (5.6)
Have you ever been taught about disaster planning?	256 (48.2)		275 (51.8)
Have ever performed a disaster drill(s) or workshop(s) in your facility or city?	166 (31.3)		365 (68.7)
A disaster is an imbalance between the demands that caused by an events and an available resources?	319 (60.1)		212 (39.9)
A disaster can occur either from natural or man-made causes?	377 (71.0)		154 (29.0)
Did you think, one day your country/city might be affected by disaster?	454 (85.5)		77 (14.5)
Did you think, one day your facility might be affected by disaster?	372 (70.1)		159 (29.9)
A disaster planning is to prepare to what might be needed to be done, how to be done, before and after disaster?	323 (60.8)		208 (39.2)
The surrounding hazards that most likely causing disaster to your facility most be identified and dealt with?	378 (71.2)		153 (28.8)
A disaster management it is includes both a health or non-health professional employees in the facility?	334 (62.9)		197 (37.1)
A disaster management it is an integral collaborative action of different agencies such as the hospitals, local health authority, civil defense and others?	347 (65.3)		184 (34.7)
Attitude items			
Training in disaster planning should be taught in your country	agree	disagree	No sure
Training in disaster planning is necessary in each health facilities.	451 (84.9)	24 (4.6)	56 (10.5)
It is necessary to have an emergency plan in your facility, city or country for any anticipated hazards.	438 (82.5)	26 (4.7)	67 (12.5)
It is necessary to have a disaster management committee in your facilities?	377 (71.0)	23 (4.3)	131 (24.7)
It is necessary to know your duty(s) and role(s) during disaster response in your facility.	340 (64.0)	35 (6.5)	156 (29.5)
To improve disaster management, is a training through the stimulation exercises, drills or workshops should be provided.	411 (77.4)	25 (4.7)	95 (17.9)

improvement. Only 32% of health professionals were knowledgeable about disaster management, with 53.5% and 14.5% expressing fair and poor knowledge respectively Fig. 3a.

This unsatisfactory outcome status was reported in some studies conducted worldwide for the same purpose [19, 20, 22–25]. For instance, studies conducted via a non-probability sampling method on selected tertiary hospitals in Lagos, Nigeria [19] and Nairobi, Kenya [20]. Healthcare and non-healthcare professionals in the hospitals were evaluated and the overall level of knowledge among the staff was 47.8% and 36% in Lagos and Nairobi

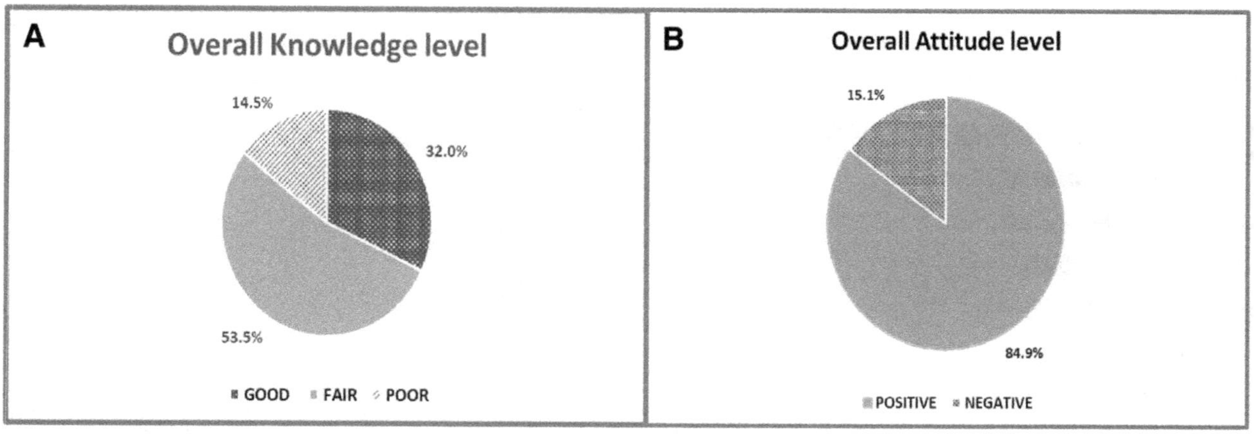

Fig. 3 The overall scores of the respondents toward emergency and disaster preparedness; **a** Knowledge status of the respondents. **b** The attitude level of the respondents

Table 3 Health professionals correctly answering the knowledge section test based on an educational and experience categories

Disaster knowledge related questions		Educational level				Experience period			
		Total	Graduate	Post graduate	*P* value	Less than 5 years	5 – 10 years	More than 10 years	*P* value
Q1	Background of disaster	501 (94.4)	331 (93.5)	170 (96.0)	0.232	249 (94.7)	167 (95.4)	85 (91.4)	0.376
Q2	Disaster planning background	256 (48.2)	140 (39.5)	116 (56.5)	< 0.001*	114 (43.3)	89 (50.9)	53 (57.0)	0.054
Q3	Disaster training background	166 (31.3)	92 (26.0)	74 (41.8)	< 0.001*	71 (27.0)	58 (33.5)	37 (39.8)	0.059
Q4	Disaster concept	319 (60.1)	201 (56.8)	118 (66.4)	0.028*	150 (57.0)	112 (64.0)	57 (61.3)	0.334
Q5	Sources of disaster	377 (70.1)	235 (66.4)	142 (80.2)	0.001*	176 (66.9)	134 (76.6)	67 (72.0)	0.090
Q6	Country vulnerability to disaster	454 (85.5)	287 (81.1)	167 (94.4)	< 0.001*	224 (85.2)	151 (86.3)	79 (84.9)	0.936
Q7	Facility vulnerability to disaster	372 (70.1)	233 (65.8)	139 (78.5)	0.003*	174 (66.2)	131 (74.9)	67 (72.0)	0.135
Q8	Concept of disaster planning	323 (60.8)	200 (56.5)	123 (69.5)	0.004*	151 (57.4)	113 (64.6)	59 (63.4)	0.275
Q9	Hazard vulnerability analysis	378 (71.2)	233 (65.8)	145 (81.9)	< 0.001*	169 (64.3)	130 (74.3)	79 (84.9)	< 0.001*
Q10	Response team	334 (62.9)	201 (56.8)	133 (75.1)	< 0.001*	155 (58.9)	117 (66.9)	62 (66.7)	0.173
Q11	Mutual collaboration	347 (65.3)	214 (60.4)	133 (75.1)	0.001*	160 (60.8)	127 (72.4)	60 (64.5)	0.040*

*Statistically significant

Table 4 Health professionals correctly answering the knowledge section test based on the specialty and professional career categories

Disaster knowledge related questions		Specialties					Career			
		Total	Physician	NPM staff$	Health Admin	*P* value	Medical Teacher	Practitioner	Managers	*P* value
Q1	Background of disaster	501 (94.4)	249 (95.8)	218 (92.0)	34 (100)	0.064	49 (94.2)	371 (94.2)	81 (95.3)	0.919
Q2	Background disaster planning	256 (48.2)	151 (58.1)	86 (36.3)	19 (55.9)	< 0.001*	35 (67.3)	175 (44.4)	46 (54.1)	0.004*
Q3	Background Disaster training	166 (31.3)	98 (37.7)	52 (21.9)	16 (47.1)	< 0.001*	22 (42.3)	112 (28.4)	32 (37.6)	0.049
Q4	Disaster concept	319 (60.1)	163 (62.7)	133 (56.1)	23 (67.6)	0.212	24 (46.2)	240 (60.9)	55 (64.7)	0.079
Q5	Sources of disaster	377 (71.0)	194 (74.6)	158 (66.7)	25 (73.5)	0.141	30 (57.7)	286 (72.6)	61 (71.8)	0.083
Q6	Country vulnerability to disaster	454 (85.5)	237 (91.1)	191 (80.6)	26 (76.4)	0.001*	47 (90.4)	334 (84.8)	73 (85.9)	0.555
Q7	Facility vulnerability to disaster	372 (70.1)	196 (75.4)	158 (66.7)	18 (52.9)	0.008*	43 (82.7)	272 (69.0)	57 (67.1)	0.104
Q8	Concept of disaster planning	323 (60.9)	177 (68.1)	122 (51.5)	24 (70.6)	< 0.001*	37 (71.2)	241 (61.2)	45 (52.9)	0.102
Q9	Hazard vulnerability analysis	378 (71.2)	199 (76.5)	153 (64.6)	26 (76.5)	0.010*	45 (86.5)	266 (67.5)	67 (78.8)	0.004*
Q10	Response team	334 (62.9)	185 (71.2)	126 (53.2)	23 (67.6)	< 0.001*	39 (75.0)	242 (61.4)	53 (62.4)	0.162
Q11	Mutual collaboration	345 (65.0)	185 (71.2)	141 (59.5)	21 (61.8)	0.022*	40 (76.9)	253 (64.2)	54 (63.5)	0.180

***Statistically significant, $ Non-physician medical staff**

Table 5 Health professionals agreed to an attitude section test based on their educational and experience level categories

	Disaster management attitude related questions	Educational level				Experience period			
		Total	Graduate	Post graduate	P value	Less than 5 years	5 - 10 years	More than 10 years	P value
Q12	Disaster training in country.	451 (84.9)	295 (83.4)	156 (88.1)	0.145	218 (82.9)	148 (84.6)	85 (91.4)	0.141
Q13	Disaster training in facility	438 (82.5)	284 (80.3)	154 (87.0)	0.053	211 (80.2)	149 (85.1)	78 (83.9)	0.385
Q14	Availability of emergency plan	377 (71.0)	241 (68.1)	136 (76.8)	0.036*	184 (70.0)	118 (67.4	75 (80.6)	0.066
Q15	Disaster management committee	340 (64.0)	209 (59.0)	131 (74.0)	0.001*	161 (61.2)	118 (67.4)	61 (65.6)	0.391
Q16	Roles and responsibility	411 (77.4)	265 (74.9)	146 (82.5)	0.048*	197 (74.9)	144 (82.3)	70 (75.3)	0.168
Q17	Hand on exercises vs lectures in disaster training	440 (82.9)	279 (78.8)	161 (90.9)	< 0.001*	203 (77.2)	152 (86.9)	85 (91.4)	0.002*

*statistically significant

respectively. A study in Shanghai, China [22] used a probability sampling for medical professionals and medical students and random sampling for community residents. Two different tools were conducted and it concluded that health professionals were more knowledgeable than medical students. Community residents displayed very poor knowledge. However, educational level showed statistical significance in their knowledge level towards disaster management. In Madinah, KSA [24], a study carried out on two batches of postgraduate nursing students with at least ten years prior working experience. The sample was obtained via a non-probability method and the findings revealed that the knowledge and training levels were below acceptable levels.

In contrast to the present results, international studies showed that staff had good enough knowledge regarding disaster management [25, 26]. Pre World Cup South Africa in 2010, a study conducted in a teaching tertiary hospital in Johannesburg [25] showed an overall acceptable knowledge base. Although the results were acceptable, it was recommended that there was room for improvement among the training staff. This came up despite the fact that staff undergo regular training courses in disaster management and the hospital had a disaster committee with an already implemented action plan for emergencies. In Mecca, Saudi Arabia, a non-probability based study targeted all registered nurses working in the emergency departments of all four public hospitals in Mecca [26]. Results showed that most emergency nurses appeared to be confident and knowledgeable about their roles in responding effectively to mass gathering disasters. However, their knowledge of other disaster types was still insufficient despite their frequent training in the hospitals. Thus, both hospital and university-based training programs were recommended.

In the current study, a significant difference in knowledge level was exhibited between postgraduates and graduates regardless of the length of experience. More than 90 % of responses to knowledge items presented were statistically different in relation to the educational level of the respondents. In contrary, more than 90 % of responses to knowledge test were not statistically different, based on the length of experience ($P < 0.05$) Table 3. It seems that graduated participants had limited exposure to training programs. One possible explanation for this is the lack of disaster training programs in medical schools and during the continuing medical education (CME) programs in the health facilities. On the

Table 6 Health professionals agreed to an attitude section test based on the specialty and professional career categories

	Disaster management attitude related questions	Total	Specialties				Career			
			Physician	NPM staff$	Health Admin	P value	Medical Teacher	Practitioner	Managers	P value
Q12	Disaster training in country.	451 (84.8)	223 (85.8)	196 (82.7)	32 (94.1)	0.191	47 (90.4)	335 (85.0)	69 (81.1)	0.342
Q13	Disaster training in facility	438 (82.5)	221 (85.0)	185 (78.1)	32 (94.1)	0.023*	44 (84.6)	322 (81.7)	72 (84.7)	0.773
Q14	Emergency plan	377 (71.0)	190 (73.1)	166 (70.0)	21 (61.8)	0.357	43 (82.7)	268 (68.0)	66 (77.6)	0.031*
Q15	Disaster management committee	340 (64.0)	178 (68.5)	142 (59.9)	20 (58.8)	0.113	41 (78.8)	240 (60.9)	59 (69.4)	0.021*
Q16	Roles and responsibility	441 (77.4)	212 (81.5)	180 (75.9)	19 (55.9)	0.003*	41 (78.8)	308 (78.2)	62 (72.9)	0.559
Q17	Hand on exercises vs lectures in disaster training	440 (82.9)	232 (89.2)	177 (74.7)	31 (91.2)	< 0.001*	47 (90.1)	316 (80.2)	77 (90.5)	0.022*

*statistically significant, $ Non-physician medical staff

other hand, findings showed that some programs were conducted for postgraduates. Nonetheless, the study did not specify whether the postgraduate programs were held within or outside the country. Therefore, this is still an issue that needs to be particularly addressed and further study is suggested.

Health administrators even with the good background to disaster and emergencies as reflected in Q1 and Q3, did not meet their expected proficiency in disaster management. They underestimated the risk analysis, the importance of the mutual aids and multidisciplinary collaboration role in disaster planning. Therefore, training programs in leadership skills might enhance the provision of health administrator's capacity with respect to disaster. Physicians enjoyed higher knowledge level than other specialties. In agreement with these findings, there was a study which reported a similar outcome [22]. Managers also displayed insufficient knowledge in disaster management especially in the related items (Q7, Q9, Q10, and Q11). Meanwhile, medical teachers in general, appeared knowledgeable when compared to the managers and practitioners. However, they appeared to have a misunderstanding of disaster concepts and origins (Q4, Q5) and this lag could be attributed to the lack of disaster medicine faculties and/or instructors.

We can argue that the main reason for a shortcoming in Yemeni health professional's knowledge regarding disaster management is the paucity of the formal training programs or lack of disaster medicine from the medical school curriculum. It explored merely some short-term courses focusing on specific disaster responses. Furthermore, 35.9% of the study subjects had heard about disaster from the media and only 14.7% through undergraduate school lessons. Moreover, only 41% of respondents had ever been trained in disaster medicine. Of those who had received training, a higher percentage 15.7% attended courses through NGOs and 13.6% through online programs compared to the negative role of formal institutions and facilities.

The present study revealed a positive attitude of respondents and exhibited their readiness to learn disaster management and desire to be prepared. These findings were reported in some international published studies [19, 21–25]. The respondents felt that their facilities should have an emergency plan with a disaster committee supervising the implementation of this plan. Furthermore, they should know their assignments when the plan has activated. The current study revealed a higher percentage of respondents agreeing that training is necessary for the country and in their facilities (84.8%, 82.5%) respectively. Moreover, 82.9 % confirmed that drills, workshops, or other simulations exercises must be conducted in their workplaces and they are perceived as being appropriate for disaster training.

In 1997, the Yemen government authorized the Supreme Council of Civil Defense (SCCD) of the Ministry of Interior to lead the disaster management in the country [27]. SCCD focused mainly on reactive responses and post-disaster relief [28]. In 2006, after a national flood disaster SCCD developed a national plan for emergencies and disasters, but it does not meet the needs. So there exists, a requirement for a national authority which will revise legislation and policies in regards to disaster management. The national authority should lead and oversee an emergency and disaster preparedness including training in the country.

Indeed, education and training are key elements of disaster preparedness [29]. Thus, for the strengthening of health professional's ability in regards to an emergency and disaster management, provision of formal educational programs is necessary. Long-term training programs that have a comprehensive curriculum are more standardized than short courses [30]. Government has to establish undergraduate or postgraduate degree-based courses on disaster medicine either inside the country or overseas on scholarships. Blended learning programs, a mix of online lectures and classroom discussions followed by hands-on field workshops, drills or large-scale exercises are suggested. Operational-based exercises incorporating the key personnel of multi-agencies, which focus on leadership skills, team collaboration, communication and resources allocation decision-making rather than individual based performance, are necessary.

Additionally, based on the study findings, traumatic MCIs are frequent events that could cause a burden to healthcare providers, particularly surgical teams. Therefore, field first responders have to be trained in incident command system (ICS) and mass causality triage [31]. Other courses such as basic and advanced disaster life support (BDLS, ADLS) and prehospital trauma life support (PHTLS), advanced trauma life support (ATLS) are to be considered.

The government has to enforce disaster-planning training as a part of the orientation and CME programs of each health facilities. Stakeholders have to establish an emergency HICS, and plan for any disaster that could happen. Furthermore, the staff must be trained regularly to enhance their performance in order to respond effectively to such disasters [32]. The community also has to be integrated to disaster management. Public awareness of disaster risks, effects, and response when disaster strikes are key to a community surviving [33]. Moreover, to support the formal response efforts in disaster response, the government has to launch training programs for public volunteers. For that, search, rescue, evacuation and basic first aids skills courses are suggested. Aftermath disaster, mental support of the stressed victims is important [4]. Thus, psychological first aid skills courses have to be considered. Finally, study findings reported that infectious casualties found a common issue facing healthcare providers in their workplaces; hence, providing training programs in infection control measures, personnel protective equipment (PPE), surveillance, early warning and case-tracking systems are a must.

Conclusion

A considerable number of Yemeni health professionals presented as 'unknowledgeable', with limited opportunities for training despite their beliefs towards disaster management. There was a gross lack of formal teaching and training programs in emergency and disaster medicine. Therefore, disaster-training programs are urgently needed, with specific emphasis on key personnel such as health administrators, facility managers, medical teachers, first responders and public health providers. It is recommended that disaster medicine be augmented either in the curriculum of undergraduate medical schools or in postgraduate university-based programs as well as in the continuing medical educations CME programs of MoPHP and health facilities of Yemen.

Limitations

Several limitations were met in the current study. One limitation was the interest of the community to such research and internet availability. These issues have been addressed; authors used both online and paper forms to get a large enough sample for the study. Another issue was the size and technique of sampling used since there was no available data to get comparable proportional figures of health professionals, the limited time, funding and unsafe access to cities due to the ongoing war. Thus, researchers used the non-probability purposive sampling, using both an online and paper surveys to collect a large amount of data and to generalize the survey to the unvisited provinces to minimize the selective bias as much as possible.

The generalizability of findings has taken in the author's concern. For the same reasons, all health professionals and provinces in Yemen will not get an equal chance to participate. Authors focused on the main urban cities i.e. Sana'a and Aden in addition to the feasible cities. Therefore, we can say the overall findings can reflect the current knowledge of the country. The origin of training among the taught respondents; was not specified in the questionnaire's items as to whether the training was held inside or outside the country. Thereby, it does not reflect the provided actual size of formal programs. Finally, the items' content of the questionnaire. Since there was no emergency plan applicable in all health facilities to be tested in this survey, the authors just included the basic principles in disaster management in the questionnaire.

Abbreviations

CME: Continuing Medical Educational; HICS: Hospital Incident Command System; ICS: Incident Command System; MCIs: Mass Causality Incidents; MoPHP: Ministry of Public Health and Population; NOGs: Non-Governmental Organizations; PHC: Primary Healthcare Centers; SCCD: Supreme Council of Civil Defense; WHO: World Health Organization

Acknowledgements

We would like to acknowledge and thank the study participants for their cooperation. A great appreciation to Associate Prof: Dr. Iman Ba Saddik, the Chairperson of Research and Ethical Committee of the Faculty of Medicine and Health Sciences, University of Aden. Great thanks also to Dr. Mohammad Alsabri, Dr. Galal Aleassai and Dr. Waleed Awad for their support and advice during setting the study. Deep gratitude goes to data Collectors, Dr. Bakeel Fadel, Dr Wegdan Ali, Dr. Muner Alshaikh and Mr Hafez Nasr.

Authors' contributions

WN conceived the study and developed the questionnaire. WN, HBS contributed in study concept and design. WN contributed in data acquisition, analysis and interpretation. HBS supervised the process of data analysis and interpretation. WN wrote the manuscript draft. HBS reviewed and approved the draft for publication. WN took the responsibility for the paper and drafted the manuscript. All authors read and approved the final manuscript.

Competing interests

The authors declare that they have no competing interests.

Author details

[1]King Khalid Hospital Najran, King Abdul-Aziz Road, Najran, Kingdom of Saudi Arabia. [2]Faculty of Medicine and Health Sciences, Aden University, Aden, Yemen.

References

1. Songer T. Epidemiology of Disasters. Definition of disaster. http://www.pitt.edu/~epi2170/lecture15/sld007.htm. Accessed 25 June 2017.
2. International Federation of Red Cross and Red Crescent Society. World Disasters Report 2014 – Data. http://www.ifrc.org/en/publications-and-reports/world-disasters-report/world-disasters-report-2014/world-disasters-report-2014%2D%2D-data/. Accessed 12 June 2017.
3. UNISDR. PreventionWeb. Yemen disaster and risk profile. http://www.preventionweb.net/countries/yem/data/. Accessed 26 May 2017.
4. Zhang Z, Wang W, Shi Z, et al. Mental Health Problems among the Survivors in the Hard-Hit Areas of the Yushu Earthquake. PLoS ONE. 2012; 7(10):e46449. https://doi.org/10.1371/journal.pone.0046449.
5. Pietrzak RH, Tracy M, Galea S, et al. Resilience in the Face of Disaster: Prevalence and Longitudinal Course of Mental Disorders following Hurricane Ike. PLoS ONE. 2012;7(6):e38964. https://doi.org/10.1371/journal.pone.0038964.
6. World Bank Group. Climate Portal. Yemen Dashboard Natural Hazards 2016. http://sdwebx.worldbank.org/climateportalb/home.cfm?page=country_profile&CCode=YEM&ThisTab=NaturalHazards. Accessed 26 May 2017.
7. World Health Organization. Yemen: Snap Shot of Health Facilities based Reported Deaths and Injuries. 19 March 2015 - 15 July 2017 http://applications.emro.who.int/docs/YEM/COPub_YEM_2017_19865_EN.pdf?ua=1. Accessed 20 Mar 2018.
8. World Health Organization. Media center. http://www.who.int/mediacentre/news/releases/2017/cholera-yemen-mark/en/. Accessed 19 Mar 2018.
9. World Health Organization. Regional Office for Eastern Mediterranean. http://www.emro.who.int/images/stories/zoonoses/Cholera_situation_update_Yemen_February_2018.pdf?ua=1. Accessed 19 Mar 2018.
10. INFORM 2017 Risk Index. Yemen disaster and risk profile. Prevention web. http://www.preventionweb.net/countries/yem/data/. Accessed 10 July 2017.

11. You C, Chen X, Yao L. How China responded to the May 2008 Earthquake during the emergency and rescue period. J Public Health Policy. 2009;30:379–93.
12. Ingrassia PL, Foletti M, Djalali A, Scarone P, Ragazzoni L, et al. Education and training initiatives for crisis management in the European Union:a web-based analysis of available programs. Prehospital Disaster Med. 2014;29(2): 115–26. https://doi.org/10.1017/S1049023X14000235.
13. Naser WN, Ingrassia PL, Aladhrae S, Abulraheem WA. A Study of Hospital Disaster Preparedness in South Yemen. Prehosp and Disaster Med J. 2018;19 https://doi.org/10.1017/S1049023X18000158
14. Aladhrai SA, Corte FD, Dejalali A, Ingrassia PL, et al. An Impact of the 2011 Revolution on Hospital Disaster Preparedness in Yemen. Disaster Med Public Health Prep. 2015;9(4):396–402.
15. Naing L, Winn T, Rusli BN. Practical Issues in Calculating the Sample Size for Prevalence Studies. Arch Orofac Sci. 2006;1:9–14.
16. Daniel WW. Biostatistics: A Foundation for Analysis in the Health Sciences. 7th ed. New York: Wiley; 1999.
17. Dykema J, Elver K, Schaeffer NC, et al. Survey fundamentals. A guide to designing and implementing surveys. Office of Quality Improvement, University of Wisconsin System Board of Regents, Madison, US. 2010. http://www.quality.wisc.edu.
18. Ozmen F. The level of preparedness of the schools for disasters from the aspect of the school principals. Elazig, Turkey. Disaster Prev Manag. 2006;15:383–95.
19. Adenekan BA, Balogun MR, Inem V. Knowledge, attitude, and practices of emergency health workers toward emergency preparedness and management in two hospitals in Lagos. J Clin Sci. 2016;13:23–8.
20. Kiongo J. Disaster preparedness among members of staff at Kenyatta national hospital, Nairobi County, Kenya. 2015.
21. Moabi R. Knowledge, attitudes and practices of health care workers regarding disaster preparedness at Johannesburg hospital in Gauteng province, South Africa. Nov. 25, 2008.
22. Su T, Han X, Chen F, Du Y, Zhang H, et al. Knowledge Levels and Training Needs of Disaster Medicine among Health Professionals, Medical Students, and Local Residents in Shanghai, China. PLoS ONE. 2013;8(6):e67041.
23. Berhanu B, Abrha H, Ejigu Y, et al. Knowledge, Experiences and Training Needs of Health Professionals about Disaster Preparedness and Response in Southwest Ethiopia: a cross sectional study. Ethiop J Health Sci. 2016;26(5):415–26.
24. Ibrahim FA. Nurses Knowledge, Attitudes, Practices and Familiarity Regarding Disaster and Emergency Preparedness–Saudi Arabia. Am J Nurs Sci. 2014;3(2):18–25. https://doi.org/10.11648/j.ajns.20140302.12.
25. Ahayalimudin N, Ismail A, Saiboon IM. Disaster management: a study on knowledge, attitude and practice of emergency nurse and community health nurse. BMC Public Health. 2012;12(Suppl 2):A3. https://doi.org/10.1186/1471-2458-12-S2-A3.
26. Alzahrani F, Kyratsis Y. Emergency nurse disaster preparedness during mass gatherings: a cross-sectional survey of emergency nurses' perceptions in hospitals in Mecca, Saudi Arabia. BMJ Open. 2017;7:e013563. https://doi.org/10.1136/bmjopen-2016-013563.
27. Rep. of Yemen, Ministry of Interior. Supreme Council of Civil Defense. Disaster management Unit. National Emergency Plan 2006. Sana'a, Yemen.
28. Global Facility for Disaster Reduction and Recovery. Country profile. Yemen 2015.https://www.gfdrr.org/sites/default/files/publication/country-profile-2016-yemen.pdf. Accessed 27 Mar 2018.
29. Daily E, Padjen P, Birnbaum M. A review of competencies developed for disaster healthcare providers: limitations of current processes and applicability. Prehospital and Disaster Med. 2010;25(5):387–95.
30. Peleg K, Michaelson M, Shapira SC, Aharonson-Daniel L. Principles of Emergency Management in Disasters. Adv Ren Replace Ther J. 2003;10(2): 117–21. https://doi.org/10.1053/jarr.2003.50019.
31. Algaali KYA, Djalali A, Della Corte F, Ismail MA, Ingrassia PL. Postgraduate education in disaster health and medicine. Front Public Health. 2015;3:185. https://doi.org/10.3389/fpubh.2015.00185.
32. Lynn M, Gurr D, Memon A, et al. Management of conventional mass casualty incidents: ten commandments for hospital planning. J Burn Care Res. 2006;27(5):649–58.
33. United Nations International Strategy for Disaster Reduction. Hyogo Framework for Action 2005–2015: Building the resilience of nations and communities to disasters (HFA). Kobe: UNISDR; 2005.

23

Pain score, desire for pain treatment and effect on pain satisfaction in the emergency department

Judith E. van Zanden[1*], Susanne Wagenaar[1], Jozine M. ter Maaten[2], Jan C. ter Maaten[1] and Jack J. M. Ligtenberg[1]

Abstract

Background: Pain management in the Emergency Department has often been described as inadequate, despite proven benefits of pain treatment protocols. The aim of this study was to investigate the effectiveness of our current pain protocol on pain score and patient satisfaction whilst taking the patients' wishes for analgesia into account.

Methods: We conducted a 10-day prospective observational study in the Emergency Department. Demographics, pain characteristics, Numeric Rating Scale pain scores and the desire for analgesics were noted upon arrival at the Emergency Department. A second Numeric Rating Scale pain score and the level of patient satisfaction were noted 75–90 min after receiving analgesics. Student T-tests, Mann-Whitney U tests and Kruskall-Wallis tests were used to compare outcomes between patients desiring vs. not desiring analgesics or patients receiving vs. not receiving analgesics. Univariate and multivariate logistic regression models were used to investigate associations between potential predictors and outcomes.

Results: In this study 334 patients in pain were enrolled, of which 43.7% desired analgesics. Initial pain score was the only significant predictive factor for desiring analgesia, and differed between patients desiring (7.01) and not desiring analgesics (5.14). Patients receiving analgesics (52.1%) had a greater decrease in pain score than patients who did not receive analgesics (2.41 vs. 0.94). Within the group that did not receive analgesics there was no difference in satisfaction score between patients desiring and not desiring analgesics (7.48 vs. 7.54). Patients receiving analgesics expressed a higher satisfaction score than patients not receiving analgesics (8.10 vs. 7.53).

Conclusions: This study pointed out that more than half of the patients in pain entering the Emergency Department did not desire analgesics. In patients receiving analgesics, our pain protocol has shown to adequately treat pain, leading to a higher satisfaction for emergency health-care at discharge. This study emphasizes the importance of questioning pain score and desire for analgesics to prevent incorrect conclusions of inadequate pain management, as described in previous studies.

Keywords: Pain management, Emergency department, Oligoanalgesia, Pain satisfaction, Numeric rating scale

* Correspondence: j.e.van.zanden@umcg.nl
[1]Department of Emergency Medicine, University of Groningen, University Medical Center Groningen, Groningen, The Netherlands
Full list of author information is available at the end of the article

Background

As pain is a common complaint of patients visiting the Emergency Department (ED) [1], its early recognition and appropriate treatment is important. Experience of pain is one of the criteria on which quality of care in the ED is reviewed and a key factor in preventing unintentional, avoidable harm.

Since Marks and Sachar published a landmark paper about undertreatment of pain in the ED [2], this became a frequently investigated subject. The benefits of pain treatment protocols have been proven [3], yet pain management in the ED has often been described as inadequate [1, 4, 5]. This raises the question whether undertreatment of pain is caused by inadequate adherence to pain protocols, or, that 'oligoanalgesia' – a term to describe the phenomenon of undertreatment of pain – is overstated, as Green postulated in the Annals of Emergency Medicine [6]. Another question is whether pain should always be treated, given the fact that not all patients in pain desire analgesics [7, 8]. To our knowledge, a prospective study on the effects of protocolized pain treatment on pain score and patient satisfaction, while taking desire for analgesics into account, has not been previously published.

The main goal of our study was to prospectively investigate the effectiveness of our current pain protocol on pain score and patient satisfaction in our ED; the desire for analgesia by the patient is hereby taken into account. 'Effectiveness' of pain treatment was defined as a decrease in pain score and increased level of satisfaction with care. A pain score reduction of > 2 Numeric Rating Scale (NRS) was considered clinically relevant [9, 10]. Secondary goals were to evaluate arguments for refusing analgesics and reasons for not receiving analgesics, despite patients' expressed desire for pain relief. We hypothesized that patients receiving analgesics would have a stronger decrease in pain score and a higher score of patient satisfaction compared to patients who did not receive analgesics.

Methods

This study had a prospective, observational design and was conducted at the ED of the University Medical Center Groningen (UMCG). The ED of this tertiary teaching hospital has an annual volume of approximately 32.000 patients, of which around 22.000 are estimated to be non-trauma patients. At the onset of the study, an analgesic protocol was present in the ED (Fig. 1). Data was obtained by study personnel filling out a comprehensive questionnaire for patients > 18 years old visiting the ED. This study was approved by the institutional review board of the UMCG. All patients signed the informed consent to participate in this study.

All patients with complaints of recent pain (< 3 months) were questioned. Exclusion criteria were patients < 18 years, no recent pain (< 3 months), patients in a life-threatening situation, patients with impaired mental status or neuropsychiatric diseases leading to inability to fill in the questionnaire (e.g. patients suffering from delirium, dementia or psychosis), a language barrier or absence of informed consent.

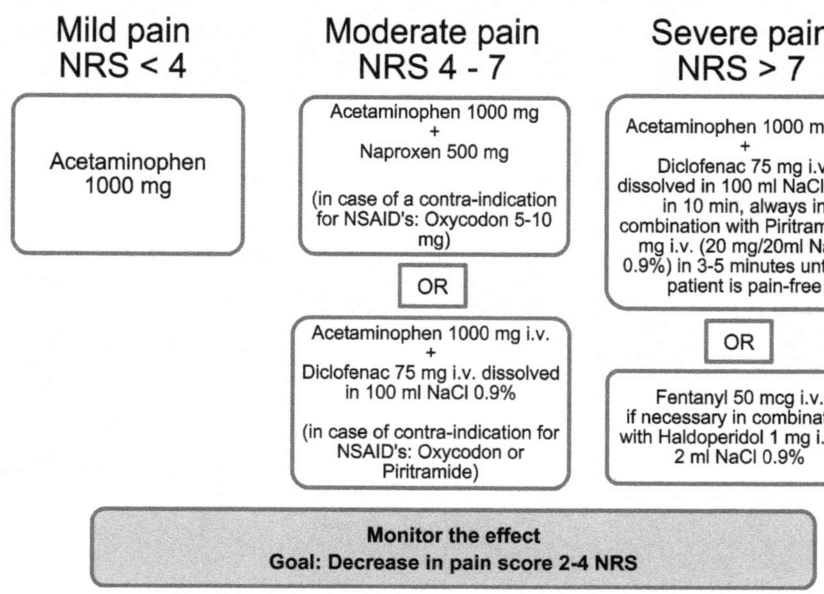

Fig. 1 The University Medical Center Groningen pain protocol

We used a manual questionnaire for a continuous period of 10 days, 24 h a day, to collect data for every patient visiting the ED.

During their stay, all patients were questioned twice. Immediately after triage of the patient, data was collected on demographics (age, sex), triage colour code (Table 1), allergy for analgesics, medical specialty of referral, pain characteristics (location, duration, type and character of pain) and pain score at that time, using the Numeric Rating Scale, ranging from 0 (no pain) to 10 (worst pain the patient can imagine). We checked whether the patient had already received analgesics before arriving at the hospital, e.g. self-medication or analgesics given by the general physician or ambulance staff. Furthermore, we asked whether the patient desired pain management. In case there was no desire for analgesics, the patient was asked about the reason. The second part of the questionnaire was filled in 75–90 min after taking the initial questionnaire. First, we checked if the patient had received analgesics in the ED and the type and dose of analgesics given. An analgesic was defined as any drug prescribed with the aim to reduce pain, such as acetaminophen, nonsteroidal anti-inflammatory drugs (NSAID) and opioids, as described in the analgesic ladder of the World Health Organization (WHO) [11]. Besides that, in accordance with previous articles published on this subject, drugs having a possible indirect effect on pain level were also included. Those were nitroglycerin for chest pain, proton pump inhibitors (PPI) for abdominal pain and benzodiazepines [7, 8]. If the patient did not receive any analgesics but had previously indicated a desire to receive analgesics, we asked the patient and the nurse why analgesics were not administered. The patient was asked again to rate pain severity on the Numeric Rating Scale. Lastly, the patient was asked to express their satisfaction on how their entire pain management was executed, rated on a Numeric Rating Scale, ranging from 0 (very dissatisfied) to 10 (very satisfied).

Primary outcomes were change in pain score and patient satisfaction score. Secondary outcomes were reasons to refuse analgesics and identifying why patients did not receive analgesics, despite desire for pain relief.

Table 1 Triage colour code, as used in the University Medical Center Groningen

Urgency	Name	Colour	Maximum waiting time
1	Immediately	Red	0 min
2	Highly urgent	Orange	10 min
3	Urgent	Yellow	60 min
4	Standard	Green	120 min
5	Not urgent	Blue	240 min

After completion of the study, all blinded questionnaires were manually entered in SPSS and checked by two investigators.

Statistical analysis

Binominal and categorical data are presented as frequencies of occurrence and percentages. Continuous variables are presented as means and standard deviations (SD). The student T-test or Mann-Whitney U test was used to compare means between patients desiring vs. not desiring analgesics or patients receiving vs. not receiving analgesics. To compare between multiple groups, the Kruskall-Wallis test was used, followed by post hoc Mann-Whitney U tests. *P*-values were described to demonstrate differences between groups, with $p < 0.05$ considered significant.

To investigate associations between potential predictors and outcomes, logistic regressions were conducted. Factors that showed to be significant in univariate logistic regressions were included in a multivariate logistic regression model. Associations are presented by odds ratios (OR) and confidence intervals (CI). *P*-values of < 0.05 were again considered significant. All analyses were performed using IBM SPSS Statistics version 22.

Results

The total number of patients that visited the ED during the 10 days of inclusion was 797 (Fig. 2). Of those, 199 patients had no recent pain. Furthermore, 93 patients were excluded for being < 18 years old, 12 patients were excluded for being in a life-threatening situation, 28 patients had an altered mental status or neuropsychiatric disease, in 13 patients a language barrier was present, 14 patients did not give informed consent and 1 patient could not be questioned due to a too high infection risk. In addition, 14 patients were excluded because they participated earlier in the study, 74 patients were discharged before completing the questionnaire and 15 patients were not questioned because of organizational issues. In total, 463 patients were excluded from the study.

Characteristics of study subjects

The total number of patients included during the 10-day study was 334. The mean age was 49 years and 53% were male. The overall mean initial pain score was 5.96 NRS (SD 2.28). Half of the patients had already taken analgesics before entering the ED (50.9%) and 5.1% of the patients indicated to have an allergy for an analgesic. Patient and pain characteristics are outlined in Table 2.

Effect of pain protocol on pain score

Of the 334 enrolled patients, 146 (43.7%) patients desired analgesics upon arrival at the ED. Initial pain scores were higher in patients with a desire for

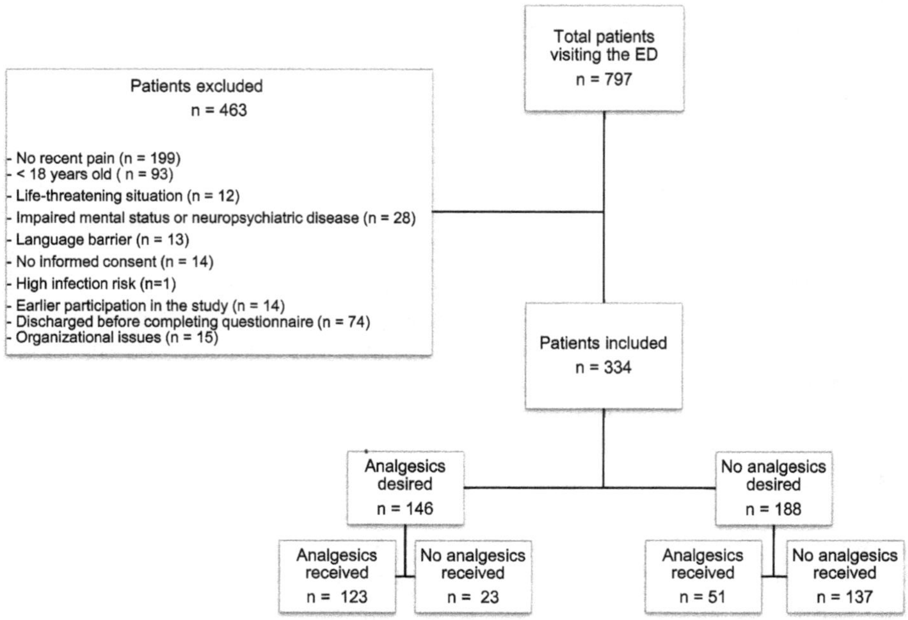

Fig. 2 Consort diagram of patient disposition through the study

analgesics compared to patients who did not wish analgesics (NRS score 7.01 [95% CI 6.70–7.33] vs. NRS score 5.14 [95% CI 4.82–5.45], Table 2). Desire for analgesics did not depend on factors such as gender, age, specialty of referral, pain character, pre-ED analgesics or known analgesic allergy. The variables triage colour code, pain location, pain duration and pain pattern (constant or intermittent pain) showed significant differences between the two groups (Table 2). Patients assigned to a group with a more urgent colour code were more likely to desire analgesics and patients with chest pain were less likely to desire analgesics. The duration of pain showed a trend towards medium pain duration (6–12 h) and a desire for analgesics. Patients suffering from constant pain were more likely to desire analgesics compared to patients experiencing intermittent pain (OR 1.89 [95% CI 1.10–3.26]).

The factors triage colour code, pain location, pain pattern and mean initial pain score were univariately significantly associated with the desire for analgesics and were the eligible factors for the multivariate model. In multivariate analysis, only the initial pain score was a significant predictive factor for desiring analgesia (Table 3).

Of all the patients in pain, 174 patients (52.1%) received analgesics. The most commonly prescribed analgesics were acetaminophen (50.2%), NSAID's (13.9%) and opioids (21.2%) (Table 4).

The number of patients receiving analgesics was greater than the number of patients who initially desired analgesics (174 vs. 146 patients). Of the 188 patients that initially refused analgesics, 51 patients had required and received analgesics at the time of the second questionnaire. Of the patients initially desiring analgesics, 23 patients did not receive them (Fig. 2). In order to accurately present the results, those two groups were temporarily excluded. In total, 260 patients (123 patients that desired and received analgesics and 137 patients that refused and did not receive analgesics) were included in the following analyses. Patients who received analgesics during their stay in the ED had significantly higher initial pain scores than those who did not receive analgesics (NRS score 7.09 [95% CI 6.76–7.42] vs. NRS score 4.82 [95% CI 4.46–5.19]). Pain scores measured 75–90 min after arrival decreased significantly in patients who received analgesics, with a reduction of 2.41 NRS (95% CI 2.02–2.79). The pain score of patients who received analgesics decreased more than patients who did not receive analgesics; the group of patients not receiving analgesics showed a reduction in pain score of 0.94 NRS ([95% CI 0.62–1.25], Table 5).

Effect of the pain protocol on patient satisfaction

Overall, all patients included in this study expressed a relatively high satisfaction of 7.83 (95% CI 7.66–7.99) for pain management. The majority of patients (67.1%) was satisfied (patient satisfaction score between 6 and 8 NRS), and 25.7% of the patients were even highly satisfied (patient satisfaction score 9–10). Only 7.2% of all patients included were dissatisfied (patient satisfaction score < 6 NRS).

Table 2 Patient and pain characteristics with subdivision in desire for analgesics

Patient factors	Desire for analgesics ($n = 146$)	No desire for analgesics ($n = 188$)	p-value
Gender			
Male ($n = 177$)	72 (40.7%)	105 (59.3%)	0.235
Female ($n = 157$)	74 (47.1%)	83 (52.9%)	
Mean age (SD)	48.38 (18.44)	49.06 (18.39)	0.675
Triage colour code			
Blue ($n = 7$)	2 (28.6%)	5 (71.4%)	0.010
Green ($n = 130$)	45 (34.6%)	85 (65.4%)	
Yellow ($n = 175$)	84 (48%)	91 (52%)	
Orange (n = 18)	13 (72.2%)	5 (27.8%)	
Red ($n = 4$)	2 (50%)	2 (50%)	
Specialty of referral			
Traumatology ($n = 78$)	38 (48.7%)	40 (51.3%)	0.121
Internal medicine ($n = 50$)	22 (44%)	28 (56%)	
Emergency medicine ($n = 26$)	12 (46.2%)	14 (53.8%)	
Cardiology ($n = 45$)	12 (26.7%)	33 (73.3%)	
Abdominal surgery ($n = 32$)	17 (53.1%)	15 (46.9%)	
Orthopedics ($n = 32$)	9 (28.1%)	23 (71.9%)	
Lung diseases ($n = 16$)	7 (43.8%)	9 (56.3%)	
Neurology (n = 15)	9 (60%)	6 (40%)	
Other ($n = 40$)	20 (50%)	20 (50%)	
Pain location			
Upper extremities ($n = 47$)	18 (38.3%)	29 (61.7%)	0.033
Lower extremities ($n = 54$)	23 (42.6%)	31 (57.4%)	
Abdomen ($n = 75$)	42 (56%)	33 (44%)	
Head/face ($n = 24$)	13 (54.2%)	11 (45.8%)	
Back ($n = 12$)	7 (58.3%)	5 (41.7%)	
Chest (n = 54)	14 (25.9%)	40 (74.1%)	
Neck (n = 3)	1 (33.3%)	2 (66.7%)	
More than 1 location (n = 47)	23 (48.9%)	24 (51.1%)	
Other (n = 18)	5 (27.8%)	13 (72.2%)	
Pain duration			
< 2 h ($n = 68$)	32 (47.1%)	36 (52.9%)	0.047
2–6 h ($n = 52$)	27 (51.9%)	25 (48.1%)	
6–12 h ($n = 31$)	19 (61.3%)	12 (38.7%)	
12 h – 3 days (n = 78)	32 (41.0%)	46 (59.0%)	
> 3 days ($n = 105$)	36 (34.3%)	69 (65.7%)	
Pain pattern			
Constant ($n = 259$)	122 (47.1%)	137 (52.9%)	0.020
Intermittent (n = 75)	24 (32%)	51 (68%)	
Pain character			
Sharp ($n = 121$)	58 (47.9%)	63 (52.1%)	0.425
Pressing ($n = 66$)	27 (40.9%)	39 (59.1%)	
Nagging ($n = 62$)	31 (50%)	31 (50%)	

Table 2 Patient and pain characteristics with subdivision in desire for analgesics *(Continued)*

Patient factors	Desire for analgesics (*n* = 146)	No desire for analgesics (*n* = 188)	p-value
Burning (n = 18)	5 (27.8%)	13 (72.2%)	
Cramping (n = 7)	3 (42.9%)	4 (57.1%)	
More than 1 answer (*n* = 48)	19 (39.6%)	29 (60.4%)	
Other (n = 12)	3 (25%)	9 (75%)	
Mean initial pain score (SD)	7.01 (1.94)	5.14 (2.19)	0.029
Pre-ED analgesics			
Yes (*n* = 170)	83 (48.8%)	87 (51.2%)	0.055
No (*n* = 164)	63 (38.4%)	101 (61.6%)	
Analgesia allergy			
Yes (n = 17)	8 (47.1%)	9 (52.9%)	0.775
No (*n* = 317)	138 (43.5%)	179 (56.5%)	

P-values show differences of the whole factor group in relation to desire vs. no desire for analgesia

After only analyzing patients who received analgesics in compliance with their initial wish, results show that patients receiving analgesics were significantly more satisfied than patients who did not receive analgesics (satisfaction score 8.06 [95% CI 7.80–8.31 vs. 7.54 [95% CI 7.24–7.84]).

Reasons for refusing analgesics

The most common reason for not wanting analgesics, even though in pain, was bearable pain (57.4%), wanting to know the diagnosis first (10%) and using analgesics before visiting the ED (8%).

Reasons for not receiving analgesics and the effect on patient satisfaction levels

As stated before, not all patients received analgesia according to their initial wish. Of the 146 patients desiring pain management, 23 patients did not receive analgesics. After performing subgroup analyses on patient satisfaction scores, results show that within the group that did not receive analgesics, patients who initially desired analgesics were not more dissatisfied than patients that did not desire analgesics (mean patient satisfaction score 7.48 [95% CI 6.90–8.06] vs. 7.54 [96% CI 7.24–7.84], Fig. 3). This result is important in investigating whether analgesics were incorrectly withheld from patients. In this cohort, the main reasons for not receiving analgesics included receiving an alternative non-pharmacological pain treatment such as splinting or applying ice or heat (31%), crowding in the ED (13%) and the clinical judgement of the nurse (13%). After correction for non-pharmacological pain treatment, 6.6% of the 334 patients in pain did not receive analgesics or a non-pharmacological pain treatment, despite their expressed desire.

Discussion

Pain management is an important criterion of quality of care given in the ED and its adequacy has therefore been often discussed in literature.

According to our initial hypothesis, our study shows that the pain score in patients who received analgesics decreased more than in patients who did not receive analgesics. Patients who received analgesics were also significantly more satisfied than patients who did not receive analgesics. Those differences are in our study unlikely to be attributed to 'undertreatment of pain' in patients that did not receive analgesics. An important question in investigating 'undertreatment of pain' or 'oligoanalgesia' is whether all patients in pain desire analgesia. Previous research shows that nearly half of the patients in pain decline analgesia, which is in agreement with our results [7, 8]: of all the patients entering the ED in pain, less than half desired analgesics in our study. In those patients, 'bearable pain' was the most common reason for refusing analgesics. More urgent cases, medium pain duration of 6–12 h and constant pain were factors more associated with desiring analgesics, describing possible reasons why and when analgesics are desired.

Of patients that did not receive analgesics, the majority (86%) did not desire analgesics. Also, there was no difference in satisfaction between those patients and patients that did not receive analgesics despite their wish, suggesting that analgesics were not incorrectly withheld from patients. According to Allione et al., almost 10% of the patients do not receive analgesics despite their expressed desire [8], however, the reason for this was

Table 3 Factors associated with a desire for analgesics (univariate and multivariate analysis)

	Univariate analysis		Multivariate analysis	
Variable	OR (95% CI)	p-value	OR (95% CI)	p-value
Gender		0.236		
Male	Reference			
Female	1.30 (0,84–2.01)			
Age	0.10 (0.99–1.01)	0.737		
Triage colour code		0.021		0.139
Blue	0.40 (0.03–5.15)		1.23 (0.07–0.76)	
Green	0.53 (0.72–3.89)		1.65 (0.19–4.61)	
Yellow	0.92 (0.13–6.70)		2.98 (0.34–5.83)	
Orange	2.60 (0.28–3.81)		6.05 (0.54–8.08)	
Red	Reference		Reference	
Specialty of referral		0.14		
Traumatology	Reference			
Internal medicine	0,83 (0.41–1.69)			
Emergency medicine	0.90 (0.37–2.20)			
Cardiology	0.38 (0.17–0.85)			
Abdominal surgery	1.19 (0.52–2.72)			
Orthopedics	0.41 (0.17–1.00)			
Lung diseases	0.82 (0.28–2.42)			
Neurology	1.58 (0.51–4.86)			
Other	1.05 (0.49–2.26)			
Pain location		0.040		0.078
Upper extremities	Reference		Reference	
Lower extremities	1.20 (0.54–2.66)		1.29 (0.53–3.09)	
Abdomen	2.05 (0.97–4.32)		1.68 (0.74–3.79)	
Head/face	1.90 (0.70–5.15)		2.94 (0.97–8.93)	
Back	2.26 (0.62–8.19)		1.99 (0.48–8.21)	
Chest	0.56 (0.24–1.31)		0.68 (0.27–1.70)	
Neck	0.81 (0.07–9.54)		0.45 (0.03–6.67)	
More than 1 location	1.54 (0.68–3.51)		2.29 (0.92–5.71)	
Other	0.62 (0.19–2.03)		0.62 (0.17–2.21)	
Pain duration		0.051		
< 2 h	1.70 (0.91–3.18)			
2–6 h	2.07 (1.05–4.07)			
6–12 h	3.04 (1.33–6.94)			
12 h – 3 days	1.33 (0.73–2.44)			
> 3 days	Reference			
Pain pattern		0.021		0.314
Constant	1.89 (1.10–3.26)		1.38 (0.74–2.58)	
Intermittent	Reference		Reference	
Pain character		0.447		
Sharp	Reference			
Pressing	0.75 (0.41–1.38)			
Nagging	1.09 (0.59–2.00)			

Table 3 Factors associated with a desire for analgesics (univariate and multivariate analysis) *(Continued)*

	Univariate analysis		Multivariate analysis	
Burning	0.42 (0.14–1.24)			
Cramping	0.82 (0.18–3.80)			
More than 1 answer	0.71 (0.36–1.40)			
Other	0.36 (0.08–1.40)			
Mean initial pain score	1.54 (1.36–1.74)	0.000	1.56 (1.37–1.77)	0.000
Pre-ED analgesics		0.056		
No	Reference			
Yes	1.53 (0.99–2.36)			
Analgesia allergy		0.775		
No	Reference			
Yes	1.15 (0.43–3.07)			

not described. Our study showed that receiving a non-pharmacological pain treatment was the most common reason for not receiving analgesics. After correcting for non-pharmacological pain treatment, only 6.6% of the patients did not receive analgesia or a non-pharmacological pain treatment despite their expressed desire for pain relief. Not correcting for the patients' wish for analgesia might lead to low rates of analgesic administration and thus to incorrect conclusions with regard to inadequate pain management, reporting undertreatment percentages ranging from 20 to 50% as described before in literature [12].

Nevertheless, it has to be mentioned that despite the statistically significant differences, one might wonder if a difference of 0.52 in patient satisfaction score is clinically relevant. Previous studies have investigated the association between pain scores and patient satisfaction and stated that pain relief on itself is not the only factor affecting patient satisfaction [13, 14]. McNeill et al. showed a negative correlation between pain scores and patient satisfaction [15], while Svensson et al. showed a high patient satisfaction score despite high pain scores [16]. Phillips et al. concluded from their study that patient satisfaction should be addressed as an independent variable in assessing pain management [12].

Table 4 Overview of prescribed types of analgesics

Administered drug	No. of patients ($n = 174$)
Acetaminophen	64 (36.8%)
NSAID	4 (2.3%)
Opioid	19 (10.9%)
Acetaminophen + NSAID	23 (13.2%)
Acetaminophen + NSAID + opioid	4 (2.3%)
Acetaminophen + opioid	25 (14.4%)
NSAID + opoid	1 (0.6%)
Nitroglycerin	9 (5.1%)
Benzodiazepine	1 (0.6%)
Others	24 (13.8%)

Another important limitation of many earlier studies on 'oligoanalgesia' is their retrospective nature. Since pain perception is a subjective phenomenon, the presence or severity of pain should be determined by asking the patient at the moment of pain itself. Estimating the pain score, without asking the patient or asking the patient in retrospective, will not reliably reveal the real severity of pain [17]. Also, the number of patients receiving analgesics has more often been investigated, but rarely the actual effects of analgesics on lowering the pain score. A review of literature on oligoanalgesia stated that inconsistency and inadequacy of pain management is caused by multiple reasons including a lack of education in pain management, inadequate management programs to evaluate pain management, the clinicians' attitude towards opioids and disbelief of pain reporting [18]. A generally accepted pain protocol is therefore important, providing guidelines aiming to prevent an inconsistency in pain treatment. Our study showed an overall pain reduction of 2.17 NRS in the group of patients treated with analgesia according to our pain protocol. Since a pain reduction of > 2 NRS is considered clinically relevant [9, 10], the current pain protocol can be considered adequate.

Limitations of the study

Measuring severity of pain among ED patients can be challenging since pain perception is considered a subjective phenomenon. A retrospective way of investigating pain management will not provide a reliable picture [17]. However, a prospective way also has its limitations. The questionnaires were filled in by researchers questioning the patient. Some patients may have been inclined to

Table 5 Reduction in pain score in patients receiving analgesics vs. patients not receiving analgesics

	Analgesics received (n = 123)	No analgesics received (n = 137)	p-value
Initial pain score (95% CI)	7.09 (6.76–7.42)	4.82 (4.46–5.19)	0.00
Pain score after 75–90 min (95% CI)	4.68 (4.23–5.14)	3.89 (3.46–4.32)	0.013
Δ Pain score (95% CI)	2.41 (2.02–2.79)	0.94 (0.62–1.25)	0.00

provide responses based on an expectation of a correct response; thus skewing data. Secondly, the study was conducted under optimal circumstances of a working pain protocol. The presence of the researchers in the work field might have induced a 'Hawthorne effect', reminding nurses to pay more attention to pain management. Some patients expressed their desire for analgesics only to the researcher. In this case, the nurses were informed for ethical reasons. Further research will focus on the adherence to the pain management protocol under ordinary working circumstances and overcrowding.

An important challenge in investigating patient satisfaction on pain management was the subgroup of patients where no analgesics were given. For that reason, all patients were asked to rate the overall management routine regarding pain treatment in the Emergency Department, and not only the effect of the therapeutics itself. Nevertheless, it is possible that less attention was given to patients who initially did not desire analgesics, possibly causing the differences in satisfaction scores between the two groups. Patient satisfaction score was expressed as one overall grade in our questionnaire. Thus, specific reasons for expression of (dis)satisfaction regarding e.g. waiting time and communication, were not investigated.

This study is limited to a single, tertiary university hospital in Groningen, the north of the Netherlands. ED's of all Dutch hospitals adhere to the same guidelines for pain management [19]. Therefore, pain protocols used in other Dutch hospitals can be considered as comparable. However, e.g. patient demographics can differ between ED's. Our results should therefore not be generalized to other, dissimilar settings.

Conclusions

In summary, our results show that less than half of the patients in pain entering the ED desire analgesics. Patients receiving analgesics were adequately treated according to the pain protocol, showing a clinically relevant reduction in pain score and higher satisfaction scores at discharge compared to patients who did not receive analgesics. Patients who did not receive analgesics despite their expressed wish were not incorrectly withheld from pain treatment, since satisfaction scores were comparable to patients who did not desire and did not receive analgesics. Additionally, most of the patients who did not receive pain medication despite desiring

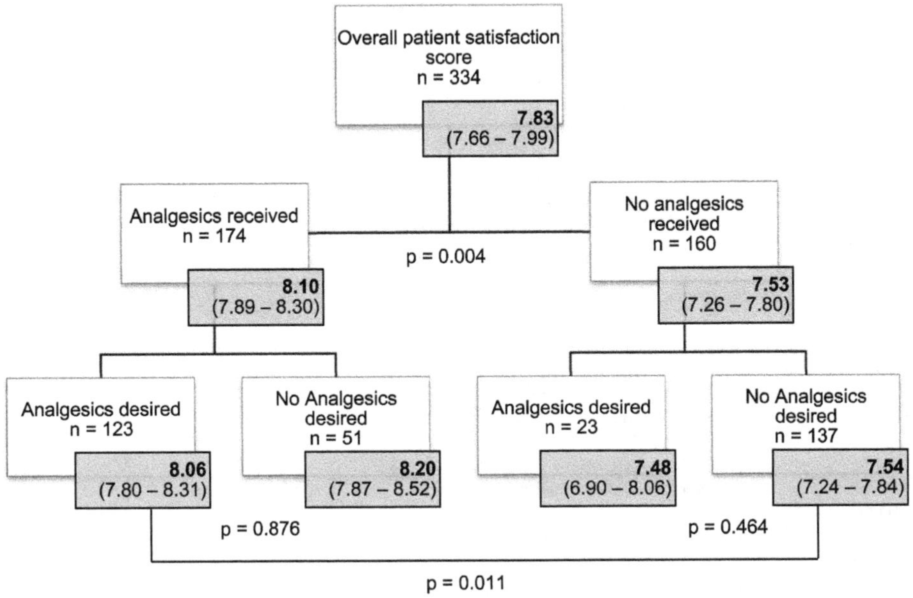

Fig. 3 Patient satisfaction scores

analgesics, received a non-pharmacological pain treatment. This study demonstrates that in this ED setting with a pain protocol in use, pain is adequately treated, and emphasizes the importance of taking the patients' wish for analgesia into account when investigating 'oligoanalgesia' in the ED.

Abbreviations

CI: Confidence Interval; ED: Emergency Department; NRS: Numeric Rating Scale; NSAID: Nonsteroidal Anti-Inflammatory Drugs; OR: Odds Ratio; PPI: Proton pump inhibitor; SD: Standard Deviation; UMCG: University Medical Center Groningen; WHO: World Health Organization

Acknowledgements

The authors are very grateful to all doctors and nurses from the Emergency Department at the University Medical Center Groningen hospital, who contributed to this study.

Funding

Not applicable.

Authors' contributions

JZ and JCM conceived the study and designed the trial. JL and JCM supervised the conduct of the trial and data collection, performed by JZ and SW. JJM provided statistical advice analyzing the data. JZ analyzed the data and drafted the article. All authors read and approved the final manuscript.

Competing interests

The authors declare that they have no competing interests.

Author details

[1]Department of Emergency Medicine, University of Groningen, University Medical Center Groningen, Groningen, The Netherlands. [2]Department of Cardiology, University of Groningen, University Medical Center Groningen, Groningen, The Netherlands.

References

1. Tanabe P, Buschmann M. A prospective study of ED pain management practices and the patient's perspective. J Emergency Nursing. 1999;25(3):171–7.
2. Marks RM, Sachar EJ. Undertreatment of medical inpatients with narcotic analgesics. Ann Intern Med. 1973;78(2):173–81.
3. Stephan F-P, Nickel CH, Martin JS, Grether D, Delport-Lehnen K, Bingisser R. Pain in the emergency department: adherence to an implemented treatment protocol. Swiss Med Wkly. 2010;140(23–24):341–7.
4. Wilson JE, Pendleton JM. Oligoanalgesia in the emergency department. Am J Emerg Med. 1989;7(6):620–3.
5. Selbst SM, Clark M. Analgesic use in the emergency department. Ann Emerg Med. 1990;19(9):1010–3.
6. Green SM. There is oligo-evidence for oligoanalgesia. Ann Emerg Med. 2012;60(2):212–4.
7. Singer AJ, Garra G, Chohan JK, Dalmedo C, Thode HC. Triage pain scores and the desire for and use of analgesics. Ann Emerg Med. 2008;52(6):689–95.
8. Allione A, Melchio R, Martini G, Dutto L, Ricca M, Bernardi E, et al. Factors influencing desired and received analgesia in emergency department. Intern Emerg Med. 2011;6(1):69–78.
9. Farrar JT, Portenoy RK, Berlin JA, Kinman JL, Strom BL. Defining the clinically important difference in pain outcome measures. Pain. 2000;88(3):287–94.
10. Farrar JT, Young JP, LaMoreaux L, Werth JL, Poole RM. Clinical importance of changes in chronic pain intensity measured on an 11-point numerical pain rating scale. Pain. 2001;94(2):149–58.
11. World Health Organization. Cancer pain relief with a guide to opioid availability. Second ed; 1996.
12. Phillips S, Gift M, Gelot S, Duong M, Tapp H. Assessing the relationship between the level of pain control and patient satisfaction. J Pain Res. 2013;6:683–9.
13. Stahmer SA, Shofer FS, Marino A, Shepherd S, Abbuhl S. Do quantitative changes in pain intensity correlate with pain relief and satisfaction? Acad Emerg Med Off J Soc Acad Emerg Med. 1998;5(9):851–7.
14. Müller-Staub M, Meer R, Briner G, Probst M-T, Needham I. Measuring patient satisfaction in an emergency unit of a Swiss university hospital: occurrence of anxiety, insecurity, worry, pain, dyspnoea, nausea, thirst and hunger, and their correlation with patient satisfaction (part 2). Pflege. 2008;21(3):180–8.
15. McNeill JA, Sherwood GD, Starck PL, Nieto B. Pain management outcomes for hospitalized Hispanic patients. Pain Management Nursing. 2001;2(1):25–36.
16. Svensson I, Sjöström B, Haljamäe H. Influence of expectations and actual pain experiences on satisfaction with postoperative pain management. Eur J Pain. 2001;5(2):125–33.
17. Nagurney JT, Brown DFM, Sane S, Weiner JB, Wang AC, Chang Y. The accuracy and completeness of data collected by prospective and retrospective methods. Acad Emerg Med Off J Soc Acad Emerg Med. 2005;12(9):884–95.
18. Rupp T, Delaney KA. Inadequate analgesia in emergency medicine. Ann Emerg Med. 2004;43(4):494–503.
19. VMS. Vroege herkenning en behandeling van pijn - VMSzorg. 2009.

24

Platelet indices and outcome after cardiac arrest

Antonella Cotoia[1,2], Federico Franchi[1], Chiara De Fazio[1], Jean-Louis Vincent[1], Jacques Creteur[1] and Fabio Silvio Taccone[1*]

Abstract

Background: Platelet variables, including platelet distribution width (PDW) and mean platelet volume (MPV), have been associated with outcome in critically ill patients. We evaluated these variables in patients after cardiac arrest (CA).

Methods: All adult CA patients admitted to the intensive care unit (ICU) over an 8-year period (2006–2014) and treated with targeted temperature management were included. We retrieved all data concerning CA characteristics as well as platelet count, PDW and MPV on the first 2 days of admission. Unfavorable 3-month neurological outcome was defined as a cerebral performance category score of 3–5.

Results: We included 384 patients (age 62 [52–75] years; 270/384 male): 231 patients (60%) died within 30-days and 246 patients (64%) had an unfavorable 3-month neurological outcome. On admission, platelet count, PDW and MPV were 87 [126–261] $*10^3$cells/mm^3, 17 [16.3–17.3]% and 8.3 [7.6–9.2] µm^3, respectively. Platelet count decreased significantly over the first 2 days, whereas PDW and MPV did not change significantly. There were no significant differences between the values on admission or time-courses of platelet count, PDW or MPV between survivors and non-survivors or between patients with unfavorable and favorable neurological outcome.

Conclusions: In our cohort of post-CA patients, PDW and MPV were not associated with outcome.

Keywords: Platelet distribution width, Cardiac arrest, Hypothermia, Platelet indices

Background

Despite improvements in the management of patients with cardiac arrest (CA), outcomes remain poor, mainly because of associated cardiogenic shock and post-anoxic brain damage [1]. Moreover, the ischemia/reperfusion injury occurring after the return of spontaneous circulation (ROSC) can contribute to a systemic inflammatory response, similar to that observed in septic patients, which may contribute to organ injury [1–4]. The activation of multiple inflammatory pathways results in platelet activation and an imbalance between endogenous coagulation and fibrinolysis pathways [4, 5]; however, these abnormalities are not easily characterized in clinical practice. In the last few years, there has been increasing interest in platelet variables, such as platelet distribution width (PDW), an indicator of variation in platelet size, and mean platelet volume (MPV), for the diagnosis of various conditions associated with altered platelet counts, including sepsis [6, 7]. These indices, which can be obtained easily from routine blood analysis, have been associated with the occurrence of organ dysfunction during sepsis and an increase in PDW greater than 18% considered as an expression of platelet activation, both being correlated with mortality [8–10].

PDW and MPV have not been widely studied in survivors of CA [11]. It would be interesting to better characterize the prognostic role of these two biomarkers, as they could be used in the future to identify patients with platelet hyperfunction or increased platelet aggregation after CA, who may require for more aggressive antiplatelet therapy, or those with the highest risk of organ dysfunction or systemic reperfusion injury, who might be treated with specific therapeutic approaches.

We therefore investigated the changes in PDW and MPV over time in CA patients treated with targeted temperature management (TTM) and their relationship with outcome.

* Correspondence: ftaccone@ulb.ac.be
[1]Department of Intensive Care, Erasme Hospital, Université libre de Bruxelles, Brussels, Belgium
Full list of author information is available at the end of the article

Methods

The local Ethical Committee (Comité d'Ethique Hospitalo-Facultaire Erasme-ULB) approved the study (Protocol P2017/264), but the need for informed consent was waived because of the retrospective analysis of data. Non-traumatic patients with Glasgow coma scale < 9, surviving for at least 24 h after in-hospital or out-of-hospital CA and admitted to the intensive care unit (ICU) were included in an institutional database (December 2006 to October 2014) and considered eligible for the study. Exclusion criteria were missing data on blood count on admission.

All patients were treated with TTM (target temperature: 32–34 °C) for 24 h, according to our standardized protocol that has been described elsewhere [12]. Briefly, cooling is started immediately after ICU admission with a combination of cold fluid bolus (20–30 ml/kg of a crystalloid solution in 30 min) and a circulating water blanket device (Medi-Therm II, Gaymar, USA). Target temperature is initially measured using a rectal temperature probe or a blood temperature monitoring in case an invasive haemodynamic monitoring (PiCCO, Pulsion, Munich, Germany) is initiated. Sedation is based on the use of midazolam (0.03–0.1 mg/kg/h) and analgesia on morphine (0.1–0.3 mg/kg/h) infusions. Cisatracurium is administered to control shivering in the induction phase (bolus of 0.15 mg/kg) and, if needed, as a continuous infusion thereafter (1–3 mcg/kg/min). After 24 h of cooling, rewarming is obtained passively at a rate of 0.3–0.5 °C/h and sedation discontinued when body temperature reaches 37 °C. Patients are kept in a 30° semi-recumbent position; ventilation is set to keep $PaCO_2$ between 35 and 45 mmHg and SpO_2 > 94–96%. Blood glucose is kept between 110 and 150 mg/dL and mean arterial pressure maintained > 65–70 mmHg using fluids, dobutamine and/or norepinephrine, as appropriate. Intra-aortic balloon counterpulsation (IABP) or extracorporeal membrane oxygenation (ECMO) are used in cases of severe cardiogenic shock.

In case of persisting deep coma associated with bilateral absence of the N20 response to somatosensory evoked potentials (on day 2–3 after arrest), and/or status myoclonus with malignant EEG (i.e. burst suppression or suppressed background) and/or refractory status epilepticus, decisions to withdraw life-support were made after interdisciplinary discussion and occurred not before 48–72 h after normothermia (> 37°) was restored and sedative agents were stopped.

We collected data on demographics, comorbidities and CA characteristics. The platelet count (normal range: 155–350*10^3cells/mm^3), PDW (normal range: 15–18%) and MPV (normal range: 6.4–10 μm^3) values were obtained on ICU admission and for two subsequent days from the routine daily blood count measured using the UniCel DXH 800 Coulter Cellular Analysis System (Beckman Coulter International S.A., Nyon, France). Thrombopenia was defined as a platelet count of < 150*10^3cells/mm^3 while high PDW and MPV in case of values > 18% and 10 μm^3, respectively. Blood lactate and C-reactive protein (CRP) levels on admission were also recorded. Treatments with vasoactive/inotropic drugs and continuous renal replacement therapy were noted. Shock was defined as the need for vasopressor agents for more than 6 h. The development of infections during the ICU stay was recorded; survival was recorded at 30-days after admission in ICU. Neurological evaluation was assessed using the cerebral performance category score (CPC) during follow-up visits or by telephone interview 3 months after CA [13]. Unfavorable neurological outcome was considered as a CPC 3–5.

Statistical analysis

Data were analyzed using SPSS 24.0 for Windows (SPSS Inc., Chicago, IL). We used the Shapiro-Wilk test and stratified distribution plots to verify the normality of distribution of continuous variables. Continuous variables are presented as median [25–75 percentile] and number (%) as appropriate. Differences between groups (survivors vs. no survivors, and unfavorable vs. favourable outcome) were assessed using Student's T test, Mann-Whitney test, χ^2 test, or Fisher's exact test, as appropriate. Time-courses of platelet parameters were analyzed using a two-way ANOVA for repeated measurement with Bonferroni *post-hoc* correction. A two-tailed test was performed and a p value < 0.05 was considered to be significant.

Results

From a total of 445 eligible CA patients admitted over the study period, 43 died within a few hours after hospital admission without blood sampling and 18 were excluded for missing PDW/MPV data, leaving 384 patients for the final analysis (mean age: 62 [52–75]; male gender, n = 270 [70%] - Table 1). The total duration of ICU stay was 4 [2–8] days; 231 patients died within day 30 (60%) and 246 (64%) patients had an unfavorable outcome.

On admission, the platelet count was 193 [131–266] *10^3cells/mm^3, PDW 17.0 [16.3–17.3]% and MPV 8.3 [7.6–9.2] μm^3 (Table 1). Platelet counts decreased significantly over the next 2 days to 160 [97–215] on day 1 and 147 [87–202] *10^3cells/mm^3 on day 2, $p <$ 0.001), whereas PDW and MPV remained stable. Thrombopenia was observed in 108 (28%) patients on admission and in 146 (38%) and 203 (53%) on day 1 and 2, respectively. High PDW and MPV were observed in 78 (20%) and 62 (16%) patients on admission, in 80 (21%) and 64 (17%) patients on day 1 and in 82 (21%) and 67 (17%) patients on day 2, respectively.

Table 1 Characteristics of study population according to favourable (FO) and unfavourable (UO) neurological outcome

	All (*n* = 384)	Survivors (*n* = 153)	Non-survivors (*n* = 231)	*P* Value	FO (*n* = 138)	UO (*n* = 246)	*P* Value
Age, years	62 [52–75]	58 [49–70]	66 [54–78]	< 0.001	58 [50–69]	66 [53–77]	< 0.001
Weight, kg	77 [67–85]	78 [70–87]	75 [65–85]	0.360	78 [70–88]	75 [65–85]	0.076
Male, n (%)	270 (70)	114 (75)	156 (67)	0.110	103 (75)	167 (68)	0.165
Comorbidities							
Chronic hypertension, n (%)	175 (46)	71 (46)	104 (45)	0.790	63 (46)	112 (45)	0.981
Diabetes, n (%)	95 (25)	33 (22)	62 (26)	0.241	28 (20)	67 (27)	0.130
Chronic heart failure, n (%)	81 (21)	30 (20)	51 (22)	0.561	29 (21)	52 (21)	0.977
Coronary artery disease, n (%)	168 (44)	60 (39)	108 (47)	0.145	56 (40)	112 (45)	0.348
Neurological disease, n (%)	64 (16)	17 (11)	47 (20)	0.028	14 (10)	50 (20)	0.011
Liver cirrhosis, n (%)	21 (6)	4 (3)	17 (7)	0.045	4 (3)	17 (7)	0.097
COPD/asthma, n (%)	66 (17)	23 (15)	43 (18)	0.362	20 (14)	46 (19)	0.294
Presentation rhythm, n (%)							
VF-VT, n (%)	151 (39)	89 (55)	62 (27)	< 0.001	83 (60)	68 (27)	< 0.001
Unknown, n (%)	23 (6)	8 (5)	15 (6)	0.941	6 (4)	17 (7)	0.875
Out of hospital CA, n (%)	215 (56)	84 (55)	131 (57)	0.675	76 (55)	139 (56)	0.739
Time to ROSC, min	15 [7–25]	12 [5–20]	18 [10–25]	0.002	12 [5–20]	17 [10–25]	0.005
Epinephrine, mg	3 [2–6]	2 [1–4]	4 [2–7]	< 0.001	2 [1–4]	4 [2–7]	< 0.001
Witnessed CA, n (%)	323 (84)	138 (90)	185 (80)	0.006	124 (90)	199 (81)	0.021
Bystander CPR, n (%)	255 (66)	138 (90)	117 (50)	0.001	107 (77)	148 (60)	0.001
Cardiac origin of arrest, n (%)	230 (60)	105 (69)	125 (54)	0.004	97 (70)	133 (54)	0.002
During ICU stay							
AKI, n (%)	231 (60)	77 (50)	154 (67)	0.001	69 (50)	162 (66)	0.002
Vasopressor use, n (%)	278 (72)	97 (63)	181 (78)	0.001	88 (64)	190 (77)	0.005
Dobutamine use, n (%)	202 (53)	77 (50)	125 (54)	0.252	69 (50)	133 (54)	0.321
Hypothermia, n (%)	339 (88)	131 (85)	208 (90)	< 0.001	119 (86)	220 (89)	0.435
Sepsis, n (%)	118 (31)	45 (29)	73 (32)	0.649	40 (29)	78 (31)	0.579
IABP, n (%)	28 (7)	8 (5)	20 (8)	0.206	7 (5)	21 (8)	0.210
ECMO, n (%)	53 (14)	20 (13)	33 (14)	0.736	19 (14)	34 (14)	0.988
CRRT, n (%)	60 (16)	25 (16)	35 (15)	0.754	22 (16)	38 (15)	0.898
Shock, n (%)	207 (54)	66 (43)	141 (61)	0.001	61 (44)	146 (59)	0.004
Steroid therapy, n (%)	74 (19)	24 (16)	50 (22)	0.147	23 (17)	51 (21)	0.333
RBC transfusion, n (%)	99 (26)	42 (28)	57 (24)	0.543	37 (27)	62 (25)	0.730
Blood sample on admission							
Creatinine, mg/dL	1.2 [0.9–1.6]	1.1 [0.9–1.6]	1.3 [0.9–1.7]	0.095	1.1 [0.9–1.6]	1.2 [0.9–1.7]	0.082
Lactate, mg/dL	4.4 [2.8–7.9]	3.9 [2.5–5.6]	4.9 [3.1–8.7]	< 0.001	3.9 [2.5–5.7]	4.6 [6.0–8.5]	0.003
CRP, mg/L	11.0 [3.6–53.2]	9.0 [2.9–49.3]	12.5 [4.0–59.0]	0.039	7 [2.3–33.1]	15.1 [4.3–64.5]	0.001
PLT, *10^3cells/mm^3	193 [131–266]	196 [133–269]	193 [133–261]	0.654	197 [134–264]	194 [130–268]	0.499
MPV, μm^3	8.3 [7.6–9.2]	8.4 [7.7–9.2]	8.4 [7.6–9.3]	0.770	8.3 [7.7–9.2]	8.4 [7.6–9.3]	0.864
PCT, %	0.2 [0.1–0.2]	0.2 [0.1–0.2]	0.2 [0.1–0.2]	0.675	0.2 [0–1-0.2]	0.2 [0.1–0.2]	0.774
PDW, %	17.0 [16.3–17.3]	17.0 [16.2–17.3]	17.0 [16.4–17.4]	0.422	16.8 [16.2–17.3]	16.9 [16.4–17.4]	0.628
ICU length of stay, days	4 [2–8]	7 [4–13]	4 [2–7]	< 0.001	6 [4–12]	4 [2–8]	< 0.001

CA cardiac arrest, *CPR* cardiopulmonary resuscitation, *ROSC* return of spontaneous circulation, *VF/VT* ventricular fibrillation/ventricular tachycardia, *AKI* acute kidney injury, *ICU* intensive care unit, *IABP* intra-aortic balloon pump counterpulsation, *ECMO* extracorporeal membrane oxygenation, *CRRT* continuous renal replacement therapy, *COPD* chronic obstructive pulmonary disease, *RBC* Red Blood Cells, *MV* mechanical ventilation, *CRP* C-reactive Protein, *PLT* Platelet count, *MPV* Mean platelet volume, *PCT* Plateletcrit, *PDW* Platelet Distribution Width

Compared to survivors, non-survivors were older, had less frequently had a witnessed arrest, bystander CPR, a cardiac origin of the arrest and an initial shockable rhythm, and had longer resuscitation times and higher epinephrine doses (Table 1). They also had higher admission lactate and CRP concentrations, more frequently received vasopressor therapy, and had a shorter ICU length of stay.

There were no significant differences between survivors and non-survivors in admission platelet counts (196 [133–269] vs. 193 [133–261] $*10^3$cells/mm^3, $p = 0.65$), PDW (17.0 [16.2–17.3] vs. 17.0 [16.4–17.4]%, $p = 0.42$) and MPV (8.4 [7.7–9.2] vs. 8.4 [7.6–9.3] μm^3, $p = 0.77$). The platelet count decreased significantly during the first 2 days of admission in survivors and non-survivors, whereas PDW and MPV remained stable in the two groups (Figs. 1a, 2a-b). Similar results were found when comparing patients with favourable and unfavourable outcomes (Table 1, Fig. 1b), between patients with in-hospital and out-of-hospital CA and between male and female gender (data not shown). Also, the number of patients with thrombopenia, high PDW or high MPV was similar between survivors and non-survivors or those with favourable and unfavourable neurological outcome on admission, as on day 1 and 2.

Discussion

The platelet count decreased during the first 48 h after CA, but the PDW and MPV did not change; moreover, changes in platelet count, PDW and MPV were not associated with patient outcome.

Post-CA syndrome is associated with a decrease in the number of platelets more than an alteration in their function [2]; the etiology of the reduced platelet count may be related to a systemic inflammatory response, triggered by the ischemia/reperfusion injury occurring after the return of spontaneous circulation, and promoting the systemic activation of platelets [14]. The decrease in platelet count was unlikely to be associated with the

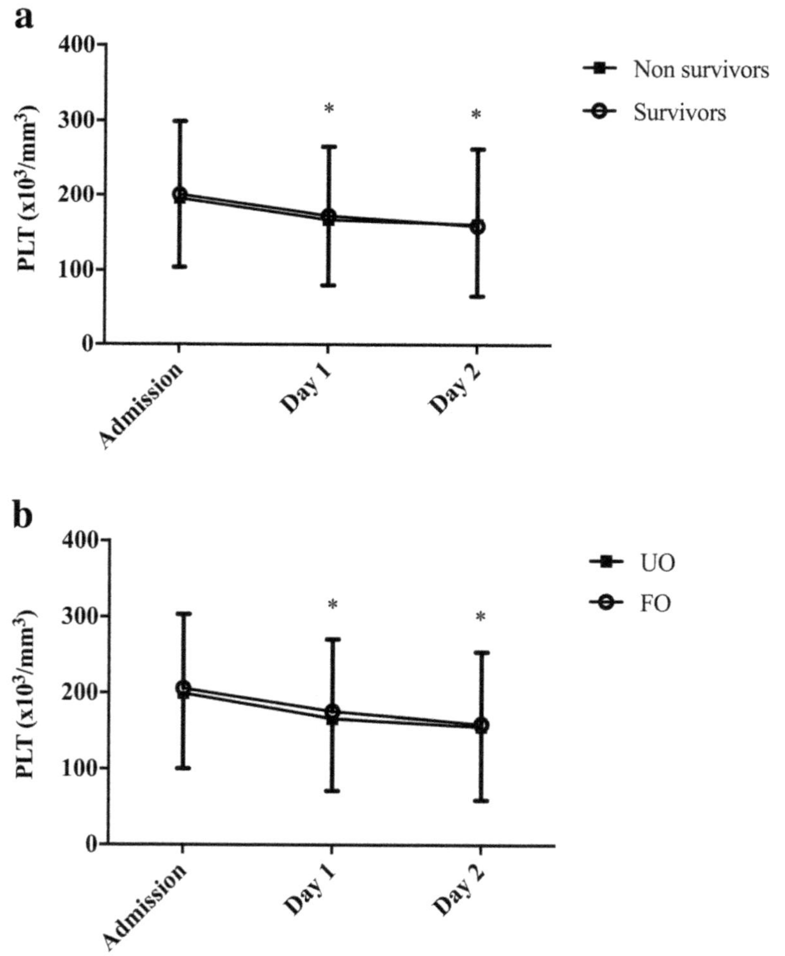

Fig. 1 a Time-course of platelet count (PLT) in survivors and non-survivors and **b**) time-course of platelet count (PLT) in patients with favorable (FO) and unfavorable (UO) neurological outcome. Data are presented as mean ± SD. * = Significant difference at day 1 and 2 compared to baseline in both survivors and non-survivors, and in patients with favourable and unfavourable neurological outcome ($p < 0.001$)

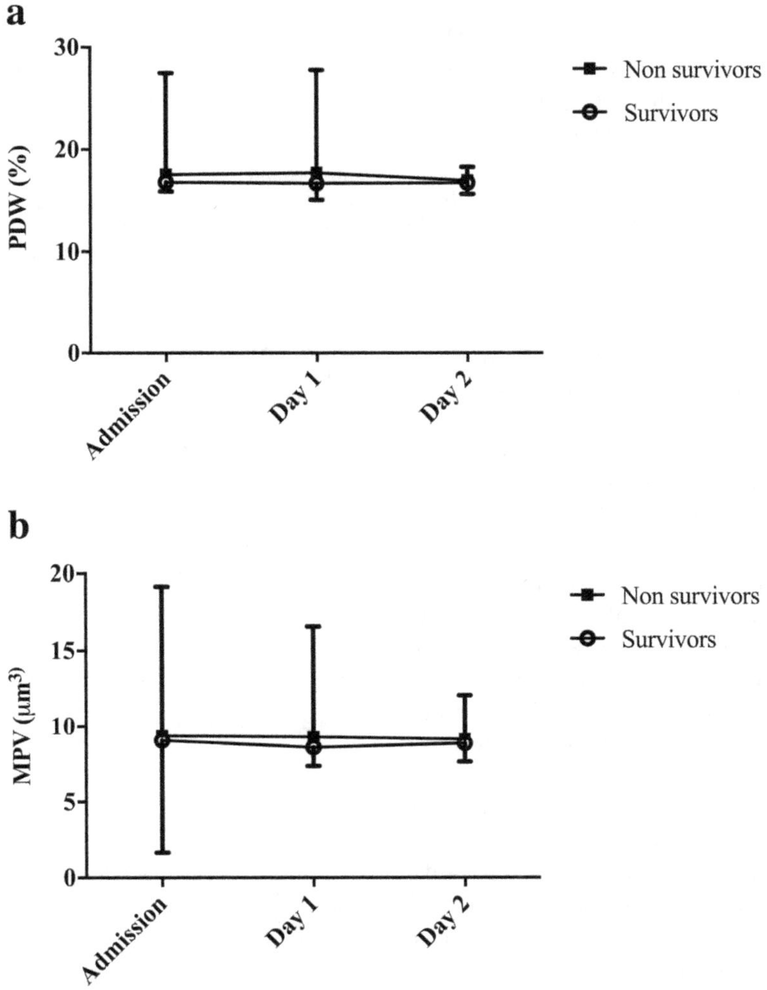

Fig. 2 a Platelet distribution width (PDW) values and **b**) Mean platelet volume (MPV) in survivors and non-survivor. Data are presented as mean ± SD. Repeated measures analysis showed no difference in PDW and MPV values over time between survivors and non-survivors ($p > 0.05$)

TTM, because platelet count, activation and/or aggregation are not influenced by a moderate decrease in body temperature to 32–34 °C [15]. The prognostic role of platelet count and/or thrombopenia has been rarely described in CA patients; in one study, Nobile et al. showed no differences in the occurrence of haematological failure (i.e. platelet count $< 50*10^3$cells/mm^3) among survivors and non-survivors after CA ($n = 469$) [16], but patients with OHCA had a greater incidence of hematologic failure than those with IHCA, both on ICU admission (7% vs. 2%; $p = 0.04$) and during the ICU stay (14% vs. 7%, $p = 0.009$).

Herein, changes in PDW or MPV during could represent an important but yet unreported component of the post-CA syndrome [14]. Several studies have reported the prognostic value of PDW or MPV in critically ill patients, focusing on the fact that an increase in these variables reflects the variation in platelet size caused by platelet activation [9, 17–19]. In our study, the lack of association between these variables and outcomes may suggest that the platelet activation occurring as a result of ischemia/reperfusion injury following CA differs from that induced by sepsis or other forms of critical illness. While no study on PDW in CA patients has been published so far, Chung et al. investigated whether MPV was associated with 30-day neurologic outcome and mortality after CA. In 184 patients with OHCA, increased 30-day mortality and poor neurological outcome rate were associated with MPV on admission [20]. Further studies are needed to investigate this phenomenon by including additional tests of platelet activation and aggregation and/or thromboelastometric measurements [21, 22]. Indeed, activated platelets are enlarged, and contain vasoactive and prothrombic factors that aggravate systemic inflammation and endothelial dysfunction. Nevertheless, it is possible that PDW and MPV are not sensitive enough to detect these changes in platelet function. In one study, CA secondary to coronary occlusion had the highest degree of platelet hyperfunction, which was tested under high shear rates with the collagen adenosine diphosphate closure time, when compared to other causes of arrest [5]. This condition of platelet hyperfuncion or increased aggregability indicated a pro-coagulopathic state in the post-cardiac arrest phase, which may contribute to the formation of microthrombi (i.e. microvascular dysfunction), but also to early stent thrombosis (i.e. post-arrest acute myocardial infarction) [23]. Thus, future studies should better characterize platelet activity in order to identify patients with enhanced clot formation and who might potentially benefit from a more rapid and aggressive antiplatelet therapy.

Our study has several limitations. First, due to the retrospective design of the study, we do not have all the variables potentially influencing these platelet indices, such as the use of antiaggregants (before arrest or after hospital admission), and the presence of hematological or autoimmune diseases or a previous infectious process, in particular for in-hospital CA. Moreover, some other confounders (i.e. gender, chronic inflammatory diseases, recent trauma or surgery) may also have influenced our findings. Second, we did not specifically collect data on coagulation parameters (such as activated partial thromboplastin time or D-dimers), although these may have been altered by specific therapies (e.g., unfractioned heparin or thrombolysis) administered in CA patients. Also, the combination of intravenous and/or oral platelet drug inhibitors, which was not available for this cohort, may also have affected our results; future studies on the use of different drugs after percutaneous coronary interventions should prospectively evaluate whether PDW and MPV are affected by such interventions and whether this phenomenon would be drug- and/or dose-related. Third, we did not look at specific organ dysfunctions and their relationship with platelet count, PDW or MPV. Forth, only few patients survived with an unfavourable neurological outcome. This may reflect local practices, as decision of withdrawal of life sustaining therapies is very often shared with patients' family in case of persistent and severe neurological impairment. Certainly, this approach prevented any additional analysis comparing survivors with good to these with poor neurological outcome. Fifth, only patients who received TTM were included in this cohort, although moderate hypothermia is not likely to influence the results. Finally, we could not record the exact time between blood sampling and laboratory analyses. In one study, Vagdatli et al. observed a remarkable decrease in PDW over time together with the absence of platelet activation, even in healthy subjects [24]; as such, samples taken outside working hours or not rapidly addressed to the laboratory for analyses may have underestimated the real PDW value and potentially biased our findings.

Conclusions

Platelet count decreased during the first 48 h after CA, while PDW and MPV did not change. Platelets reduction, PDW and MPV were not associated with patient outcome.

Abbreviations

CA: Cardiac arrest; CPC: Cerebral performance category score; CRP: C-reactive protein; ICU: Intensive care unit; MPV: Mean platelet volume; PDW: Platelet distribution width; ROSC: Return of spontaneous circulation; TTM: Targeted temperature management

Authors' contributions

AC: data collection, writing the manuscript and statistical analysis, FF: data collection and statistical analysis, CDeF: development of the study, data collection, JLV: interpretation of the data, writing the manuscript, JC: interpretation of the data, writing the manuscript, FST: interpretation of the data, writing the manuscript. AC, FF, CD, JLV, JC, FST approved the final manuscript.

Competing interests

The authors declare that they have no competing interests.

Author details

[1]Department of Intensive Care, Erasme Hospital, Université libre de Bruxelles, Brussels, Belgium. [2]Department of Anaesthesiology and Intensive Care, University of Foggia, Foggia, Italy.

References

1. Adrie C, Monchi M, Laurent I, Um S, Yan SB, Thuong M, et al. Coagulopathy after successful cardiopulmonary resuscitation following cardiac arrest: implication of the protein C anticoagulant pathway. J Am Coll Cardiol. 2005;46:21–8.
2. Roberts BW, Kilgannon JH, Chansky ME, Mittal N, Wooden J, Parrillo JE, et al. Multiple organ dysfunction after return of spontaneous circulation in Postcardiac arrest syndrome. Crit. Care Med. 2013;41:1492–501.
3. Bro-Jeppesen J, Kjaergaard J, Wanscher M, Nielsen N, Friberg H, Bjerre M, et al. The inflammatory response after out-of-hospital cardiac arrest is not modified by targeted temperature management at 33°C or 36°C. Resuscitation. 2014;85:1480–7.
4. Weidman JL, Shook DC, Hilberath JN. Cardiac resuscitation and coagulation. Anesthesiology. 2014;120:1009–14.
5. Spiel AO, Frossard M, Mayr FB, Kliegel A, Janata A, Uray T, et al. Pronounced platelet hyperfunction in patients with cardiac arrest achieving restoration of spontaneous circulation. Crit. Care Med. 2009;37:975–9.
6. Kim CH, Kim SJ, Lee MJ, Kwon YE, Kim YL, Park KS, Ryu HJ, Park JT, Han SH, Yoo TH, Kang SW, Oh HJ. An increase in mean platelet volume from baseline is associated with mortality in patients with severe sepsis or septic shock. PLoS One. 2015;10(3):e0119437.
7. Ates S, Oksuz H, Dogu B, Bozkus F, Ucmak H, Yanıt F. Can mean platelet volume and mean platelet volume/platelet count ratio be used as a diagnostic marker for sepsis and systemic inflammatory response syndrome? Saudi Med J. 2015;36:1186–90.
8. Gurbel PA, Gattis WA, Fuzaylov SF, Gaulden L, Hasselblad V, Serebruany VL, et al. Evaluation of platelets in heart failure: is platelet activity related to etiology, functional class, or clinical outcomes. Am Heart J. 2002;143:1068–75.
9. Gildo J, Monteiro DM, Oliveira D De, Torres C, Cleide M, Clementino F, et al. Atherosclerosis: Open Access Evaluation of Platelet Parameters as Prognostic Analysis in Cardiac Intensive Care Unit Patients. Atherosclerosis. 2017;2:1–6.
10. Ranjith MP, Divya R, Mehta VK, Krishnan MG, KamalRaj R, Kavishwar A. Significance of platelet volume indices and platelet count in ischaemic heart disease. J Clin Pathol. 2009;62:830–3.
11. Steblovnik K, Blinc A, Bozic-Mijovski M, Kranjec I, Melkic E, Noc M. Platelet reactivity in comatose survivors of cardiac arrest undergoing percutaneous coronary intervention and hypothermia. EuroIntervention. 2015;10:1418–24.
12. Tujjar O, Mineo G, Dell'Anna A, Poyatos-Robles B, Donadello K, Scolletta S, et al. Acute kidney injury after cardiac arrest. Crit. Care. 2015;19:169.

13. Anonymous. Randomized clinical study of thiopental loading in comatose survivors of cardiac arrest. Brain resuscitation clinical trial I study group. N Engl J Med. 1986;314:397–403.
14. Nolan JP, Neumar RW, Adrie C, Aibiki M, Berg RA, Böttiger BW, et al. Post-cardiac arrest syndrome: epidemiology, pathophysiology, treatment, and prognostication. Resuscitation. 2008;79:350–79.
15. Högberg C, Erlinge D, Braun OÖ. Mild hypothermia does not attenuate platelet aggregation and may even increase ADP-stimulated platelet aggregation after clopidogrel treatment. Thromb J. 2009;7:2.
16. Nobile L, Taccone FS, Szakmany T, Sakr Y, Jakob SM, Pellis T, et al. The impact of extracerebral organ failure on outcome of patients after cardiac arrest: an observational study from the ICON database. Crit Care. 2016;20(1):368.
17. Wiwanitkit V. Plateletcrit, mean platelet volume, platelet distribution width: its expected values and correlation with parallel red blood cell parameters. Clin Appl Thromb. 2004;10:175–8.
18. Guclu E, Durmaz Y, Karabay O. Effect of severe sepsis on platelet count and their indices. Afr Health Sci. 2013;13:333–8.
19. Gao Y, Li Y, Yu X, Guo S, Ji X, Sun T, et al. The impact of various platelet indices as prognostic markers of septic shock. PLoS One. 2014:9.
20. Chung SP, Yune HY, Park YS, You JS, Hong JH, Kong T, et al. Usefulness of mean platelet volume as a marker for clinical outcomes after out-of-hospital cardiac arrest: a retrospective cohort study. J Thromb Haemost. 2016;14(10): 2036–44.
21. Jeppesen AN, Kirkegaard H, Ilkjær S, Hvas AM. Influence of temperature on thromboelastometry and platelet aggregation in cardiac arrest patients undergoing targeted temperature management. Crit Care. 2016;20:118.
22. Mirabella L, Cotoia A, Colacicco G, Tullo L, Salatto P, Mollica G, et al. Reference values for coagulation assessment in full-term newborns. Minerva Anestesiol. 2017;83:369–74.
23. Tilemann L, Mohr SK, Preusch M, Chorianopoulos E, Giannitsis E, Katus HA, Müller OJ. Platelet function monitoring for stent thrombosis in critically Ill patients with an acute coronary syndrome. J Interv Cardiol. 2018;31(3):277–83.
24. Vagdatli E, Gounari E, Lazaridou E, Katsibourlia E, Tsikopoulou F, Labrianou I. Platelet distribution width: a simple, practical and specific marker of activation of coagulation. Hippokratia. 2010;14(1):28–32.

25

Evaluation of public awareness, knowledge and attitudes towards basic life support

Samiha Jarrah[1], Mahfuz Judeh[2] and Mohannad Eid AbuRuz[1,3*]

Abstract

Background: Out-of-hospital cardiac arrest is a major cause of mortality worldwide. When basic life support techniques are implemented quickly, the chance of survival is doubled. Therefore, this study evaluated public awareness, knowledge and attitudes towards basic life support in Jordan.

Methods: A descriptive, cross-sectional design with a convenience sample of 300 Jordanian adults aged over 18 years, recruited from three metropolitan areas in the northern, middle and southern regions.

Results: A total of 87 participants (29%) stated that they have received training about cardiopulmonary resuscitation (CPR). Among them, 20 participants (23%) received their training through the media. The highest response rate for cardiac arrest signs was chest pain ($n = 129$, 43%). Participants who received training had greater knowledge of the three signs of consciousness evaluation. The numbers of participants who received training and performed chest compression, mouth-to-mouth ventilation, and both compression and ventilation were higher than those who did not receive training. Overall, 256 participants (88.3%) reported that they would perform CPR on someone from their family without hesitation. The most important concern about performing CPR was making a mistake.

Conclusions: Improving knowledge about cardiopulmonary resuscitation is an important topic, which can be achieved by training the general population. Media can play an important role in this issue.

Keywords: Attitudes, Awareness, Jordan, Knowledge, Life support, Public

Background

Public awareness is of great importance, especially for life-saving information and skills. Globally, many countries emphasize related topics in educational institutions and workplaces. Death from sudden cardiac arrest remains very common worldwide [1, 2]. Approximately 50,000 people per year can survive until professional help arrives when basic life support (BLS) measures are performed properly. Out-of-hospital cardiac arrest (OHCA) causes 350,000 deaths each year in Europe [3]. In the US, the mortality rate due to OHCA is more than 90%, causing 276,000 deaths annually [4]. When the first person to witness OHCA uses an automated external defibrillator (AED), the chance of survival doubles. However, this instrument is used in only 4% of cases [5, 6].

The performance of BLS is usually done in chains that can be improved by educational programs. The success rate of BLS can be improved when it is performed by lay people before professional help arrives. This is usually motivated and enhanced by increasing public knowledge, attitudes and understanding of the application of the BLS techniques. Different studies have been conducted worldwide to ascertain the general level of knowledge, attitudes, and awareness about BLS in community settings. The rate was approximately 70% in Slovenia, which was considered a high percentage, reflecting a particular policy whereby training is an obligatory part of learning to drive in the country [7]. However, the percentage of this country's population with up-to-date knowledge was very low at 2%. On the other hand, the

* Correspondence: mohannadeid@yahoo.com; m_aburuz@asu.edu.jo
[1]Faculty of Nursing, Applied Science Private University, Amman, Jordan
[3]Amman, Jordan
Full list of author information is available at the end of the article

rate was 78% among teachers in Belgium, demonstrating the impact of teaching [8].

BLS training rates vary worldwide, including the following rates: Washington, DC 78% [9], Poland 75% [10], West Australia 64.1% [11], Japan 58% [12], Turkey 40.3% [1], Ireland 28% [13], New Zealand 27% [14], and Hong Kong 21% [15]. The rates also differ according to the specific area where the study was done. For example, in an urban region of Arizona, the rate was 63.2%, but this dropped to 55.4% in a rural region [16].

Studies evaluating knowledge, attitude and awareness about BLS in Middle Eastern countries, including Jordan, are limited. In a study evaluating knowledge and attitudes towards cardiopulmonary resuscitation (CPR) among university students in Riyadh, Saudi Arabia, it was found that 31% did not have prior CPR knowledge [17]. Of those with previous knowledge, 85% felt that it was inadequate. The most common sources of information were television and movies. Approximately 13% of individuals had encountered a situation that required the use of CPR, while only 14% of them performed it. This was mostly due to lack of knowledge (48.2%). Overall, 88% of students would have liked to learn how to perform CPR. The authors concluded that the general attitude towards CPR was positive, but the knowledge on the topic was insufficient [17]. Thus, more focus should be placed on the improvement of CPR skills. In addition, more studies are needed to assess knowledge and attitudes towards CPR in the community.

Methods

The purpose of the current study was to evaluate public awareness, knowledge and attitudes towards BLS in Jordan.

Research Questions: (1) What is the level of awareness among Jordanian lay people regarding BLS? (2) What is the level of knowledge Jordanian lay people have about BLS? (3) Do Jordanian lay people have positive attitudes towards BLS? (4) Does previous training about BLS have an effect on the level of awareness, knowledge, and attitudes towards BLS?

Design, Sample, and Setting: A cross-sectional design with a convenience sampling method was used in this study. The participants who met the following inclusion criteria were included: (a) Jordanian nationality, (b) aged 18 years and above, (c) able to read and write Arabic, (d) signed informed consent, and (e) not graduated from or studying at any medical field colleges (medicine, pharmacy, nursing, dentistry, and laboratory). Those individuals were excluded because their university programs have mandatory courses about BLS training.

Data were collected from three major cities in the northern, middle, and southern areas of Jordan to be representative of the country as a whole. Three research assistants collected the data, one for each area. They approached the participants every day from 8 am to 8 pm in shopping malls and public areas, which are similar in the three cities. The research assistants explained the study and the purposes to the participants, and if they agreed to participate, they signed the informed consent form and answered the questionnaire.

To make sure that the sample size was sufficient, a power analysis was performed using an online G*power sample size calculator. Research questions 1–3 were answered by descriptive statistics. Research question number 4 was answered by chi-squared test. Using this information and the assumptions of a power of .8, type 1 error of 0.05, and a medium effect size, the sample size needed was 107 participants. Therefore, we recruited 300 participants to allow for attrition and dropout.

Measurement

The researchers designed a questionnaire specifically for this study. This questionnaire was based on the latest American Heart Association (AHA) guidelines for BLS and was written in Arabic [18]. The questionnaire included two parts. Part one collected information about participants' sociodemographic characteristics (i.e., age, gender, marital status, education, and employment). Part two assessed their knowledge, attitudes and awareness about BLS. This latter part consisted of 22 questions about signs and symptoms of cardiac arrest, previous CPR experience, compression location and rate, if the participants were concerned about making mistakes when performing CPR, and people to whom they would provide CPR (Additional file 1).

Procedure of data collection and ethical consideration

The study was approved by the Institutional Review Board committee at the Applied Science Private University (Faculty 018). The principal investigator met with all research assistants and explained the purpose of the study and the questionnaire. Research assistants explained the study to the participants. They also ensured the participants that they had the right not to participate and to withdraw at any time. After this explanation, if the participants agreed to participate, they were asked to sign an informed consent form and to complete the questionnaire. The study was completely anonymous and no identifiers were required. Data were coded and entered into a password-protected computer, accessible only to the principal investigator and co-investigators.

Data analysis

Data analysis was done using SPSS version 21. Description of the sample was performed by descriptive statistics, including n (%) or mean ± SD. A chi-squared test was used to determine if there were differences between those who received training and those who did not regarding the identification of cardiac arrest, action performed when witnessing cardiac arrest, and practical application of CPR. Any p value < .05 was considered statistically significant. All statistically non-significant results were reported as not significant (NS).

Results

Demographic characteristics

A total of 400 participants were invited to participate, of whom 300 agreed and filled out the questionnaire completely, comprising the sample of the study. The participants were distributed between males and females, with a mean age of 33.55 years. More than half of the sample was married and had a high school and university degree. A detailed description of the participants' characteristics is presented in Table 1.

CPR training

Among the whole sample, only 87 participants (29%) stated that they had received CPR training. Most of those received their training at school ($n = 33$, 37.9%), followed by university ($n = 26$, 29.9%), and the media (television and internet) ($n = 20$, 23%).

Table 1 Demographic characteristics of the participants ($N = 300$)

Characteristic	Mean ± SD/ n (%)
Age	33.6 ± 11.0
Gender	
Male	139 (46.3)
Female	161 (53.7)
Marital status	
Married	181 (60.4)
Single	109 (36.3)
Divorced	10 (3.3)
Educational Level	
Elementary school	7 (2.3)
Preparatory school	45 (15)
Secondary school	92 (30.7)
Diploma	44 (14.7)
University	90 (30)
Post graduate	22 (7.3)
Job	
Governmental sector	79 (26.3)
Private sector	86 (28.7)
Self-employed	21 (7.0)
Retired	19 (6.3)
House wife	35 (11.7)
Student	35 (11.7)
Farmer	4 (1.3)
Not employed	21 (7.0)

Signs of cardiac arrest

The response rates for the signs of cardiac arrest are presented in Table 2. The highest rates were for (1) chest pain ($n = 129$, 43%), (2) respiratory standstill ($n = 119$, 39.7%), (c) loss of consciousness ($n = 114$, 38%), and (d) difficulty breathing ($n = 107$, 35.7%).

Recognizing cardiac arrest

Table 3 shows comparisons between those who had received training about CPR and those who had not regarding cardiac arrest signs, including (a) consciousness evaluation, (b) respiratory evaluation, and (c) circulation evaluation. Based on the table, participants who received training were more likely to know the three signs of consciousness evaluation than those who did not. For respiratory evaluation, the number of participants who received training and did not know that "no steam coming up in front of the mouth of the victim" was an incorrect answer was lower than the number of participants who did not receive training and did not know this answer. For circulation evaluation, the number of participants who had CPR training and could correctly feel a pulse in the vessels of the neck was higher than the number who did not receive training and could feel a pulse.

Seventy participants had witnessed a sudden cardiac arrest (23.3%). Among those, 42.8% called the ambulance, 20% told someone to call for help, 10% gave chest compression, 10% gave mouth-to-mouth breathing, 8.6% gave both chest compression and mouth-to-mouth breathing, and 8.6% just watched and left. The number of participants who received training and performed chest compression, mouth-to-mouth ventilation, and both massage and ventilation was higher than the number who performed these actions and did not receive training (Table 4).

Table 2 Response rates for the signs of cardiac arrest

Sign	[a]n (%)
Chest pain	129 (43.0)
Respiratory standstill	119 (39.7)
Loss of consciousness	114 (38.0)
Difficulty in breathing	107 (35.7)
Cyanosis	76 (25.3)
Discontinuation of circulation	62 (20.7)
Nausea	47 (15.7)
The individual is not moving	45 (15.0)
Others	10 (3.3)

[a]More than one participant gave more than one answer

Table 3 Identification of cardiac arrest

Finding	Received training n (%)	Did not receive training n (%)	Total n (%)	*P* value
Consciousness Evaluation				
No response when called[a]	47 (15.7)	84 (28)	131 (43.7)	.015
No response when touched[a]	32 (10.7)	78 (26)	110 (36.7)	NS
No movement[a]	32 (10.7)	64 (21.3)	96 (32.0)	NS
Those who knew the 3 findings correctly	18 (6.0)	16 (5.3)	34 (11.3)	0.04
Those who knew 2 of the findings correctly	21 (7.0)	31 (10.3)	52 (17.3)	.036
Those who knew one of the findings correctly	78 (26.0)	181 (60.3)	259 (86.3)	NS
Respiratory Evaluation				
No respiratory movement[a]	36 (12.0)	94 (31.3)	130 (43.3)	NS
No respiratory sound[a]	31 (10.3)	63 (21.0)	94 (31.3)	NS
No air coming out from the mouth[a]	29 (9.7)	70 (23.3)	99 (33)	NS
No steam coming up in front of the mouth of the victim[b]	13 (4.3)	55 (18.3)	68 (22.7)	.027
Those who knew the 3 findings correctly	11 (3.7)	23 (7.7)	34 (11.3)	NS
Those who knew 2 of the findings correctly	13 (4.3)	43 (14.3)	56 (18.7)	NS
Those who knew one of the findings correctly	72 (24.0)	161 (53.7)	233 (77.7)	NS
Circulation Evaluation				
Lack of circulation signs[a]	25 (8.3)	73 (24.3)	98 (32.7)	NS
Not feeling a pulse in the vessels of the neck[a]	50 (16.7)	92 (30.7)	142 (47.3) (47.3).017	.017
Not feeling a pulse in the vessels of the arm[a]	91 (30.3)	28 (9.3)	119 (39.7)	NS
Those who knew the 3 findings correctly	4 (1.3)	13 (4.3)	17 (5.7)	NS
Those who knew 2 of the findings correctly	13 (4.3)	32 (10.7)	45 (15)	NS
Those who knew one of the findings correctly	86 (28.7)	211 (70.3)	297 (99.0)	NS

[a]True reply, NS: Not significant
[b]False reply

CPR knowledge and skills

Overall, 37% of the sample knew how to perform chest compression if they witnessed a sudden cardiac arrest. Moreover, 74.3% indicated that they could give both chest compression and ventilation. Regarding mouth-to-mouth ventilation, 47.7% of the sample said that they would perform it if they witnessed a sudden arrest. The number of participants who received training about CPR and knew the correct answers regarding the meaning of chest compression, heart rate, and the massage/ventilation ratio was higher than the number who knew the correct answers and did not receive training (Table 5).

CPR attitude

When the participants were asked "To whom would you provide CPR without hesitation?" the responses were as follows: 265 (88.3%) someone from the family, 110 (36.7%) friends, and 90 (30%) neighbors.

Concerns regarding CPR

The three most important concerns regarding CPR application for family members were (1) making a mistake ($n = 185$, 61.7%), (2) causing bone fractures ($n = 51$, 17%), and (3) stopping the heart ($n = 49$, 16.3%). The three most important concerns regarding CPR applications for strangers were (1) making a mistake ($n = 177$, 59%), (2) punishment because of legal reasons ($n = 87$, 29%), and (3) causing harm to organs ($n = 72$, 24%).

Discussion

CPR knowledge and skills are of great importance to the public and communities, as they are life-saving skills from which all members of society benefit. There have been no previous studies in Jordan concerning public knowledge and attitudes towards CPR. The participants were chosen from diverse and representative parts of Jordan, from among the lay population and different backgrounds. The participants' characteristics in this study were comparable to those in other similar and related studies [1]. Regarding CPR training, the results showed that 29% of the participants stated that they had received CPR training, higher than that reported in Hong Kong (21%) [15] and mainland China (25.6%) [19] and comparable to data reported elsewhere, including 27% in New Zealand [14] and 28% in Ireland [13]. Reported percentages from other countries, including

Table 4 Classification of participants who witnessed sudden cardiac arrest by training

Action	Received training n(%)	Did not receive training n (%)	Total n (%)	*P* value
Conduct only chest compression	5 (7.1)	2 (2.9)	7 (10.0)	.007
Conduct only mouth-to-mouth ventilation	5 (7.1)	2 (2.9)	7 (10.0)	.007
Conduct both, chest compression and ventilation	5 (7.1)	1 (1.4)	6 (8.6)	.01

Australia [11], Poland [10], and the US [9] were higher, with percentages of 58, 75 and 79%, respectively. In general, Jordan has a lower percentage of trained people in comparison to other countries, indicating that more focus is needed to train the public in life-saving skills to bring Jordan in line with international norms.

The results of this study reflect that the main sources of information and training are schools, followed by universities, and finally, the media (i.e., television and the internet). Studies conducted in nearby countries, such as Saudi Arabia, indicate that the most common sources of information on CPR are television and movies [17]. Although schools and universities are of great importance to increase information, the media can reach a broader population and can also cover a large number of people to raise more awareness. Inclusion of such simple training programs by trained personnel could have positive outcomes for public health and communities.

Participants in this study who received training were knowledgeable regarding the evaluation of the three signs of consciousness. Regarding respiratory evaluation, the number of participants who received training and did not know that "no steam coming up in front of the mouth of the victim means they have stopped breathing" is an incorrect answer was lower than that among those who did not receive training. For circulation evaluation, the number of participants who received CPR training and knew how to correctly feel the pulse in the vessels of the neck was higher than the number with this knowledge who did not receive training. These results highlight the importance of training programs and ensuring that necessary information is both fully understood and practiced by trainees.

The response rates for the signs of cardiac arrest showed that the highest rates were for chest pain, respiratory standstill, loss of consciousness and difficulty breathing. Similar data were reported in a study conducted in Turkey, in which respondents indicated that the highest rates were for signs of cardiac arrest (60.7%), followed by 49.3% who answered cessation of circulation, and finally cessation of breathing (40.7%) [1]. Therefore, chest pain and circulation are given first priority by lay people, who then look for respiration. This is in line with the new guidelines of the AHA (to perform chest compression, then attend to breathing, and finally circulation).

In this study, the participants who witnessed sudden cardiac arrest comprised 23.3% of the total sample. Among those, nearly half stated that they called the ambulance, and the rest with equal or lower percentages responded that they called for help, gave chest compression, and gave mouth-to-mouth breathing. The lowest responses were for chest compression and mouth-to-mouth breathing and 'just watched and left'. These results reflect the nature of Jordanian culture and how people are willing to help each other, especially during emergency situations. However, it is culturally insensitive to give mouth-to-mouth breathing, especially between men and women.

In this study, the numbers of participants who received training and mentioned that they performed chest compression, mouth-to-mouth ventilation, and both massage and ventilation were greater than those who performed these actions and did not receive training. The majority of the respondents (74.3%) indicated that they can give both chest compression and ventilation. The number of participants who received training about CPR and knew the correct answers regarding the meaning of chest compression, heart rate, and the massage/ventilation ratio was higher than the number who knew the correct answers and did not receive training. Training sessions were beyond the scope of the current study; we merely asked participants if they had attended

Table 5 Practical application of CPR between those who received training and those who did not

Item	Received training n(%)	Did not receive training n(%)	Total n (%)	*P* value
Chest compression meaning[a]	37 (12.3)	51 (17.0)	88 (29.3)	.001
Massage rate[a]	37 (12.3)	41 (13.7)	78 (26)	.000
Massage location[a]	31 (10.3)	56 (18.7)	87 (29)	NS
Massage depth[a]	29 (9.7)	77 (25.7)	106 (53.3)	NS
Massage/ventilation ratio[a]	33 (11.0)	30 (10.0)	63 (21.0)	.000

NS not significant
[a]Numbers reflect correct answers

training or not. However, such information forms the basics of any CPR training course, even if it is learned through the media. These results indicate the importance of training programs, which empower people to provide help in emergency situations.

A high percentage of participants in this study showed no hesitation to provide CPR to their family members; the next highest percentage was to friends and finally, to neighbors. Concerns regarding CPR applications for family and strangers were classified in priority order. For family members, the highest percentage of concern was making mistakes (61.7%), and the lowest was punishment because of legal reasons (15%). Concerns regarding performing CPR on strangers were classified in priority order from making a mistake, to concern of punishment because of legal reasons (59%), with the least concern about causing a bone fracture (18.3%). The lowest priority concern for performing CPR to both family and strangers was contamination by blood or vomit. This indicates that life-saving attempts for family members and strangers will be given high priority, with apprehension about making mistakes being the most important concern. These results indicate the high necessity of education and training programs for the community.

Chair et al. [15] mentioned that people with full-time jobs and higher levels of education were more likely to have received CPR training. Respondents stating they had received CPR training were more willing to try it if needed at home (odds ratio = 3.3; 95% confidence interval, 2.4–4.6; $P < 0.001$), and on strangers in the street (4.3; 3.1–6.1; $P < 0.001$) in case of emergencies. Overall, the CPR knowledge of the respondents was low (median = 1, out of 8). More than 90% of the sample in this study was employed, and more than half of the sample also had diplomas and higher degrees of education. These characteristics support the idea of a greater willingness to conduct CPR among educated and employed people.

In their study, Chen et al. [19] described the concerns regarding CPR applications for family members and strangers. The questionnaire included individual information, current status of bystander CPR training, and individuals' willingness and attitudes towards performing CPR. The authors found that 25.6% of lay people received CPR training, the majority (98.6%) of whom would perform CPR on their family members, but fewer (76.3%) were willing to perform it on strangers. Most respondents (53.2%) were worried about legal issues. When laws were implemented to protect bystanders who give first aid, the number of laypersons who were not willing to perform CPR on strangers dropped from 23.7 to 2.4%. Although the number of people in China who knew CPR was increasing over time, CPR training was still much less common than in many developed countries. The barriers as mentioned by the authors were that laypersons were not well trained, and they feared being prosecuted for unsuccessful CPR. The authors also recommended a need for more accredited CPR training courses, and they noted that laws should be passed to protect bystanders who provide assistance.

There are some centers providing CPR training for lay persons in different areas in Jordan, including in the north, middle, and south. However, to date, there is no legislation on the part of the Ministry of Health and the Ministry of Interior to protect laypersons in case they perform CPR on victims and mistakes occur. For this reason, some people will hesitate to provide CPR if the victim is not one of their family members. The relevant government bodies should be informed about such results in order to improve outcomes and decrease mortality and morbidity after cardiac arrest, especially OHCA.

Conclusion and recommendations

The results of this study indicate the importance of continuing to train the population in CPR knowledge and skills; specifically, CPR education programs and evaluations of their effectiveness are needed. The media can play a role in increasing the knowledge of the public, hence the authors recommend promoting the training programs in the media, utilizing cheap and effective technologies such as social media to reach the general population, as well as providing more formal instruction through schools and universities. In addition, national bylaws should protect those who provide assistance to people with heart failure in such cases.

Limitations

The major limitation of this study was the use of a cross-sectional design with a convenience sampling method. Moreover, we used the 2010 AHA criteria and did not ask about the timing for when participants received their training.

Abbreviations

AED: Automated external defibrillator; AHA: American Heart Association; BLS: Basic life support; CPR: Cardiopulmonary resuscitation; OHCA: Out-of-hospital cardiac arrest; SPSS: Statistical package for social sciences

Acknowledgments

We wish to thank research assistants who helped in the data collection for this research project.

Funding

The authors are grateful to the Applied Science Private University, Amman, Jordan, for the full financial support granted to this research project including data collection, analysis, and the financial support granted to cover the publication fees of this research article.

Authors' contributions
SJ Was the primary investigator and contributed in all facets of the study including study conception/design, data collection, data analysis, and was the lead author for all drafts of the manuscript. MJ contributed to study conception/design, data analysis, and edited all drafts of the manuscript. MEA contributed to study conception/design, was the primary data analyst, and edited all drafts of the manuscript. All authors read and approved the final manuscript.

Competing interests
The authors declare that they have no competing interests.

Author details
[1]Faculty of Nursing, Applied Science Private University, Amman, Jordan. [2]Applied Science Private University, Amman, Jordan. [3]Amman, Jordan.

References
1. Ozbilgin S, Akan M, Hanci V, Aygun C, Kuvaki B. Evaluation of public awareness, knowledge and attitudes about cardiopulmonary resuscitation: report of Izmir. Turk J Anaesthesiol Reanim 2015;43(6):396–405. Epub 2016/07/02. doi: https://doi.org/10.5152/TJAR.2015.61587. PubMed PMID: 27366536; PubMed Central PMCID: PMC4894183.
2. Puttgen HA, Pantle H, Geocadin RG. Management of cardiac arrest patients to maximize neurologic outcome. Curr Opin Crit Care 2009;15(2):118–124. Epub 2009/07/07. doi: https://doi.org/10.1097/MCC.0b013e328326077c00075198-200904000-00008. PubMed PMID: 19578322.
3. Berdowski J, Berg RA, Tijssen JG, Koster RW. Global incidences of out-of-hospital cardiac arrest and survival rates: Systematic review of 67 prospective studies. Resuscitation. 2010;81(11):1479–1487. Epub 2010/09/11. doi: https://doi.org/10.1016/j.resuscitation.2010.08.006. PubMed PMID: 20828914.
4. Benjamin EJ, Blaha MJ, Chiuve SE, Cushman M, Das SR, Deo R, et al. Heart Disease and Stroke Statistics-2017 Update: A Report From the American Heart Association. Circulation. 2017;135(10):e146-e603. Epub 2017/01/27. doi: https://doi.org/10.1161/CIR.0000000000000485. PubMed PMID: 28122885; PubMed Central PMCID: PMC5408160.
5. Berdowski J, Blom MT, Bardai A, Tan HL, Tijssen JG, Koster RW. Impact of onsite or dispatched automated external defibrillator use on survival after out-of-hospital cardiac arrest. Circulation. 2011;124(20):2225–2232. Epub 2011/10/19. doi: https://doi.org/10.1161/CIRCULATIONAHA.110.015545. PubMed PMID: 22007075.
6. McNally B, Robb R, Mehta M, Vellano K, Valderrama AL, Yoon PW, et al. Out-of-hospital cardiac arrest surveillance --- cardiac arrest registry to enhance survival (CARES), United States, October 1, 2005--December 31, 2010. MMWR Surveill Summ 2011;60(8):1–19. Epub 2011/07/29. PubMed PMID: 21796098.
7. Rajapakse R, Noc M, Kersnik J. Public knowledge of cardiopulmonary resuscitation in Republic of Slovenia. Wien Klin Wochenschr 2010;122(23–24):667–672. Epub 2010/12/07. doi: https://doi.org/10.1007/s00508-010-1489-8. PubMed PMID: 21132393.
8. Mpotos N, Vekeman E, Monsieurs K, Derese A, Valcke M. Knowledge and willingness to teach cardiopulmonary resuscitation: a survey amongst 4273 teachers. Resuscitation. 2013;84(4):496–500. Epub 2013/02/05. doi: https://doi.org/10.1016/j.resuscitation.2013.01.023. PubMed PMID: 23376584.
9. Sipsma K, Stubbs BA, Plorde M. Training rates and willingness to perform CPR in King County, Washington: a community survey. Resuscitation 2011; 82(5):564–567. Epub 2011/01/25 https://doi.org/10.1016/j.resuscitation.2010.12.007. PubMed PMID: 21257253.
10. Rasmus A, Czekajlo MS. A national survey of the polish population's cardiopulmonary resuscitation knowledge. Eur J Emerg Med 2000;7(1):39–43. Epub 2000/06/06. PubMed PMID: 10839378.
11. Celenza T, Gennat HC, O'Brien D, Jacobs IG, Lynch DM, Jelinek GA. Community competence in cardiopulmonary resuscitation. Resuscitation 2002;55(2):157–165. Epub 2002/11/05. PubMed PMID: 12413753.
12. Kuramoto N, Morimoto T, Kubota Y, Maeda Y, Seki S, Takada K, et al. Public perception of and willingness to perform bystander CPR in Japan. Resuscitation. 2008;79(3):475–481. Epub 2008/09/23. doi: https://doi.org/10.1016/j.resuscitation.2008.07.005. PubMed PMID: 18805615.
13. Jennings S, Hara T.O, Cavanagh B, Bennett K. A national survey of prevalence of cardiopulmonary resuscitation training and knowledge of the emergency number in Ireland. Resuscitation. 2009;80(9):1039–1042. Epub 2009/07/10. doi: https://doi.org/10.1016/j.resuscitation.2009.05.023. PubMed PMID: 19586705.
14. Larsen P, Pearson J, Galletly D. Knowledge and attitudes towards cardiopulmonary resuscitation in the community. N Z Med J 2004;117(1193): U870. Epub 2004/05/11. PubMed PMID: 15133520.
15. Chair SY, Hung MS, Lui JC, Lee DT, Shiu IY, Choi KC. Public knowledge and attitudes towards cardiopulmonary resuscitation in Hong Kong: telephone survey. Hong Kong Med J. 2014;20(2):126–133. Epub 2014/03/15. doi: https://doi.org/10.12809/hkmj134076. PubMed PMID: 24625387.
16. Coons SJ, Guy MC. Performing bystander CPR for sudden cardiac arrest: behavioral intentions among the general adult population in Arizona. Resuscitation. 2009;80(3):334–340. Epub 2009/01/23. doi: https://doi.org/10.1016/j.resuscitation.2008.11.024. PubMed PMID: 19157675.
17. Al-Turki YA, Al-Fraih YS, Jalaly JB, Al-Maghlouth IA, Al-Rashoudi FH, Al-Otaibi AF, et al. Knowledge and attitudes towards cardiopulmonary resuscitation among university students in Riyadh, Saudi Arabia. Saudi Med J. 2008;29(9): 1306–1309. Epub 2008/09/25. PubMed PMID: 18813417.
18. Al-Najjar T, Al-Khouli AT, Dakak FM, Awad JA, Naseef MA, Kentab OY. Arabic Version of Basic Life Support for Health Care Providers. 1st ed; 2011.
19. Chen M, Wang Y, Li X, Hou L, Liu J, Han F. Public knowledge and attitudes towards bystander cardiopulmonary resuscitation in China. Biomed Res Int 2017;2017:3250485. Epub 2017/04/04. doi: https://doi.org/10.1155/2017/3250485. PubMed PMID: 28367441; PubMed Central PMCID: PMC5359437.

Delayed intracranial hemorrhage in elderly anticoagulated patients sustaining a minor fall

Nolan Mann[1], Kellen Welch[1], Andrew Martin[1], Michael Subichin[1], Katherine Wietecha[2], Lauren E. Birmingham[1*], Tiffany D. Marchand[1] and Richard L. George[1]

Abstract

Background: Falls are a common cause of hospitalization, morbidity, and mortality among the elderly in the United States. Evidence-based imaging recommendations for evaluation of delayed intracranial hemorrhage (DICH) are not generally agreed upon. The purpose of this project was to evaluate the incidence of DICH detected by head computer tomography (CT) among an elderly population on pre-injury anticoagulant or antiplatelet (ACAP) therapy.

Methods: Data from a Level 1 Trauma Center trauma registry was used to assess the incidence of DICH in an elderly population of patients (≥65 years) who sustained a minor fall while on pre-injury ACAP medications. Counts and percentages are reported.

Results: Data on 1076 elderly trauma patients were downloaded, of which 838 sustained a minor fall and 513 were found to be using a pre-injury ACAP medication. One patient (0.46%) with a DICH was identified out of 218 patients who received a routine repeat head CT. Aspirin and warfarin were the most common pre-injury ACAP medications and 19.27% (42/218) of patients were found to be using multiple ACAP medications.

Conclusions: Universal screening protocols promote immediate-term patient safety, but do so at a great expense with respect to health expenditures and increased radiation exposure. This analysis highlights the need for an effective risk assessment tool for DICH that would reduce the burden of unnecessary screenings while still identifying life-threatening intracranial hemorrhages in affected patients.

Keywords: Intracranial hemorrhage, Head injury, Elderly, Fall, Delayed intracranial hemorrhage

Background

Falls are recognized as one of the primary causes of injury and death in the elderly population [1]. In 2015, 6359 per 100,000 elderly adults (aged 65 and older) experienced an unintentional nonfatal fall, costing the U.S. health care system approximately $31 billion [2, 3]. Intracranial injury as a result of falling is a concern in any patient that falls, but is of principal concern in the elderly population, and even more so among those who use anticoagulant and antiplatelet (ACAP) medications. Individuals taking pre-injury ACAP medications have a two-fold increase in the risk of intracranial injury after blunt head injury [4–6]. Furthermore, elderly adults are the most common age cohort prescribed ACAP medications, making them more susceptible to this risk [6].

Rates of immediate traumatic intracranial hemorrhage following a traumatic injury identified by head CT scan vary in the literature, ranging from 5.1–29.1% [7–13]. In the event that an immediate intracranial hemorrhage has been ruled out, delayed intracranial hemorrhage (DICH) among injured elderly patients on ACAP therapy still remains a concern [14, 15]. Prior studies have concluded that rates of DICH in elderly injured patients on pre-injury ACAP medications are low, ranging from 0 to 6% [8, 9, 13, 16–19]. Most of these analyses have considered limited panels of ACAP medications and have not

* Correspondence: lbirming@kent.edu
[1]Summa Health System- Department of Surgery, Akron Campus, Akron, OH, USA
Full list of author information is available at the end of the article

addressed patients taking multiple ACAP medications. Even in cases where a DICH is detected, neurosurgical operative intervention has been shown to be infrequent [17, 19, 20].

Performing a repeat head computed tomography (CT) after an initial negative head CT is one strategy to evaluate delayed intracranial hemorrhage. Evidence has shown that most DICHs occur within 6–24 h of injury [21, 22], although a recent large multicenter prospective study found that delayed hemorrhages occurred up to 5 days after injury [19]. There is no clear consensus on whether or not to routinely perform repeat head CTs in elderly patients with minor injuries on ACAP therapies, although this is the standard practice in many European trauma centers [23]. Low rates of DICH and even lower rates of subsequent neurosurgical operative intervention have caused many to question the value of the routine repeat head CT [19]. Yet, others still see it as a valuable tool to diagnose DICH, especially since there are no known predictors of DICH [18, 24].

The primary aim of this analysis was to quantify the frequency of DICH in an elderly cohort presenting following a minor fall while taking pre-injury ACAP medications. Prior studies have typically included only specific ACAP medications—most commonly warfarin and clopidogrel. This analysis includes a multitude of ACAP medications which is more reflective of our population. Additionally, this analysis used patients who fell and were admitted to a trauma service as the primary inclusion criteria, rather than discharge diagnosis codes that are assigned retrospectively to select patients for inclusion. This more closely resembles prospective clinical decision-making.

Methods

This was a retrospective analysis utilizing data from the trauma registry of a Midwestern College of Surgeons verified Level 1 Trauma Center and electronic medical record system. Head CT utilization, results, and medication data were abstracted from the medical record, while all other data elements came from the trauma registry. Data from January 2014–December 2015 was utilized. The present study is not regulated by our institution's Institutional Review Board as it is not considered human subjects research per the federal definition. Our institutional office of research administration has deemed and approved this to be a quality improvement project and approved the publication of the results.

Inclusion criteria comprised of being 65 years or older, admission to the trauma service, sustaining a minor fall as defined by the National Trauma Data Standard (NTDS) as a fall from less than 10 ft [25], having a documented head CT scan in the trauma registry, actively taking an anticoagulant or antiplatelet medication at the time of presentation to the emergency room, and having both an initial and routine repeat head CT performed prior to discharge. In order to be admitted to the trauma service at the institution where this analysis was performed evidence of cranio-facial trauma must be present. Many prior studies have relied on discharge diagnoses to limit the analysis to only those patients with documented head injuries whereas the present analysis is limited to those patients who had evidence of cranio-facial trauma without relying on subsequent administrative data. While the populations are very similar, the current analysis does not rely on discharge diagnoses to define the population, but rather, clinical observation that occurred during the trauma-related visit. A wide variety of ACAP therapies included were: warfarin (Coumadin and Marevan), dabigatran (Pradaxa), apixaban (Eliquis), rivaroxaban (Xarelto), dipyridamole (Aggrenox), Enoxaparin (lovenox), heparin, aspirin, clopidogrel (Plavix), prasugrel (Effient), ticlopidine (Ticlid), and ticagrelor (Brilinta). Figure 1 demonstrates how patients were identified for the analysis.

Several demographic variables were exported from the trauma registry including age, sex, race, hospital length of stay, presence of alcohol, injury severity score (ISS), and the initial Glasgow Coma Score (GCS). Data was analyzed using SAS 9.3 (Cary, N.C.).

The primary outcome was the prevalence of DICH identified on repeat head CT scan. DICH was defined as the

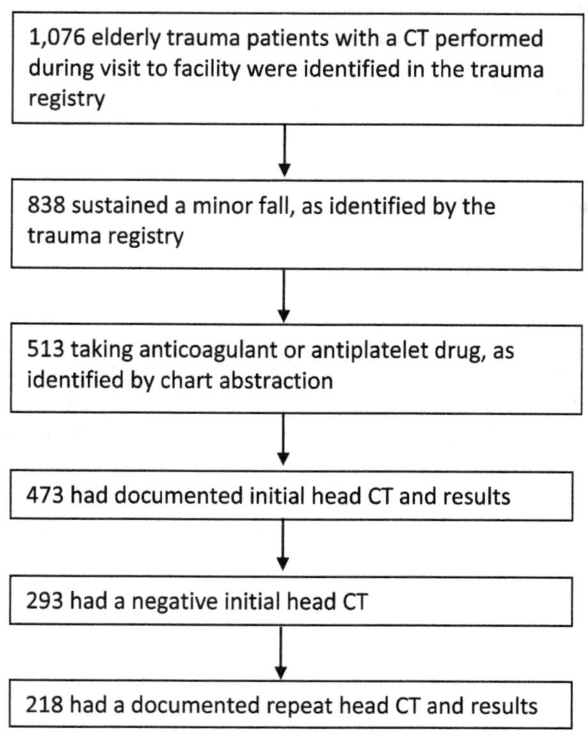

Fig. 1 Patient Flow Diagram

presence of subdural hematoma, epidural hematoma, subarachnoid hemorrhage, parenchymal contusion, or intraventricular hemorrhage evidenced on repeat head CT after an initial negative head CT. Secondary outcomes included neurosurgical interventions and mortality for patients with DICH and adherence to the departmental practice guideline. The departmental practice guideline is that a routine repeat head CT should be performed for any patient 65 years of age or older with a negative initial head CT who presents within 6 h of a minor fall, while on a pre-injury ACAP medication.

Results

Trauma registry data was exported on 1076 patients admitted to the trauma service aged 65 years or older during the study period with at least one head CT. Eight hundred thirty-eight (838) were identified as minor fall patients and 513 were found to be taking pre-injury ACAP medications. Figure 1 presents the patient flow diagram. The average age of the sample population was 81.3 years of age. Most cases had injury severity classified as minor (80.28%) or moderate (15.60%). The vast majority of GCS scores fell into the lowest-risk range, which can still be indicative of mild traumatic brain injury. Demographics are presented in Table 1.

Table 2 summarizes ACAP medication utilization. The most commonly used ACAP medication was aspirin (54.13%), followed by warfarin (33.03%) and clopidogrel (Plavix) (16.51%).

Approximately one-fifth (19.27%, 42/218) of patients presented to the emergency department (ED) on more than one pre-injury ACAP medication. Aspirin and clopidogrel (Plavix) was the most common combination, followed by aspirin and warfarin (Coumadin or Marevan) (Table 3). Out of all ACAP medications, aspirin was most commonly used in combination with another medication, followed by warfarin (Coumadin or Marevan). Two patients presented to the ED on three separate ACAP medications.

Out of 513 eligible patients for an initial head CT, 473 (92.22%) received an initial head CT. Two-hundred ninety-three (293) patients had negative initial head CT (61.95%). Of the 293 patients eligible for a routine repeat head CT, 218 were documented with results (74.40%). Of the 293 eligible for a routine repeat head CT, 24 were documented as not ordered because the patient arrived more than 6 h after being injured, 2 were not ordered because the patient expired, and 49 were not ordered for an unspecified reason. One positive routine repeat head CT was identified (0.46%) out of 218. The single patient with a positive repeat head CT survived to discharge without neurosurgical intervention or significant morbidity.

Table 1 Demographics of Elderly Minor Fall Patients Admitted to the Trauma Service on Pre-injury ACAP Therapy who Received a RRHCT ($n = 218$)

Characteristic	Mean (SD)
Age	81.6 (7.65)
	Mean (IQR)
Length of stay, days	2 (1–4)
	n (%)
Sex	
Female	127 (58.26%)
Male	91 (41.74%)
Race	
Black	9 (4.13%)
White	206 (94.50%)
Other	3 (1.37%)
ISS Group	
0–9 (Minor)	175 (80.28%)
10–14 (Moderate)	34 (15.60%)
15–24 (Severe)	8 (3.66%)
≥ 25 (Very Severe)	0 (0.00%)
Not documented	1 (0.46%)
Alcohol Evident	
Negative	144 (66.05%)
Trace	63 (28.90%)
Yes	9 (4.13%)
Not documented	2 (0.92%)
Glasgow Coma Scale	
3–8	5 (2.30%)
9–12	6 (2.75%)
13–15	202 (92.65%)
Not documented	5 (2.30%)

Discussion

This study identified one patient with a DICH out of 218 patients who received routine repeat head CTs. This patient required no neurosurgical intervention and no change in clinical management. The patient had an ISS of 22 and was taking apixaban (Eliquis) prior to injury. No additional risk factors were identified in this patient.

The lack of surgical intervention in the identified patient is consistent with prior studies that have reported very low levels of surgical intervention in this patient population [8, 19, 26]. Additionally, this analysis identified that 49 patients did not receive a routine repeat head CT. These patients were analyzed further, and it was determined that approximately half of the patients arrived more than 6 h after their injury, thus should not have received a routine repeat head CT, per the departmental guideline. Given that some head CTs were still

Table 2 Anticoagulation and Antiplatelet Pre-injury Use (n = 218)

ACAP Therapy	n (%)
Warfarin (Coumadin and Marevan)	
Yes	72 (33.03%)
No	146 (66.97%)
Dabigatran (Pradaxa)	
Yes	6 (2.75%)
No	212 (97.25%)
Apixaban (Eliquis)	
Yes	11 (5.05%)
No	207 (94.95%)
Rivaroxaban (Xarelto)	
Yes	13 (5.96%)
No	205 (94.04%)
Dipyridamole (Aggrenox)	
Yes	4 (1.83%)
No	214 (98.17%)
Enoxaparin (lovenox)	
Yes	2 (0.92%)
No	216 (99.08%)
Heparin	
Yes	0 (0.00%)
No	218 (100.00%)
Ticagrelor (Brilinta)	
Yes	0 (0.00%)
No	218 (100.00%)
Aspirin	
Yes	118 (54.13%)
No	100 (45.87%)
Clopidogrel (Plavix)	
Yes	36 (16.51%)
No	182 (83.49%)
Prasugrel (Effient)	
Yes	0 (0.00%)
No	218 (100.00%)
Ticlopidine (Ticlid)	
Yes	0 (0.00%)
No	218 (100.00%)

Table 3 Number of Patients Taking Multiple Pre-injury ACAP Therapies

ACAP Therapy	N
Aspirin + clopidogrel (Plavix)	16
Warfarin (Coumadin or Marevan) + aspirin	14
Apixaban (Eliquis) + aspirin	2
Dabigatran (Pradaxa) + aspirin	2
Rivaroxaban (Xarelto) + clopidogrel (Plavix)	2
Warfarin (Coumadin or Marevan) + Enoxaparin (lovenox)	2
Warfarin (Coumadin or Marevan) + clopidogrel (Plavix)	1
Warfarin (Coumadin or Marevan) + aspirin + clopidogrel (Plavix)	1
Dipyridamole (Aggrenox) + clopidogrel (Plavix) + aspirin	1
Dipyridamole (Aggrenox) + aspirin	1

missed, a larger quality improvement project was conducted to reduce practice variation with respect to repeat head CT ordering in this population.

The literature demonstrates variation in rates of DICH among elderly injured populations (0.3% versus results up to 6%) [8, 19]. One reason for this may be differences in inclusion criteria that can potentially vary (e.g., injury type, age, etc.). Some states, including the state where this analysis was conducted, have specific geriatric trauma triage guidelines established to help protect elderly patients from undertriage which may have the effect of increasing the denominator for elderly patients screened for DICH [27]. Undertriage occurs when patients are taken to facilities that do not have the resources required to treat their acute health problems, and can lead to poor patient outcomes and poor resource utilization [27, 28]. Elderly populations have been found to be at greater risk of undertriage which is why some states have moved to triage models where age is a criteria for referral to a level I trauma center and trauma activation [28]. Furthermore, it is possible that rates of DICH diagnosed by CT have decreased due to increased overall usage of CT scans of the head in minor trauma (increasing the denominator to include more minor patients).

There continues to be significant debate in the literature regarding best clinical practices with respect to screening for DICH in elderly patients with minor injuries on ACAP therapies. Overutilization of CT scans is undesirable from a financial perspective and raises concerns over radiation exposure, although this concern is somewhat reduced in the elderly population. While increased CT utilization has drawbacks, DICH in patients taking anticoagulant agents has historically been reported as significant contributor to both morbidity and mortality [29] however a recent large multicenter study has suggested that this risk is less pervasive [19]. In response to these reports, a 2002 initiative by the European Federation of Neurological Societies (EFNS) recommended a 24-h observation period followed by a repeat head CT for all anticoagulated patients with minor head trauma [23]. An Italian study by Menditto investigated the EFNS recommendations and reported a 6% rate of DICH in patients receiving warfarin [8]. As a result, many trauma centers in Europe have offered admission and repeat head CT to all anticoagulated patients with head trauma. This gradually became the standard at many institutions worldwide, and is the model for the practice guideline at the institution where this work was conducted.

Our findings of DICH are consistent with previous studies and highlight the need for a more efficient way to detect DICH. Current protocols using repeat CT imaging are resource intensive. One study found that the average cost to detect a single DICH was $1,016,960 when using a universal screening protocol, which has caused some to question the cost-effectiveness of this method of screening [30]. For this reason, future research into risk factors that can accurately predict DICH is imperative.

Some improvements have already taken place that have likely decreased rates of DICH. The quality, efficiency, and speed of CT imaging has improved significantly overtime. This improvement has allowed for decreased radiologic artifact, decreased motion artifact, increased number of images, and increased quality of images all in an abbreviated timeframe [31]. This allows for a more confident exclusion of pathology with CT imaging. Thus, it is possible that some previously reported DICHs were simply missed immediate intracranial hemorrhages. Furthermore, it is possible that service delivery innovations, such as geriatric consultations for geriatric trauma patients, could also improve processes and subsequent outcomes for geriatric patients [32].

Improvements in the management of patients on blood thinners may also contribute to a decrease in the overall number of DICH detected. Known risks of ACAP agents have led to a significant improvement in anticoagulant management. This has included the development of carefully monitored warfarin clinics, public awareness regarding blood thinners, and the development of new and safer anticoagulant agents. Several direct oral anticoagulants (DOACs) have been introduced (apixaban, rivaroxaban, and dabigatran). The safety of these DOACs in the trauma population has recently been assessed. DOACs have a considerably lower rate of the development of intracranial hemorrhage compared to warfarin (24% vs. 31%) [33]. While there has likely been benefit, the DOACs have few established protocols for reversal of anticoagulation, although work continues to be done in this area [33–36]. Research has shown that utilization of multiple ACAP medications is associated with increased bleeding risk [37]. The present analysis, with approximately 20% of elderly patients were utilizing more than one ACAP medication, double the rate of the recent Chenoweth et al. [19] study, still does not suggest that dual or triple pre-injury ACAP use is associated with increased risk of DICH, although our numbers were relatively small.

The volume of CT scans has increased due to the wide availability of timely CT imaging, which may have the effect of increasing the probability of detecting DICHs. In 2007, there were an estimated 75 million CT scans performed [38]. Since then, the number of CT scans performed has increased by approximately 10% per year [39]. Increased screening will likely lead to increased detection. An unintended consequence of the increase in CT utilization as a result of the EFNS repeat head CT guideline is that this increases length of stay, and as such, may result in a greater consumption of health care resources from the trauma service, or other hospital service lines which subsequently increases costs for patients. Given these considerations, a comprehensive examination of the costs and benefits associated with this screening protocol is warranted.

This analysis was not without limitations. As a retrospective analysis, the project was subject to some intrinsic limitations including the potential for missed enrollment due to possible errors in documentation and varying adherence to our institutional practice recommendations which could have resulted in selection bias. In a separate analysis for an associated lean six sigma project, factors associated with missing a RRHCT including age, gender, GCS, injury severity, aspirin-only, or warfarin utilization were examined. No factor was statistically significantly associated with missing a RRHCT in logistic regression analysis. Furthermore, in discussions with providers about why they believed RRHCT were missed, the most common responses were (1) not being aware of the departmental guideline, and (2) forgetting to adhere to the departmental guideline. For these reasons, the risk of selection bias is somewhat reduced since the evidence suggests that missing RRHCTs were missing at random. Given our usage of a trauma registry that is maintained by trained trauma registrars, the possibility of documentation errors is also somewhat reduced. Adherence to institutional practice recommendations, namely performing the repeat head CT, was the center of a larger quality improvement project aimed at reducing variation in clinical practice with respect to this guideline. The project has led to significant improvements in compliance, thus in the future it would be possible to reassess our rate of DICH with less potential for selection bias. Given the very low incidence of DICH at our institution and others, there was an inability to power and match our study to examine individual pharmacologic agents. The state in which the analysis was conducted has specific geriatric trauma triage criteria which may differ from other states, potentially limiting generalizability to trauma centers without such geriatric-specific trauma triage criteria [26]. Lastly, long-term outcomes were outside the scope of this analysis, and as such we were unable to examine long-term complications and outcomes.

A strength of this analysis is that there was greater inclusion of ACAP medications than previous studies. This project included DOACs and aspirin which many prior analyses have not included. Furthermore, this study presents utilization rates for multiple ACAP medications which is a unique contribution to the literature.

Conclusion

The incidence of DICH in geriatric patients using a broad range of ACAP therapies prior to a minor fall was very low. The rate of surgical intervention following a DICH was even lower. Some have recommended against universal DICH screening protocols, but without evidence-based guidelines that effectively stratify DICH risk, this recommendation is somewhat risky, even if the risk is a low probability event. Future research should investigate a broad spectrum of ACAP medications and work to identify risk factors for DICH so that patient safety and clinical quality are not sacrificed for operational efficiency.

Abbreviations

ACAP: Anticoagulant or antiplatelet; CT: Computed tomography; DICH: Delayed intracranial hemorrhage; DOAC: Direct oral anticoagulant; EFNS: European Federation of Neurological Societies; NTDS: National Trauma Data Standard

Acknowledgements

Summa Health System- Akron City Campus Level 1 Trauma Center.

Funding

No funding was received to conduct this research.

Authors' contributions

NM contributed to the design of the analysis, abstracted data, contributed to the writing of the manuscript and provided critical revision and final approval. KW contributed to the design of the analysis, abstracted data, contributed to the writing of the manuscript and provided final approval. AM contributed to the design of the analysis, abstracted data, contributed to the writing of the manuscript and provided final approval. MS contributed to the design of the analysis, contributed to the writing and revision of the manuscript and provided final approval. KW contributed to the design of the analysis, abstracted data, provided critical revision and approved the final manuscript. LB contributed to the design of the analysis, conducted the data analysis, abstracted data, contributed to the writing of the manuscript, provided critical review and provided final approval of the manuscript. TM contributed to the design of the study, contributed to writing, provided critical review, and provided final approval of the manuscript. RG contributed to the design of the study, contributed to writing, provided critical review, and provided final approval of the manuscript.

Competing interests

The authors declare that they have no competing interests.

Author details

[1]Summa Health System- Department of Surgery, Akron Campus, Akron, OH, USA. [2]Summa Health System- Department of Surgery, Division of Trauma Akron Campus, Akron Ohio, USA Northeast Ohio Medical University, Rootstown, OH, USA.

References

1. Johnson NB, Hayes LD, Brown K, Hoo EC, Ethier KA. Centers for disease C, prevention: CDC National Health Report: leading causes of morbidity and mortality and associated behavioral risk and protective factors--United States, 2005-2013. MMWR Suppl. 2014;63(4):3–27.
2. Centers for Disease Control and Prevention: WISQARS™ (Web-based Injury Statistics Query and Reporting System). In. Atlanta: National Center for Injury Prevention and Control; 2017.
3. Burns ER, Stevens JA, Lee R. The direct costs of fatal and non-fatal falls among older adults - United States. J Saf Res. 2016;58:99–103.
4. Li J, Brown J, Levine M. Mild head injury, anticoagulants, and risk of intracranial injury. Lancet. 2001;357(9258):771–2.
5. Mina AA, Knipfer JF, Park DY, Bair HA, Howells GA, Bendick PJ. Intracranial complications of preinjury anticoagulation in trauma patients with head injury. J Trauma. 2002;53(4):668–72.
6. Robert-Ebadi H, Le Gal G, Righini M. Use of anticoagulants in elderly patients: practical recommendations. Clin Interv Aging. 2009;4:165–77.
7. Nishijima DK, Offerman SR, Ballard DW, Vinson DR, Chettipally UK, Rauchwerger AS, Reed ME, Holmes JF. Clinical Research in Emergency S, Treatment N: Immediate and delayed traumatic intracranial hemorrhage in patients with head trauma and preinjury warfarin or clopidogrel use. Ann Emerg Med. 2012;59(6):460–8. e461–467
8. Menditto VG, Lucci M, Polonara S, Pomponio G, Gabrielli A. Management of minor head injury in patients receiving oral anticoagulant therapy: a prospective study of a 24-hour observation protocol. Ann Emerg Med. 2012; 59(6):451–5.
9. Gittleman AM, Ortiz AO, Keating DP, Katz DS. Indications for CT in patients receiving anticoagulation after head trauma. AJNR Am J Neuroradiol. 2005;26(3):603–6.
10. Haydel MJ, Preston CA, Mills TJ, Luber S, Blaudeau E, DeBlieux PM. Indications for computed tomography in patients with minor head injury. N Engl J Med. 2000;343(2):100–5.
11. Brewer ES, Reznikov B, Liberman RF, Baker RA, Rosenblatt MS, David CA, Flacke S. Incidence and predictors of intracranial hemorrhage after minor head trauma in patients taking anticoagulant and antiplatelet medication. J Trauma. 2011;70(1):E1–5.
12. Peck KA, Sise CB, Shackford SR, Sise MJ, Calvo RY, Sack DI, Walker SB, Schechter MS. Delayed intracranial hemorrhage after blunt trauma: are patients on preinjury anticoagulants and prescription antiplatelet agents at risk? J Trauma. 2011;71(6):1600–4.
13. Swap C, Sidell M, Ogaz R, Sharp A. Risk of delayed Intracerebral hemorrhage in Anticoagulated patients after minor head trauma: the role of repeat cranial computed tomography. Perm J. 2016;20(2):14–6.
14. Kaups KL, Davis JW, Parks SN. Routinely repeated computed tomography after blunt head trauma: does it benefit patients? J Trauma. 2004;56(3):475–80. discussion 480-471
15. Wang MC, Linnau KF, Tirschwell DL, Hollingworth W. Utility of repeat head computed tomography after blunt head trauma: a systematic review. J Trauma. 2006;61(1):226–33.
16. Garra G, Nashed AH, Capobianco L. Minor head trauma in anticoagulated patients. Acad Emerg Med. 1999;6(2):121–4.
17. McCammack KC, Sadler C, Guo Y, Ramaswamy RS, Farid N. Routine repeat head CT may not be indicated in patients on anticoagulant/antiplatelet therapy following mild traumatic brain injury. West J Emerg Med. 2015; 16(1):43–9.
18. Miller J, Lieberman L, Nahab B, Hurst G, Gardner-Gray J, Lewandowski A, Natsui S, Watras J. Delayed intracranial hemorrhage in the anticoagulated patient: a systematic review. J Trauma Acute Care Surg. 2015;79(2):310–3.
19. Chenoweth JA, Gaona SD, Faul M, Holmes JF, Nishijima DK. Sacremental County Prehospital Research Consortium. Incidence of delayed intracranial hemorrhage in older patients after blunt head trauma. JAMA Surg. 2018; 153(6):570-575.
20. Holmes JF, Borgialli DA, Nadel FM, Quayle KS, Schambam N, Cooper A, Schunk JE, Miskin ML, Atabaki SM, Hoyle JD, et al. Do children with blunt head trauma and normal cranial computed tomography scan results require hospitalization for neurologic observation? Ann Emerg Med. 2011;58(4):315–22.
21. Brown CV, Zada G, Salim A, Inaba K, Kasotakis G, Hadjizacharia P, Demetriades D, Rhee P. Indications for routine repeat head computed tomography (CT) stratified by severity of traumatic brain injury. J Trauma. 2007;62(6):1339–44. discussion 1344-1335
22. Eroglu SE, Onur O, Ozkaya S, Denizbasi A, Demir H, Ozpolat C. Analysis of repeated CT scan need in blunt head trauma. Emerg Med Int. 2013;2013:916253.

23. Vos PE, Battistin L, Birbamer G, Gerstenbrand F, Potapov A, Prevec T, Stepan Ch A, Traubner P, Twijnstra A, Vecsei L, et al. EFNS guideline on mild traumatic brain injury: report of an EFNS task force. Eur J Neurol. 2002;9(3):207–19.
24. Scantling D, Fischer C, Gruner R, Teichman A, McCracken B, Eakins J. The role of delayed head CT in evaluation of elderly blunt head trauma victims taking antithrombotic therapy. Eur J Trauma Emerg Surg. 2017;43(6):741-746. doi:https://doi.org/10.1007/s00068-017-0793-7. Epub 2017 Apr 24.
25. American College of Surgeons. National Trauma Data Standards. Retrived online from, https://www.facs.org/quality-programs/trauma/ntdb/ntds.
26. Kaen A, Jimenez-Roldan L, Arrese I, Delgado MA, Lopez PG, Alday R, Alen JF, Lagares A, Lobato RD. The value of sequential computed tomography scanning in anticoagulated patients suffering from minor head injury. J Trauma. 2010;68(4):895–8.
27. Locasto D. Geriatric Trauma Triage. JEMS. 2009;
28. Llompart-Pou JA, Perez-Barcena J, Chico-Fernandez M, Sanchez-Casado M, Raurich JM. Severe trauma in the geriatric population. World J Crit Care Med. 2017;6(2):99–106.
29. Qureshi AI, Mendelow AD, Hanley DF. Intracerebral haemorrhage. Lancet. 2009;373(9675):1632–44.
30. Li J. Admit all anticoagulated head-injured patients? A million dollars versus your dime. You make the call. Ann Emerg Med. 2012;59(6):457–9.
31. Fornell D. Technology Improvements in Current Generation CT Systems. In: Imaging Technology News (ITN). itnonline.com. Arlington Heights: Scranton Gillette Communications; 2015. http://www.itnonline.com/article/technologyimprovements-current-generation-ct-systems.
32. Fallon WF Jr, Rader E, Zyzanski S, Mancuso C, Martin B, Breedlove L, DeGolia P, Allen K, Campbell J. Geriatric outcomes are improved by a geriatric trauma consultation service. J Trauma. 2006;61(5):1040–6.
33. Kobayashi L, Barmparas G, Bosarge P, Brown CV, Bukur M, Carrick MM, Catalano RD, Holly-Nicolas J, Inaba K, Kaminski S, et al. Novel oral anticoagulants and trauma: the results of a prospective American Association for the Surgery of Trauma multi-institutional trial. J Trauma Acute Care Surg. 2017;82(5):827–35.
34. Escolar G, Fernandez-Gallego V, Arellano-Rodrigo E, Roquer J, Reverter JC, Sanz VV, Molina P, Lopez-Vilchez I, Diaz-Ricart M, Galan AM. Reversal of apixaban induced alterations in hemostasis by different coagulation factor concentrates: significance of studies in vitro with circulating human blood. PLoS One. 2013;8(11):e78696.
35. Cheung YW, Barco S, Hutten BA, Meijers JC, Middeldorp S, Coppens M. In vivo increase in thrombin generation by four-factor prothrombin complex concentrate in apixaban-treated healthy volunteers. J Thromb Haemost. 2015;13(10):1799–805.
36. Hansen ML, Sorensen R, Clausen MT, Fog-Petersen ML, Raunso J, Gadsboll N, Gislason GH, Folke F, Andersen SS, Schramm TK, et al. Risk of bleeding with single, dual, or triple therapy with warfarin, aspirin, and clopidogrel in patients with atrial fibrillation. Arch Intern Med. 2010;170(16):1433–41.
37. Pollack CV Jr, Reilly PA, van Ryn J, Eikelboom JW, Glund S, Bernstein RA, Dubiel R, Huisman MV, Hylek EM, Kam CW, et al. Idarucizumab for Dabigatran reversal - full cohort analysis. N Engl J Med. 2017;377(5):431–41.
38. Smith-Bindman R. Is computed tomography safe? N Engl J Med. 2010; 363(1):1–4.
39. Mettler FA Jr, Bhargavan M, Faulkner K, Gilley DB, Gray JE, Ibbott GS, Lipoti JA, Mahesh M, McCrohan JL, Stabin MG, et al. Radiologic and nuclear medicine studies in the United States and worldwide: frequency, radiation dose, and comparison with other radiation sources--1950-2007. Radiology. 2009;253(2):520–31.

Safety and efficiency of a redirection procedure toward an out of hours general practice before admission to an emergency department

Charles Morin[1], Jacques Choukroun[2] and Jean-Christophe Callahan[3*]

Abstract

Background: Primary care patients are often cited as a cause of Emergency Department overcrowding (ED). The aim of this study was to evaluate a physician led redirection procedure of selected patients towards an out of hours general practice (OHGP) in an Emergency Department with 55,000 admissions per year.

Methods: Observational monocentric study over a period of 2 months. Every patient redirected to the OHGP was included and subsequently contacted by telephone to answer a standardized questionnaire, in order to measure:

- Redirection rate over the entire period and during weekdays or weekends/holiday
- Rate of redirected patients who went to the OHGP
- Rate of redirected patients who consulted in an ED in the next 72 h for the same reason
- Redirected patients' satisfaction rate

Results: During the study period 9551 patients presented to the ED, of which 288 were redirected towards the OHGP (3%). The redirection rate was 1.9% during weekdays and 5.7% during weekends/holiday ($p < 0.001$). Of the redirected patients, 77% answered the telephone interview.
Ninety percent of these patients consulted the OHGP. The main reasons for not consulting were: unduly long wait, opening hours not suitable, too costly. The rate of redirected patients who consulted in an ED in the following 72 h for the same reason was 4.1%. The satisfaction rate was 79.6% among interviewed patients.

Conclusions: A physician led procedure to redirect selected patients from the ED towards an OHGP results in a low redirection rate, unlikely to have a significant effect on ED patient flow. However, the procedure is safe and well accepted by a majority of patients.

Keywords: Emergency department management, Patient redirection, Patient safety, Primary care

Background

Despite differences across health care systems, primary care patients treated in the emergency department (ED) are usually defined as lower acuity patients, unlikely to be admitted, and who could have been handled by a primary care provider outside of the ED [1]. In France, EDs can be accessed after telephonic referral by the Emergency Medical Service (SAMU), after referral by a General practitioner (GP), or by self-referral. In a one-day observational study conducted in every ED in France on the 11th of June 2013, out of 52,018 patients 58% were self-referrals and it was considered that 16.4% of all ED admissions could have been handled the same day in a primary care setting had there been the possibility [2].

Between 2002 and 2012, the number of admissions in EDs in France has increased by 30% (to 18 million admissions for a population of 65.8 million), and ED overcrowding has become a public safety issue [3].

* Correspondence: jccallahan@ch-lemans.fr
[3]Service de Réanimation Polyvalente, Centre Hospitalier du Mans, 194 Avenue Rubillard, 72000 Le Mans, France
Full list of author information is available at the end of the article

Several international studies have found a correlation between ED admissions during a period of overcrowding and excess morbidity [4–6]. Admission of low acuity patients that could have been seen in a general practice setting, while not the only factor in ED overcrowding, can have a negative impact on patient flow by diverting resources needed elsewhere [7–9]. Furthermore, low acuity patients are more likely to leave the ED without being seen [10]. An ED admission for these patients is also more costly than a general practice consult from an economic standpoint [3, 11, 12].

In France, non-emergency unscheduled care can be handled during nights, weekends and holidays by general practice physicians in out of hours general practice clinics (OHGP). These clinics are not equipped for imaging or laboratory testing. Redirecting patients presenting to the ED with complaints not requiring the level of care of an ED towards an OHGP reduces the number of admissions, especially during periods of overcrowding. This practice exists in a majority of University Hospital EDs [13]. However, there exists potential risks with such a procedure by misestimating the severity of the clinical picture presented by the patient.

Therefore, the aim of this study was to assess whether such a procedure is effective, safe, and satisfactory for the patients.

Methods

Setting and study design

We conducted a prospective observational study. All patients presenting to the adult ED of the Le Mans general hospital between February first and March 31st 2016 were screened for inclusion.

The department averages 155 admissions per day. Every patient presenting to the ED is evaluated within minutes by a triage nurse according to a pragmatic standardized triage scale. The redirection procedure towards the OHGP is summarized in Table 1.

A time stamped administrative record is created for every redirected patient. This record contains the patients age, sex, contact details and whether the patient has a declared primary care physician.

The OHGP is easily accessible on foot from the ED. It is open from 20 h00 to midnight Monday through Friday, from 12 h00 to midnight on Saturday, and from 08 h00 to midnight on Sunday and holidays.

During the study period, every adult patient redirected towards the OHGP was included in the study and received an information sheet explaining the aims of the study and a summary of the protocol. Redirected patients were contacted by telephone between 72 h and 15 days after their initial presentation to the ED in order to answer an 18 question semi-structured questionnaire. The aim of this questionnaire was to elicit answers concerning the primary and secondary complaints, patient pathway before and after the redirection, understanding and satisfaction of the redirection, whether further testing, specialist referrals or ED visits were necessary for the same complaints following the OHGP visit. Patient complaints were classified according to the International Classification of Primary Care (ICPC), developed by the World Organization of family Doctors (WONCA). Telephone interviews were conducted by a single investigator in order to limit the risk of bias.

A patient was considered as a non-responder if five calls went unanswered between 72 h and 15 days after inclusion.

Table 1 Redirection procedure towards the OHGP

Redirection is warranted after medical validation by a senior emergency physician if the following criteria are met:

- Absence of priority criteria according to the triage scale,
- The patient was not referred to the ED by a physician,
- The OHGP is easily accessible by the patient,
- The patient is covered by social security,
- Informed consent of the patient was obtained concerning the redirection. If the patient refuses the redirection he is admitted to the ED.

Outcome measures

Redirection rate was defined as the proportion of patients presenting to the ED who were subsequently redirected towards the OHGP during the study period. A secondary analysis was performed comparing the redirection rates during weekdays and during weekends or holidays. We also sought to determine the reason why a primary care physician was not consulted instead of coming to the ED.

Safety was evaluated using the rate of patients redirected towards the OHGP who were subsequently admitted in an ED in the next 72 h for the same complaint. We also analyzed the complaints, final diagnostic and treatment pathway for these patients.

Accessibility rate was defined as the proportion of redirected patients who actually consulted the OHGP. In case of non-consultation, the reason was requested.

Satisfaction was measured by the proportion of redirected patients who felt that the redirection was justified according to their primary complaint. In case of non-satisfaction, the cause was ascertained.

Data analysis

Continuous variables were presented as means and standard deviation; categorical variables were presented as absolute values and percentages. Proportions were compared with the Chi2 test using R software. Tests were bilateral with a type 1 error defined at 5%.

Using a power calculation with a type 1 error of 5%, an absolute precision of 4%, and an estimated maximum rate of readmitted patients at 72 h of 10% we calculated that at least 216 patients were necessary for analysis. In order to ascertain the generalizability of the telephonic interview results with the entire reoriented population we compared these two groups according to demographic data, whether the reorientation was performed during a weekday or not, during daytime (08 h00 to 20 h00) or not, and whether a treating physician was declared. The only difference between variables to reach statistical significance was the proportion of patients having a declared treating physician (77.6% in the non-responder group vs. 88.7% in the responder group, $p = 0.02$).

Results

Patient characteristics and redirection rate

Demographic data are summarized in Table 2. Between February 1st and March 31st 2016, 9551 patients presented to our ED. Of these, 288 were redirected towards the OHGP (overall redirection rate 3%). Redirection rate was 5.7% during week-ends and holidays, against 1.9% during weekdays ($p < 0.001$).

86% of redirected patients declared having a corresponding primary care physician.

Characteristics of responders

Two hundred and twenty one out of 288 reoriented patients answered the telephonic interview (76.7%).

A majority of responders (178; 80.5%) did not try to contact their GP before presenting to the ED. For 118 of these patients (53.4%) their usual GP was absent or the practice was closed. For 194 patients (87.8%), had their GP been able to see them the same day they would have chosen that option.

The most frequent primary complaints are summarized in Table 3.

Safety

Nine redirected patients were admitted to an ED in the following 72 h for the initial complaint (4.1%).

One of these patients had to be hospitalized because of an anal abscess. It was the only patient redirected to the ED from the OHGP.

Table 2 Patient demographics. SD: standard deviation

	All patients	Redirected patients
Total:	9551 (100%)	288 (3%)
Weekdays	6815 (100%)	132 (1.9%)
Week-ends and holidays	2736 (100%)	156 (5.7%)
Gender:		
Male	4897 (51.3%)	131 (45.5%)
Female	4654 (48.7%)	157 (54.5%)
Age (SD)	53 (27.7)	36 (15.4)

Table 3 Ten most common primary complaints among redirected patients

Primary complaint	Number of patients (%)
Hyperthermia	24 (10.9%)
Lumbar symptoms	23 (10.4%)
Dental or gingival symptoms	18 (8.1%)
Throat symptoms	15 (6.8%)
Dysuria	10 (4.5%)
Localized rash	10 (4.5%)
Cough	9 (4.1%)
Lower limb symptoms	8 (3.6%)
Abdominal pain	7 (3.2%)
Ear pain	7 (3.2%)

Accessibility

One hundred and ninety nine reoriented patients consulted the OHGP (accessibility rate 90%). The main reasons for not presenting to the OHGP were: excessive waiting times (9 patients), opening hours not suitable (5 patients) and consultation costs (4 patients).

Twenty nine percent of redirected patients had never heard of the OHGP before presenting to the ED.

Patient satisfaction

For 176 patients the redirection from the ED was justified according to their primary complaint (satisfaction rate 79.6%). The main causes for non-satisfaction were the absence of imaging modalities or laboratory testing in the OHGP (12 patients), absence of specialist (including dentist) consultation (8 patients), pain too important (4 patients), "should have been seen in the ED" (4 patients), and excessive waiting times (4 patients).

Discussion

The results of our study show that relatively few patients are redirected from the ED towards an OHGP, although the redirection rate is higher during week-ends and holidays. The redirection procedure is safe, with few patients requiring a follow-up in an ED in the 72 h post-redirection, and without prejudice for their level of care. Furthermore, a majority of patients believed that their redirection from the ED was justified.

Few studies have evaluated in different health care systems to what extent patients with minor ailments can be redirected from the ED towards a primary care provider. Using a redirection procedure similar to ours, Bentley found a higher redirection rate of 7% in a Scottish teaching hospital, with a sub-optimal care rate of 0.23% as a result of the redirection [14]. In our study, only one of the 221 redirected patients who could be contacted for the interview required a subsequent hospitalization, for a benign condition.

Van der Straten evaluated the use of the Manchester Triage Scale by trained nurses at an "Acute Care Post" to separate flows of patients between an ED and an OHGP [15]. Seventy one percent of patients were directed towards the GP, and out of the sub group of less urgent patients initially oriented to the GP, 6.5% were redirected towards the ED with a 1.2% hospitalization rate in the 4 weeks following the initial triage. The large difference in the triage rate towards the GP between this study and both the Scottish and our study may be explained that triage was done at an earlier stage, before ED presentation. In France and Scotland this is done by centralized telephone advice and triage services (SAMU / Centre 15 for France and NHS 24 for Scotland). Despite these differences, all three studies demonstrate that it is possible to safely redirect low acuity patients to a GP before the ED.

The low redirection rate in our study is unlikely to have a significant impact on ED flow and does not support the idea that primary care patients are a major burden on EDs. However, in the French 1 day cross-sectional study of 2013 [2], it was considered that 16.4% of all ED admissions could have been handled the same day in a primary care setting had there been the possibility. This appraisal was done at discharge from the ED by the treating emergency doctor, and thus is subject to hindsight bias. Nerveless, it raises the question whether our redirection procedure might be too selective and whether more patients could be redirected in our ED. In a systematic review, Durand found that the proportion of low-acuity ED visits ranged from 4.8 to 90% depending on studies [16]. This variability could be explained by different health care systems, the lack of consensus for defining low-acuity ED visits and also whether the categorization was done prospectively at triage or retrospectively. Additionally, there is a distinction between a low-acuity ED visit and a patient that can be safely and appropriately redirected towards a less urgent primary care facility in a timely manner. Many patients require ED care not because of the severity of their symptoms but because of the technical aspects of their care which can be managed in an ED.

In our study the redirection rate was significantly higher during week-ends and holidays than during weekdays. This could be explained either by the longer opening hours of the OHGP during week-ends or by a higher rate of low-acuity complaints among patients presenting to the ED due to the diminished accessibility of GPs during these periods. An argument in favor of this second hypothesis is that a majority of redirected patients in our study did not try to contact their primary GP because they believed he or she would be absent. Effects of an extended access to primary care facilities on ED visits are debated in the literature, with conflicting results. Whittaker found a correlation between the implementation of an extended access primary care service and a reduction of self-referring low-acuity patients by 26.4% in Manchester (United Kingdom) in 2014 [17]. In a study by Martsolf however, during the period between 2007 and 2012 in 23 American states, no association was found between the opening of a retail clinic and ED visits for low-acuity patients [18]. Despite differences in setting and methods, these studies underline the complexity of health care systems and their responses to heterogeneous primary care demands.

Our study shows that redirecting lower acuity patients toward an OHGP is unlikely to affect ED patient flow due to the low redirection rate. Despite this low redirection rate, we believe that this procedure still has its usefulness. ED and GP services should not be considered interchangeable. Each has its own specificities, and redirection should be considered as a service aimed at giving the patient the most adequate care, not as a means to lower ED flow.

In our study, 10% of redirected patients did not follow the instruction to go to the OHGP. Although none of these patients presented an unfavorable outcome, they present a challenge in the sense that not all redirected patients have benign self-limiting conditions. Furthermore, not requiring an ED consult does not mean that no medical advice is warranted. In particular, ED doctors should remember to enquire whether the patient has the ability to pay in advance the fee for the OHGP.

Limitations

This study has several limitations. As an observational study, it was not designed to measure a possible impact of a redirection procedure on traditional measures of patient flow in the ED such as mean length of stay. As a single center study, the results should not be directly generalizable to EDs in different health care systems. As there was no change in the redirection procedure, no internal comparison was possible. The study was also open to selection bias, as different care providers at triage might have different assessments of what is a complaint requiring a GP. It is possible that a certain number of patients were admitted to the ED who could have benefited from the procedure and the study was not designed to measure this. Also the number of patients who refused redirection was not measured. The data for this study was collected in February and March and any seasonal variations in pathologies that could influence the redirection rate are not accounted for. Despite the standardized nature of the telephone interview, it is subject to recall bias. For example, patient's initial feeling about the redirection might have a different opinion of the procedure after a few days depending on the evolution of their ailment. Almost a quarter of redirected patients did not respond to the telephonic interview. However, comparison of demographic data between the group of responders and non-responders did not find any significative difference, aside from whether there was a declared primary care physician.

Conclusion

In summary, a physician led procedure to redirect selected patients from the ED towards an OHGP results in a low redirection rate, unlikely to have a significant effect on ED patient flow. However, the procedure is safe with few patients requiring a follow-up in an ED in the 72 h post-redirection, and without prejudice for their level of care. Furthermore, a majority of patients believed that their redirection from the ED was justified.

Abbreviations

ED: Emergency Department; GP: General Practitioner; ICPC: International Classification of Primary Care; NHS: National Health Service; OHGP: Out of Hours General Practice Clinic; SAMU: Emergency Medical Service (Service d'Aide Médicale Urgente); WONCA: World Organization of Family Doctors

Acknowledgements

The authors would like to thank Mr. Dominique Blin, Charge Nurse, for his help with the data retrieval from the electronic health record.

Authors' contributions

CM is the principal investigator, and was responsible for data collection. The study is based on an original idea by JC. CM, JC and JCC were jointly responsible for study conception and design. CM and JCC were responsible for data analysis and interpretation. CM and JCC were responsible for writing the manuscript, with important contributions from JC. All authors read and approved the final manuscript.

Competing interests

The authors declare that they have no competing interests.

Author details

[1]Service de Médecine Polyvalente, Centre Hospitalier du Mans, 194 Avenue Rubillard, 72000 Le Mans, France. [2]Service des Urgences Adultes, Centre Hospitalier du Mans, 194 Avenue rubillard, 72000 Le Mans, France. [3]Service de Réanimation Polyvalente, Centre Hospitalier du Mans, 194 Avenue Rubillard, 72000 Le Mans, France.

References

1. Bezzina AJ, Smith PB, Cromwell D, et al. Primary care patients in the emergency department: who are they? A review of the definition of the 'primary care patient' in the emergency department. Emerg Med Australas. 2005;17:472–9. https://doi.org/10.1111/j.1742-6723.2005.00779.x.
2. DREES. Enquête nationale sur les structures des urgences hospitalières. Access at: http://www.data.drees.sante.gouv.fr/TableViewer/tableView.aspx?ReportId=1198. Accessed 13 Aug 2018.
3. Cour des comptes. Chapitre XII Les urgences hospitalières : une fréquentation croissante, une articulation avec la médecine de ville à repenser. Access at: https://www.ccomptes.fr/sites/default/files/EzPublish/rapport_securite_sociale_2014_urgences_hospitalieres.pdf. Accessed 13 Aug 2018.
4. Richardson DB, Bryant M. Association of Daily Patient Care Time with adverse events in patients who do not wait to be seen. Acad Emerg Med. 2004;11:461–2. https://doi.org/10.1197/j.aem.2004.02.227.
5. Sprivulis PC, DaSilva JA, Jacobs IG, et al. The association between hospital overcrowding and mortality among patients admitted via western Australian emergency departments. Med J Aust. 2006;184(5):208–12.
6. Richardson DB. Increase in patient mortality at 10 days associated with emergency department overcrowding. Med J Aust. 2006;184(5):213.
7. Chartier L, Josephson T, Bates K, et al. Improving emergency department flow through rapid medical evaluation unit. BMJ Qual Improv Rep. 2015;4 https://doi.org/10.1136/bmjquality.u206156.w2663.
8. Sun BC, Hsia RY, Weiss RE, et al. Effect of emergency department crowding on outcomes of admitted patients. Ann Emerg Med. 2013;61:605–11. https://doi.org/10.1016/j.annemergmed.2012.10.026.
9. Guttmann A, Schull MJ, Vermeulen MJ, et al. Association between waiting times and short term mortality and hospital admission after departure from emergency department: population based cohort study from Ontario, Canada. BMJ. 2011;342:d2983.
10. Baibergenova A, Leeb K, Jokovic A, et al. Missed opportunity: patients who leave emergency departments without being seen. Healthcare Policy. 2006; 1(4):35–42.
11. Baker LC, Baker LS. Excess cost of emergency department visits for nonurgent care. Health Aff. 1994;13(5):162–71.
12. Bamezai A, Melnick G, Nawathe A. The cost of an emergency department visit and its relationship to emergency department volume. Ann Emerg Med. 2005;45:483–90.
13. Marchetti M, Lepape M, Lauque D. La réorientation à l'accueil des services d'urgences : évaluation des pratiques professionnelles françaises. Annales Françaises de Medecine d'Urgence. 2014;4(6):349–53.
14. Bentley JA, Thakore S, Morrison W, et al. Emergency department redirection to primary care: a prospective evaluation of practice. Scott Med J. 2017; 62(1):2–10.
15. van der Straten LM, van Stel HF, Spee FJM, et al. Safety and efficiency of triaging low urgent self-referred patients to a general practitioner at an acute care post: an observational study. Emerg Med J. 2011;29:877–81. https://doi.org/10.1136/emermed-2011-200539.
16. Durand A-C, Gentile S, Devictor B, et al. ED patients: how nonurgent are they? Systematic review of the emergency medicine literature. Am J Emerg Med. 2011;29:333–45. https://doi.org/10.1016/j.ajem.2010.01.003.
17. Whittaker W, Anselmi L, Kristensen SR, et al. Associations between extending access to primary care and emergency department visits: a difference-in-differences analysis. PLoS Med. 2016;13:e1002113. https://doi.org/10.1371/journal.pmed.1002113.
18. Martsolf G, Fingar KR, Coffey R, et al. Association between the opening of retail clinics and low-acuity emergency department visits. Ann Emerg Med. 2017;69:397–403. https://doi.org/10.1016/j.annemergmed.2016.08.462.

28

Reduction in the IL-6 level at 24 h after admission to the intensive care unit is a survival predictor for Vietnamese patients with sepsis and septic shock

Pham Thi Ngoc Thao[1], Ton Thanh Tra[1*], Nguyen Truong Son[1] and Koji Wada[2]

Abstract

Background: Sepsis and septic shock are common problems in intensive care units (ICUs). The mortality of patients with sepsis or septic shock is high. We investigated if reduction in the serum concentration of the cytokines tumor necrosis factor α, interleukin (IL)-6 and IL-10, and the rate of change in the IL-6 level at 24 h after ICU admission were survival predictors for patients with sepsis and septic shock in a Vietnamese population.

Methods: This was a prospective study conducted at an ICU in Cho Ray Hospital, Vietnam, from October 2014 to October 2016. Patients diagnosed with sepsis or septic shock using validated international guidelines were enrolled. Plasma samples were collected upon (T_0) and 24 h after (T_{24}) ICU admission for measurement of cytokine concentrations. Blood tests were done to detect organ dysfunction. The duration of ICU stays, hospital stay, APACHE II and SOFA scores, and the in-hospital mortality were compared between survival and non-survival groups. Univariate logistic regression and multivariate analysis were done to determine the association between survival and IL-6 reduction at 24 h after ICU admission.

Results: A total of 123 patients were enrolled. The concentration (in pg/mL) of IL-6 at T_o was 413.3 in survivors and 530.0 in non- survivors. At T_{24}, the IL-6 level was 65.4 for survivors and 286.9 for non-survivors. The survival rate was 39.0%. At T_{24}, the concentrations of IL-6 and the reduction in IL-6 level were predictors of survival in patients with sepsis and septic shock. We found a significant association between IL-6 reduction and survival at ≥86% with Odds Ratio (OR) 5.67, 95% Confidence Interval (CI); 1.27–25.3, compared with an increase in the IL-6 rate of change.

Conclusions: Our findings suggested that a reduction in the IL-6 level of ≥86% at 24 h from ICU admission is a survival predictor for patients with sepsis and septic shock in our population.

Keywords: IL-6, Sepsis, Survival, Intensive care

* Correspondence: tonthanhtra@yahoo.com
[1]Cho Ray Hospital, 201B Nguyen Chi Thanh Street, District 5, Ho Chi Minh City, Vietnam
Full list of author information is available at the end of the article

Background

Sepsis and septic shock are common problems in intensive care units (ICUs). The corresponding mortality for sepsis and septic shock is 24.3–60.0% even in developed countries [1–5]. This mortality rate has decreased 1.3% annually since 2012 due to early diagnosis and appropriate empiric antibiotic therapy [6, 7]. However, the treatment of sepsis and septic shock remains expensive. The total hospital cost for patients with severe sepsis in the USA increased from $15.4 billion in 2003 to $24.3 billion in 2007 [8].

Monitoring of the severity of sepsis or septic shock is a considerable challenge. Most decisions about patients with sepsis and septic shock are based on clinical and laboratory findings that have limited accuracy. Biomarkers such as cytokines have been suggested to be predictors of severity and mortality in patients with sepsis and septic shock in several studies [7, 9, 10]. Acute Physiology and Chronic Health Evaluation (APACHE) II and Sequential Organ Failure Assessment (SOFA) scores have been used widely as predictors of severity in sepsis and septic shock [11].

The cytokine interleukin (IL)-6 is essential in cell development, initiation of innate immunity and cell functions in adaptive immunity [12]. In 2016, Klag T et al. studied 20 severe bacterial sepsis patients and showed that a rapid decline in IL-6 concentration after 24–48 h to or below baseline value was evidence of successful empiric antibiotic therapy, and was a survival predictor [13]. Juan et al. in Argentina showed that the IL-6 level decreased after 72 h from admission in 48 sepsis or septic shock patients, and was a survival predictor. They showed that the IL-6 at admission was 161 ± 24 pg/ml in survivors and 121 ± 17 pg/ml at 72 h after admission ($p = 0.04$) [14]. How changes in plasma levels of cytokines may be used to predict survival in patients with sepsis and septic shock for a Vietnamese population is not known. We determined to find out if reductions in the plasma concentrations of the cytokines tumor necrosis factor (TNF)-α, IL-6, and IL-10, and the rate of change of IL-6 at 24 h after ICU admission were survival predictors for patients with sepsis and septic shock at an ICU in Ho Chi Minh City, Vietnam.

Methods

We included patients admitted to the ICU at Cho Ray Hospital (Ho Chi Minh City, Vietnam) prospectively from October 2014 to October 2016. The ICU has 36 beds amongst a total of 2600 hospital beds. It cares for surgical, medical and post-operative patients. Patients who had undergone surgical procedures for severe head injury or who had open-heart surgery were excluded. There are 12 physicians and 36 nurses working in a shift system in the ICU.

Patients were eligible for inclusion if they fulfilled the criteria for the diagnosis of sepsis and septic shock defined by the American College of Chest Physicians/Society of Critical Care Medicine Consensus Conference in 2001 [15]. The doctors in charge explained to patients' relatives the research. If they agreed to be enrolled, they signed consent.

Clinical data were collected using pre-designed forms. Patients were followed up for the duration of their ICU stay and their duration of hospital stay, and their survival rate was ascertained.

Blood samples were collected at the time of ICU admission (T_0) and at 24 h after ICU admission (T_{24}). The 3 ml venous blood sample was taken and then centrifuged to separate the serum, which was stored at – 20 °C for further use. The concentrations of TNF-α, IL-6 and IL-10 were measured using an enzyme-linked immunosorbent assay. The Human IL-6 ELISA (Enzyme-Linked Immunosorbent Assay) kit was an in vitro enzyme-linked immunosorbent assay for the quantitative measurement of human IL-6 in plasma. The IL-6 enzyme-linked immunosorbent assay kit was purchased from Biochip Randox (County Antrim, United Kingdom). The blood cell analyzer was purchased from Randox company. The IL-6 rate of change at 24 h after ICU admission was measured using the following equation: IL-6 rate of change at 24 h from ICU admission = (IL-6 level at T_0 – IL-6 level at T_{24})/IL-6 level at T_0 × 100%.

The therapy for sepsis and septic shock was according to the SSC 2012 guidelines. Empiric antibiotic therapy was used according to local Hospital Antibiotic Guidelines. Renal replacement therapy was indicated in sepsis or septic shock with acute kidney injury, but no cytokine blood purification was used.

The Student's *t*-test and Mann–Whitney test were used to determine the significance of difference between survival and non-survival groups. The univariate logistic regression and multivariate regression analyses were done to identify which variables were associated with survival. We also divided the IL-6 reduction into quartiles. We adjusted for the variables with the *p*-value over 0.1 for multivariate logistic regression such as BUN, Creatinine, aPTT, pH, HCO_3^-, gender and age.

Results

One hundred and twenty-three patients were enrolled. Table 1 shows the characteristics of those patients who survived and those who died. Patients diagnosed with sepsis and septic shock admitted to the ICU who subsequently died had high APACHE II and SOFA scores. APACHE II score, SOFA score and the number of dysfunctional organs were significantly different between non-survival and survival groups ($p < 0.05$). The duration of ICU stay for survivors was longer (median 18, the interquartile range (IQR) 13–31 days) than that of non-survivors (7, IQR 3–16). Also, 98/123 (79.7%) of

Table 1 Characteristics of patients upon ICU admission and the mortality rate ($n = 123$)

Variable	Survival ($n = 48$)	Non-survival ($n = 75$)	p
Age (years), (median, IQR)	62 (46–75)	54 (43–73)	0.18**
Pre-ICU stay (days),(mean ± SD)	3.8 ± 5.7	2.9 ± 4.9	0.11**
Duration of hospitalization (days) (mean ± SD)	21.5 ± 13.8	12.7 ± 15.4	< 0.01*
Duration of ICU stay (day) (median, IQR)	18 (13–31)	7 (3–16)	0.03**
APACHE II score (mean ± SD)	18.0 ± 5.8	26.6 ± 7.9	< 0.01*
SOFA score (mean ± SD)	9.1 ± 2.9	11.6 ± 3.6	< 0.01*
Mechanical Ventilation (n, %)	32/48 (66.7)	66/75 (88.0)	< 0.01*
Days of ventilation (median, IQR)	5 (3–12)	4(1–15)	0.15**
Sites of infection	Prevalence	Mortality	
Gastrointestinal tract	56.1%	66.7%	
Respiratory tract	21.1%	61.5%	
Urinary tract	7.3%	44.4%	
Others	15.4%	47.2%	

(*) Student's *t*-test, (**) Mann–Whitney test, IQR: interquartile range, SD: standard deviation

cases had mechanical ventilation, and the median number of days of mechanical ventilation was 5 (IQR 3–12) days. The overall survival rate was 39.0%.

Table 2 shows the laboratory parameters at ICU admission and IL-6 rate of change at 24 h after ICU admission. Levels of blood–urea–nitrogen (BUN) and activated partial thromboplastin time (aPTT) were higher for non-survivors ($p = 0.02$). Levels of arterial pH and bicarbonate among non-survivors were significantly lower than those of survivors ($p = 0.04$ and 0.01 respectively). The rate of change in IL-6 level at T_{24} was significantly different between survival and non-survival groups (p = 0.04).

Figure 1 shows that the concentration of IL-6 was similar at T_0 in both groups ($p = 0.34$), but was significantly reduced at T_{24} in the survival group compared to the non-survival group ($p = 0.002$).

Table 2 Laboratory parameters upon ICU admission and IL-6 rate of change after 24 h ICU admission ($n = 123$)

Laboratory parameters	Survival ($n = 48$) Mean ± SD	Non- survival ($n = 75$) Mean ± SD	p (Student's *t*-test)
Hemoglobin (g/dL)	11.3 ± 2.3	11.0 ± 2.6	0.50
White blood cells (K/mm^3)	20.6 ± 14.2	18.1 ± 13.2	0.34
Platelets (K/mm^3)	164 ± 126	193 ± 134	0.24
Blood glucose (mg/dL)	129.3 ± 80.8	138.6 ± 77.8	0.55
Blood–urea–nitrogen (mg/dL)	35.7 ± 21.6	45.9 ± 25.1	0.02
Creatinine (mg/dL)	1.97 ± 1.5	2.47 ± 1.6	0.08
Bilirubin (mg/dL)	2.40 ± 2.4	3.34 ± 4.6	0.17
Prothrombin time (s)	16.9 ± 5.4	18.6 ± 10.0	0.27
aPTT (s)	35.9 ± 9.4	42.9 ± 20.8	0.02
pH	7.33 ± 0.1	7.28 ± 0.10	0.04
$PaCO_2$ (mmHg)	35.6 ± 7.8	33.5 ± 9.3	0.21
PaO_2 (mmHg)	120.4 ± 79.3	129.9 ± 99.6	0.58
HCO^-_3 (mmol/L)	19.0 ± 4.4	16.4 ± 5.8	0.01
C-reactive protein (mg/L)	123.3 ± 45.7	122.4 ± 60.8	0.93
Procalcitonin (ng/dL)	42.5 ± 109.8	54.4 ± 91.4	0.16
Lactate (mmol/L)	4.2 ± 2.6	5.3 ± 4.3	0.59
IL-6 rate of change	0.8 ± 4.5	−0.7 ± 0.3	0.04

aPTT, activated partial thromboplastin time; $PaCO_2$, arterial pressure of carbon dioxide; PaO_2, arterial pressure of oxygen; HCO^-_3, bicarbonate
IL-6 rate of change = (IL-6 (T_0) − IL-6 T_{24})/ IL-6 T_0

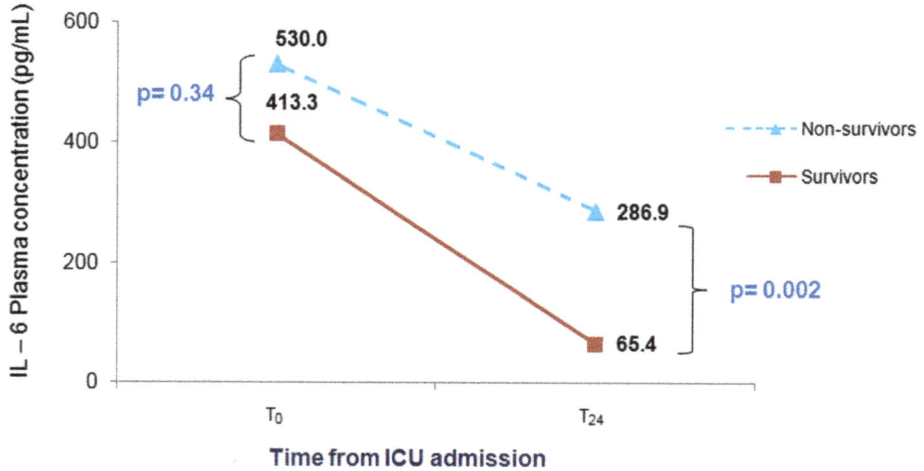

Fig. 1 The IL-6 change after 24 h of ICU admission

Table 3 shows cytokine concentrations at T_0 and T_{24} in survivors and non-survivors. There were significant differences in the levels of IL-6 ($p < 0.01$) and IL-10 (p < 0.01), and in the IL-6 rate of change at 24 h after ICU admission ($p = 0.03$).

Table 4 shows the association of IL-6 reduction rate and survival for sepsis and septic shock with logistic regression analysis. The quartiles for IL-6 reduction rate were 100% to 86%, 85% to 50%, 49% to 0%, and increased from 0%. We found a significant association between IL-6 reduction and survival at ≥86% reduction, with an Odds Ratio (OR) 5.67, 95% Confidence Interval (CI); 1.27–25.3, compared with the increase in the IL-6 rate of change. According to logistic regression, the rate of change of TNF-α and of IL-10 were not a predictor of survival.

Discussion

We aimed to investigate if reductions in the plasma concentrations of TNF-α, interleukin (IL)-6 and IL-10, and of the IL-6 rate of change at 24 h after ICU admission were survival predictors for Vietnamese patients with sepsis and septic shock. The results showed that IL-6 reduction at the level of ≥86% at 24 h from ICU admission could be a survival predictor for our patients with sepsis and septic shock. Our study showed that patients who had decreased IL-6 level after 24 h of ICU admission at ≥86% were 5.68 times more likely to survive compared to non-survivors.

IL-6 plays a key part in the systemic inflammatory response. Increased IL-6 levels in plasma have been identified in severe forms of sepsis, and correlate with an increased prevalence of mortality [4]. Levels of IL-6 and CRP were shown to be unreliable predictors for 102 critically ill patients admitted to the ICU of a tertiary hospital in Serbia [16]. In healthy adults without an ongoing inflammatory process, the IL-6 concentration ranged from 0.2 to 7.8 pg/mL, whereas the IL-6 concentration in adults with sepsis could be > 1600 pg/mL [17]. The IL-6 level is also proven as a predictor of acute kidney injury [18].

Table 3 Association of IL-6 reduction rate and survival for sepsis and septic shock ($n = 123$)

	Univariate		Multivariate	
	OR	(95%CI)	OR	(95%CI)
IL-6 reduction rate (quartile)				
Q1: 100% to 86%	5.08	(1.60–16.1)	5.67	(1.27–25.3)
Q2: 85% to – 50%	1.45	(0.52–4.11)	1.86	(0.44–7.94)
Q3: 0.49% to 0%	0.64	(0.22–1.83)	0.54	(0.14–2.02)
Q4: increased	ref		ref	

Adjusted for age, sex, BUN, Cre, aPTT, pH, HCO_3^-
ref: Reference
OR Odds Ratio, *CI* Confidence Interval
IL-6 reduction rate = (IL-6 (T_0) – IL-6 T_{24})/ IL-6 T_0
T_0: At ICU admission time
T_{24}: 24 h after ICU admission

Table 4 Association of IL-6 reduction rate and survival for sepsis and septic shock in logistic regression analysis ($n = 123$)

	Univariate		Multivariate	
	OR	(95%CI)	OR	(95%CI)
IL-6 reduction rate (quartile)				
Q1: 100% to 86%	5.08	(1.60–16.1)	5.67	(1.27–25.3)
Q2: 85% to 50%	1.45	(0.52–4.11)	1.86	(0.44–7.94)
Q3: 49% to 0%	0.64	(0.22–1.83)	0.54	(0.14–2.02)
Q4: Increased	ref		ref	

Adjusted for age, sex, BUN, Cre, aPTT, pH, HCO_3^-
ref: Reference
OR Odds Ratio, *CI* Confidence Interval
IL-6 reduction rate = (IL-6 (T_0) – IL-6 T_{24})/ IL-6 T_0
T_0: At admission time
T_{24}: 24 h after ICU admission

Reduction in IL-6 level denoted the patients' response to treatment. This finding also implies that the initial empiric antibiotic therapy was appropriate and should continue until formal culture results. Besides that, any treatment that can reduce IL-6 concentration would be supportive for these patients. Mohammad and co-workers found that, compared with the IL-6 level upon ICU admission, the IL-6 concentration at ICU discharge predicted all-cause mortality [19]. A meta-analysis in 2010 by Jaffer and colleagues, using data from human studies and experimental animal models, suggested that pro- and anti-inflammatory cytokines are released following a variety of initiating stimuli (e.g., endotoxin release, complement activation, ischemia–reperfusion injury). "Cytokine adsorption therapy" provides a potential solution to improving outcomes following systemic inflammatory response syndrome [20]. A study by Marissa and co-workers in 2010 showed that, 24 h after ICU admission, cytokine concentrations in low- and high-concentration subgroups were significantly different in the survival and non-survival groups [21]. The high cytokine concentrations 24 h after ICU admission were predictors of mortality for sepsis patients [21]. IL-6 clearance by extracorporeal membrane oxygenation and continuous renal replacement therapy has been shown to lower the mortality [22].

Sepsis and septic shock are the most common causes of death in the ICU [23, 24]. In recent years, the age of patients suffering from sepsis admitted to the ICU has been increasing [5]. The mean age of our study cohort was 58.2 ± 18.8 years, the duration of ICU stay was 6 (IQR 3–12) days, and 39.0% of patients survived. Compared with the previous studies at Cho Ray Hospital undertaken in 2013 and 2014, the mean age of our study cohort was higher and more patients died [25, 26]. These observations could have been because our patients had more severe disease, were resuscitated later, and or discharged earlier from the ICU compared with the studies carried out in 2013 and 2014. Also, Cho Ray Hospital has a post-resuscitation area where recovering ICU patients can be cared for. The prevalence of mortality was higher than that observed in other studies because our patients underwent treatment in other departments before ICU admission. Also, the APACHE II and SOFA scores upon ICU admission were high indicating severe illness.

Several cytokines could be indicators for severity and mortality for patients with sepsis and septic shock. In 2016, Stalder and colleagues evaluated 129 sepsis patients. They recorded an in-hospital mortality of 26%, and showed that plasma levels of growth arrest-specific gene 6 within 24 h of ICU admission could predict mortality for sepsis patients [27].

In our analysis, IL-10 concentration at T_{24} was also significantly different. However, the IL-10 rate of change was not calculated as IL-10 is a pre - inflammatory biomarker, and is used to diagnose sepsis rather than survival prognosis in sepsis patients [28]. Also, IL-10 is not tested as a point of care test, and is not widely used clinically.

Whether pro-inflammatory biomarkers such as C-reactive protein (CRP) or procalcitonin could be predictors for mortality remains controversial [29]. Biron and co-workers showed that a single procalcitonin concentration is not a good predictor for sepsis and septic shock, but that serial procalcitonin concentrations with high clearance of procalcitonin were reliable predictors [29]. However, a meta-analysis involving 4467 patients showed that procalcitonin-guided therapy did not lower the mortality [30].

We observed a significant increase in mean plasma levels of CRP (122.7 mg/L) and procalcitonin (49.8 ng/mL), but a significant difference between the survival group and non-survival group was not observed ($p =$ 0.931 and 0.159, respectively). Levels of CRP and procalcitonin were thus poor predictors for survival. Other studies undertaken at Cho Ray hospital have elicited similar results [25, 26]. Measurement of the concentrations of CRP and procalcitonin thus aids the diagnosis of infection, but has low accuracy for predicting survival.

In this research, our sepsis and septic shock patients were treated according to Surviving Sepsis Campaign 2012 guidelines. The empiric antibiotic therapy was based on our hospital antibiotic guideline. The research was finished before the Surviving Sepsis Campaign guidelines 2016 were published [31].

Limitations

Our study had two main limitations. First, the time to sepsis onset could not be identified accurately. In this study, we did not find how long our patients may have been affected by sepsis before their admission. Further research may be needed with more frequent monitoring of vital signs to detect early sepsis based on the new guidelines SSC 2016. Second, this research was performed at Cho Ray hospital, a tertiary teaching hospital where modern medical equipment and techniques are available. The generalizability of this finding for all Vietnamese hospitals may be limited. However, there were several hospitals which have similar levels of equipment and facilities in Vietnam, who could apply this research.

Conclusions

Our findings indicate that a reduction in IL-6 level of ≥86% at 24 h from ICU admission was a survival predictor for sepsis and septic shock patients comparing with patients who had an increasing IL-6 rate of change. This finding also supports continuing the initial empiric antibiotic therapy in sepsis and septic shock patients. Hence, in terms of clinical applications, measurement of the IL-6 level should be done upon admission, and at 24 h after ICU admission in sepsis and septic shock patients.

Abbreviations
APACHE: Acute Physiology and Chronic Health Evaluation; AUC: Area under the curve; BUN: Blood-urea-nitrogen; CRP: C-reactive protein; ICU: Intensive care unit; IL: Interleukin; IQR: Interquartile range; SOFA: Sequential Organ Failure Assessment; SSC: Surviving Sepsis Campaign; TNF: Tumor necrosis factor

Acknowledgments
We thank all staff at the Critical Care Unit, Emergency Department, Cho Ray Hospital for their outstanding support.
We also thank Professor Anthony FT Brown (University of Queensland, Australia), Dr. Gerard O'Reilly (Monash University, Australia) for their edition, revision the manuscript and technical support for this research.

Funding
No funding was received to conduct this research. The first author (PTNT) funded for this research.

Authors' contributions
PTNT and TTT conceived and designed the study, reviewed the policy, drafted and finalized the manuscript, and revised the manuscript. NTS and KW also conceived the study, conducted statistical analysis, revised and edited the manuscript. All authors have read and approved the manuscript.

Competing interests
The authors declare that they have no conflicts of interest. All authors have read and approved the manuscript.

Author details
[1]Cho Ray Hospital, 201B Nguyen Chi Thanh Street, District 5, Ho Chi Minh City, Vietnam. [2]International University of Health and Welfare, Tokyo, Japan.

References
1. Carolin F, Daniel O, Rueddel T, Hartmann M, Hartog SC, Welte T, et al. Hospital incidence and mortality rates of Sepsis. Dtsch Arztebl Int. 2016;113: 159–66.
2. Ferrario M, Cambiaghi A, Brunelli L, Giordano S, Caironi P, Guatteri L, et al. Mortality prediction in patients with severe septic shock: a pilot study using a target metabolomics approach. Sci Rep. 2016;6:2039.
3. McPherson D, Griffiths C, Williams M, Baker A, Klodawski E, Jacobson B, et al. Sepsis-associated mortality in England: an analysis of multiple cause of death data from 2001 to 2010. BMJ. 2013;3. https://doi.org/10.1136/bmjopen-2013-002586.
4. Meda AG, Grigorescu LB, Chirteş RL, Alexander A, Fodor SR. The relevance of coding gene Polymorphysms of cytokines and cellular receptors in Sepsis. The Journal of Critical Care Medicine. 2017;3:5–11.
5. Huang TC, Chuang CY, Tsai JY, Ko JW, Yu JC. High mortality in severe Sepsis and septic shock patients with do-not-resuscitate. PLoS One. 2016;11: e0159501.
6. Maija KK, Bailey M, Suzuki S, Pilcher D, Bellomo R. Mortality related to severe Sepsis and septic shock among critically ill patients in Australia and New Zealand, 2000-2012. JAMA. 2014;311:1308–16.
7. Dellinger RP, Levy MM, Rhodes A, Annane D, Gerlach H, Opal SM, et al. Surviving Sepsis campaign: international guidelines for Management of Severe Sepsis and Septic Shock: 2012. Crit Care Med. 2013;4:580–637.
8. Lagu T, Rothberg MB, Shieh MS, Pekow PS, Steingrub JS, Lindenauer PK. Hospitalizations, costs, and outcomes of severe sepsis in the United States 2003 to 2007. Crit Care Med. 2012;40:754–61.
9. Alexander K, John RS. Interleukin-6 in Sepsis and capillary leakage syndrome. J Interf Cytokine Res. 2011;32:60–5.
10. Kusunoki M, Nishi K, Wang S, Okamoto A, Hamano N, Hirota K. Effect of high-dose intravenous immunoglobulin administration on the levels of Interleukin-6 in patients with Sepsis. J Intensive Crit Care. 2017;3:1–6.
11. Chen K, Gao C, Zhou Q, Li W, Lin Z. Predictors of in-hospital mortality for sepsis patients in intensive care units. Int J Clin Exp Med. 2016;9:4029–34.
12. Gentile FL, Cuenca GA, Vanzant LE, Efron AP, McKinley B, Moore F, et al. Is there value in plasma cytokine measurements in patients with severe trauma and Sepsis? Methods. 2013;6:3–9.
13. Klag T, Cantara G, Sechtem U, Athanasiadis A. Interleukin-6 kinetics can be useful for early treatment monitoring of severe bacterial sepsis and septic shock. Infectious Disease Reports. 2016;8. https://doi.org/10.4081/idr.2016.6213.
14. Juan P, Bratti R, Brizuela YN, Albarran JN, Montrull LH. IL-6, MMP 3 and prognosis in previously healthy sepsis patients. Revista de la Facultad de Ciencias Médicas. 2017;74:99–106.
15. Banerjee D,Levy MM, Sepsis Definitions. Springer 2003;Chaper (2):1–23.
16. Dragan D, Pejovic J, Surbatovic M, Jevdjic J, Radakovic S, Veljovic M, et al. Prognostic value and daily trens of Interleukin –6 ,Neutrophil CD 64 expression, C- Reactive protein and Lipopolysaccharide- binding protein in critical ill patients: Reliable predictors of outcome or not? J Med Biochem. 2015;34:431–9.
17. Thompson KD, Huffman MK, Kraus EW, Kraus BV. Critical Appraisal of Four IL-6 Immunoassays. PLoS ONE. 2012;7. https://doi.org/10.1371/journal.pone.0030659.
18. Chawla SL, Seneff GM, Nelson RD, Williams M, Levy H, Kimmel L.P et al., Elevated plasma concentrations of IL-6 and elevated APACHE II score predict acute kidney injury in patients with severe Sepsis. Clin J Am Soc Nephrol 2007;2:22–30.
19. Mohammad N, Makhoul FB, Aronson D, Saliba W, Azzam SZ. Interleukin-6 at discharge predicts all-cause mortality in patients with sepsis. Am J Emerg Med. 2013;31:1361–4.
20. Jaffer U, Wade RG, Gourlay T. Cytokines in the systemic inflammatory response syndrome: a review. HSR Proc Intensive Care Cardiovasc Anesth. 2010;2:161–75.
21. Marissa MA, Lansang AM, Fonbuena EG, Fadreguilan E, Timbreza F, Luna DM, et al. Epidemiology and Predictors of Mortality from Sepsis in Medical Patients at UP-PGH*. Phil J Microbiol Infect Dis. 2000;29:23–32.
22. Shum HP, Yan WW, Chan TM. Extracorporeal blood purification for sepsis. Hong Kong Med J. 2016;22:478–85.
23. Giacomini GM, Valéria M, Lopes AC, Villafanha J, Lobo MS. Septic shock: a major cause of hospital death after intensive care unit discharge. Rev Bras Ter Intensiva. 2015;27:51–6.
24. Moskowitza A, Omarb Y, Chasec M, Lokhandwalad S, Patelc P, Lars W. A et al., reasons for death in patients with sepsis and septic shock. J Crit Care. 2017;38:284–8.
25. Thao PTN, The clinical presentation, laboratory findings and cytokine concentrations in severe sepsis patients The doctoral thesis at University of Medicine and Pharmacy at Ho Chi Minh City, Vietnam 2013;Vietnamese version.
26. Tra TT, Thang QB. Characteristics of Leucocytes, CRP, Procalcitonin and Interleukine concentrations in sepsis and septic shock patients to Emergency department Ho Chi Minh City. Medical Journal. 2014;1:279–83 Vietnamese version.
27. Stalder G, Que AY. Calzavarini S, Burnier L, Kosinski C, Ballabeni P et al., Study of Early Elevated Gas6 Plasma Level as a Predictor of Mortality in a Prospective Cohort of Patients with Sepsis. PLoS ONE. 2016;11. https://doi.org/10.1371/journal.pone.0163542.
28. Chuang YT, Chang TH, Chung PK, Cheng SH, Liu YC, Huang HH, et al. High levels of serum macrophage migration inhibitory factor and interleukin 10 are associated with a rapidly fatal outcome in patients with severe sepsis. Int J Infect Dis. 2014;20:13–7.
29. Biron BM, Alfred A, Joanne LL. Biomarkers for Sepsis: what is and what might be? Biomark Insights. 2015;10:7–17.

30. Schuetz P, Chiappa V, Briel M, Greenwald LJ. Procalcitonin algorithms for antibiotic therapy decisions: a systematic review of randomized controlled trials and recommendations for clinical algorithms. Arch Intern Med. 2011; 171:1322–31.

31. Rhodes A, Evans EL, Alhazzani W, Levy MM, Antonelli M, Ferrer R, et al. Surviving Sepsis campaign: international guidelines for Management of Sepsis and Septic Shock: 2016. Intensive Care Med. 2017;43:304–77.

Epidemiological and clinical profiles of acute poisoning in patients admitted to the intensive care unit in eastern Iran (2010 to 2017)

Omid Mehrpour[1,2*], Ayob Akbari[1], Firoozeh Jahani[1], Alireza Amirabadizadeh[1], Elaheh Allahyari[3], Borhan Mansouri[1] and Patrick C. Ng[2]

Abstract

Background: Acute poisoning is a common chief complaint leading to emergency department visits and hospital admissions in developing countries such as Iran. Data describing the epidemiology of different poisonings, characteristics of the clinical presentations, and the predictors of outcome are lacking. Such data can help develop more efficient preventative and management strategies to decrease morbidity and mortality related to these poisonings. This manuscript describes the epidemiology of acute poisoning among patients admitted to the intensive care unit (ICU) in Birjand, Iran.

Methods: This retrospective, cross-sectional study was conducted to characterize acute poisonings managed in the ICU during a 7-year period from March 2010 to March 2017 in a single center in Birjand, Iran. Patient characteristics, suspected exposure, the route of exposure, and outcome data were collected from hospital medical records.

Results: During the study period, 267 (64% male and 36% female) patients met inclusion criteria. Pharmaceutical medication (36.6%), opioids (26.2%) followed by pesticides (13.9%) were the most common exposures 38.2% of these cases were identified as suicide attempts. There were different frequencies in terms of xenobiotic exposure in relation to gender ($p = 0.04$) and the survival ($p = 0.001$). There was a significant difference between various xenobiotics identified as the cause of poisoning ($p = 0.001$). Mortality rate in our study was 19.5%. The incidence of outcomes was significantly higher in patients poisoned with opioids, pesticides, benzodiazepines, and tricyclic antidepressants ($p < 0.05$). The median length of hospital stay was higher in pesticide-poisoned patients ($p = 0.04$).

Conclusion: Opioids and pesticides were the most common exposures. The mortality rate of the poisoned patients in the ICU was proportionately high. The mortality rate due to opioid poisoning is a major concern and the most significant cause death due to poisoning in the region. Further monitoring and characterization of acute poisoning in Birjand, Iran is needed. These data can help develop educational and preventative programs to reduce these exposures and improve management of exposures in the prehospital and hospital settings.

Keywords: Acute poisoning, Intensive care unit (ICU), Opioids, Benzodiazepines, Pesticides

* Correspondence: omid.mehrpour@yahoo.com.au
[1]Medical Toxicology and Drug Abuse Research Center (MTDRC), Birjand University of Medical Sciences, Moallem Avenue, Birjand 9717853577, Iran
[2]Rocky Mountain Poison and Drug Center, Denver, CO, USA
Full list of author information is available at the end of the article

Background

A poison is a xenobiotic that, in the right dose, can lead to injury or death of an organism [1]. Poisoning is a common, resource intensive chief complaint resulting in thousands of hospital admissions worldwide. Acute poisoning, depending on the xenobiotic, can present in many ways. Some signs and symptoms associated with poisoning include: CNS depression, miosis, hypothermia, respiratory depression, hypotension, delirium, dysrhythmias and multisystem organ failure [2–4]. Poisoning can be categorized into intentional and accidental. Many cases of intentional poisoning occur in developing countries where resources are limited and are associated with a high degree of morbidity and mortality [3, 5, 6].

The prevalence of acute poisoning varies in relation to religious, cultural, and geographical contexts and is dynamic given the continued development and varying availability of different xenobiotics [4]. For example, in developed countries the most common cause of acute poisoning is the abuse of commercially available pharmaceuticals [7], in contrast, in developing countries, insecticides are the most common [8]. Furthermore, the availability of pharmaceuticals is regional; in Iran, prescriptions for and availability of commercially available opioids are significantly less compared to countries like the United States. In Iran, the majority of poisonings are intentional and occur mainly in the age range of 21–30 years. In this country, the mortality rate from poisoning is 8 per 1000 individuals in the general hospitalization wards and 109 per 1000 people in the intensive care unit (ICU). According to the World Health Organization (WHO), suicide and chemical substances account for nearly one million deaths annually worldwide with pesticides as a major cause [9]. Timely diagnosis of poisoning and appropriate treatment is vital to prevent morbidity and mortality.

More data on the general pattern of poisonings in each geographic region is important to address this issue. To reduce hospital morbidity and mortality, early diagnosis and rapid treatment in ED and ICU are critical for the poisoned patient. Currently, there are very few data available that detail poisonings in Eastern Iran especially in South Khorasan province. Despite this need, few studies in Iran have addressed the patterns of poisoning in the patients hospitalized in the ICU [9]. The main aim of this study was to assess the epidemiological characteristics and clinical features of acute poisoning in all adult patients admitted to the Imam Reza Hospital ICU in Birjand City, Iran from 2010 to 2017. With a deeper understanding of poisoning in Iran, more effective education and management plans can lead to more efficient recognition and management of these patients, eventually reducing morbidity and mortality associated with this potentially deadly chief complaint.

Methods

Study design

This retrospective, observational cross-sectional study was conducted to investigate the clinical characteristics and epidemiological patterns of acute poisoning leading to ICU admission. The study took place in Imam Reza Hospital in Birjand City, South Khorasan Province, Iran from March 21, 2010 to March 21, 2017 (Fig. 1). The study protocol was approved by a local institutional review board. Imam Reza Hospital, a teaching hospital affiliated with Birjand University of Medical Sciences, is the referral center for toxicology patients in the South Khorasan Province [10].

Study population

The study population consisted of all individuals diagnosed with acute poisoning admitted to the ICU of Imam Reza Hospital in Birjand City during the seven years. The inclusion criteria were: Age > 13 years and chief complaint of acute poisoning. In our center, patients less than 13 years old are usually admitted to a pediatric unit. Exclusion criteria included: Age < 13 years, history of underlying chronic disease (e.g. diabetes

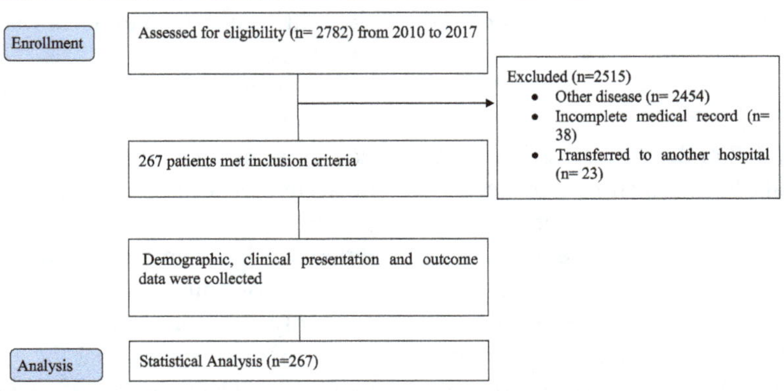

Fig. 1 Flow chart of study patient selection

mellitus and renal failure), presentation with concomitant acute pathology with intoxication (such as burns, trauma, etc.), and/or incomplete medical file.

Data gathering

Poisoned patients in the emergency department were examined and treated by the physicians on duty. Depending on the severity of symptoms, the patients were discharged after management in the emergency department, transferred to an 18-bed specialty poisoning ward, or admitted to the ICU. ICU admission decisions were made by the ICU physician on duty. Criteria for admission to the ICU included: potentially lethal exposure (for example, aluminum phosphide (AlP), strychnine, arsenic, or cyanide), seizure, deep CNS depression, respiratory distress (RR > 35 breaths/min), and hemodynamic instability (systolic arterial pressure < 80 mmHg or 20 mmHg below the patient's usual pressure) [11]. A standardized data collection sheet was used to collect demographic characteristics (age, gender, etc.), timing of presentation, the cause of poisoning (accidental, overdose, intentional), the suspected exposure (envenomation, asphyxiates, opioids (methadone, heroin, opium, opium residue), insecticides, and pharmaceutical drugs), the outcome (in-hospital mortality, discharge) and vital signs. Data was collected from patient medical records. This study was approved by the ethics committee of Birjand University of Medical Sciences with ethics code of IR.BUMS.1395.6. Administrative permissions were obtained, in order to review patient records from ethics committee of Birjand University of Medical Sciences.

Statistical analysis

Data analysis was performed by the SPSS package, version 22 (Chicago, IL, USA). Descriptive statistics including frequency, percentage, mean, and standard deviation were reported. Using Kolmogorov-Smirnov test, we examined the normality of quantitative variables distribution. Mann-Whitney and Kruskal-Wallis tests were employed to analyze quantitative variables with non-normal distribution. Chi-square and Fisher's exact tests were used to analyze qualitative data. The significance level was considered to be 0.05.

Results

During the study period, 267 of 2782 cases reviewed met inclusion criteria, 173 (64.8%) of which were male. Most of the cases [$n = 72$; 27%] occurred in summer.

Pharmaceutical drug poisoning was the most common cause of intoxication (36.6%). Of these, benzodiazepines were the most frequent, followed by tricyclic antidepressants. Opioids (26.2%) (Methadone, opium, opium residue) and Pesticide (13.9%) were also common exposures (Table 1).

Table 1 Frequency distribution of demographic variables in the studied patients

Variable		Number of cases (n)	Percentage (%)
Gender	Male	173.0	64.8
	Female	94.0	35.2
Age group (years)	20–35	167.0	62.5
	35–50	46.0	17.2
	50–65	26.0	9.5
	> = 65	28.0	10.5
Residence	Urban	183.0	69.6
	Rural	84.0	30.4
Education status	Illiterate	25.0	9.4
	Primary school	26.0	9.7
	Secondary school	43.0	16.1
	High school	32.0	11.9
	College	28.0	10.5
	Unknown	113.0	42.4
Employment status	Student	13.0	4.8
	Unemployed	68.0	25.5
	Employed	26.0	9.7
	Farmer	14.0	5.2
	Others	45.0	16.8
	Unknown	101	38.0
Season	Spring	62.0	23.2
	Summer	72.0	27.0
	Autumn	63.0	23.6
	Winter	70.0	26.2
Glasgow Coma Scale (GCS)	< 9	124.0	46.4
	9–13	51.0	19.1
	13–15	92.0	34.5

There was a difference in terms of the exposure identified between men and women ($\chi^2 = 23.25$, $p = 0.04$). Of the deceased patients, 36 (20.8%) were men and 16 (17.1%) were women. The data did not detect a significant difference in outcomes between men and women ($p = 0.45$).

One hundred two (38.2%) [Male = 60] of cases were related to suicide. Twenty two (8.2%) cases were identified as accidental poisonings. There was no significant different between male and female regarding cause of poisoning ($p = 0.16$) (Table 2). There was a significant difference between various xenobiotics identified as the cause of poisoning ($p = 0.001$), Table 3.

Seventy (26%) of cases were opioid related (Table 4). The Bonferroni test showed that the incidence of outcomes was significantly higher in patients poisoned with opioids, pesticides, benzodiazepines, tricyclic antidepressants (TCAs),

Table 2 Comparison of the frequencies of poisoning agents, route of use, causes of poisoning, and poisoning outcomes per gender

Variable	Total	Male	Female	Test result
Poisoning agent				$\chi^2 = 23.25$ $P = 0.04$
Acetaminophen	2 (0.7%)	2 (1.2%)	0 (0%)	
Tramadol	9 (3.4%)	5 (2.9%)	4 (4.3%)	
Benzodiazepines	34 (12.7%)	22 (12.7%)	12 (12.8%)	
Tricyclic antidepressants	23 (8.6%)	11 (6.4%)	12 (12.8%)	
Antipsychotics	20 (7.5%)	11 (6.4%)	9 (9.6%)	
Anticonvulsant	4 (1.5%)	4 (2.3%)	0 (0%)	
Beta Blocker	6 (2.2%)	5 (2.9%)	1 (1.1%)	
Opioids	70 (26.2%)	53 (30.6%)	17 (18.1%)	
Alcohol	4 (1.5%)	4 (2.3%)	0 (0%)	
Cannabis	3 (1.1%)	3 (1.7%)	0 (0%)	
Co-Poisoning	8 (3.0%)	5 (2.9%)	3 (3.2%)	
Aluminum phosphide	2 (0.7%)	1 (0.6%)	1 (1.1%)	
Pesticides	37 (13.9%)	19 (11.0%)	18 (19.1%)	
Others	11 (4.1%)	4 (2.3%)	7 (7.4%)	
Unknown	34 (12.7%)	24 (13.9%)	10 (10.6%)	
total	267 (100%)	173(100%)	94 (100%)	
Cause of poisoning				$\chi^2 = 5.09$ $P = 0.16$
Accidental	22 (8.2%)	12 (6.9%)	10 (10.6%)	
Suicide	102 (38.2%)	60 (34.7%)	42 (44.7%)	
Overdose	49 (18.4%)	33 (19.1%)	16 (17.0%)	
Unknown	94 (35.2%)	68 (39.3%)	26 (27.7%)	
Route of use				
Oral ingestion	215 (80.5%)	137 (79.2%)	78 (83.0%)	$\chi^2 = 0.77$ $P = 0.86$
Inhalation	11 (4.1%)	7 (4.0%)	4 (4.3%)	
Injection	3 (1.1%)	2 (1.2%)	1 (1.1%)	
Unknown	38 (14.2%)	27 (15.6%)	11 (11.7%)	
Outcome				$\chi^2 = 0.56$ $P = 0.45$
Survival	215 (80.5%)	137 (79.2%)	78 (83.0%)	
Death	52 (19.5%)	36 (20.8%)	16 (17.0%)	

and unspecified agents than in those poisoned with other medications and substances ($p < 0.05$). According to the results of this study, 52 (19.5%) of the patients admitted to the ICU died. One-hundred and ten patients (41.2%) were intubated, of whom 47 (17.6%) died and 63 (23.6%) survived. Among those discharged ($n = 215$), 12 patients left the hospital before completion of treatment and discharged against medical advice.

Table 5 shows median length of hospital stay in various types of poisoning. Kruskal-Wallis testing determined that the median length of hospital stay was significantly higher in the patients treated for pesticide poisoning than in those poisoned patients treated for poisoning from other xenobiotics ($\chi2 = 23.89$, $p = 0.04$). The median duration of hospital stay in the orally poisoned patients was 3.0 [2.0–4.0] days with the mean duration of 4.66 ± 6.74 days. In overdose patients, the median length of hospital stay was 3.0 [2.0–5.5] days with the mean duration of 4.94 ± 6.04 days. The median length of hospital stay in the deceased patients was 5.5 [2.0–13.0] days with the mean duration of 8.53 ± 8.99 days. The results of the Mann-Whitney test showed that the median length of hospital stay was significantly higher in the deceased patients than in the survived ones ($z = 4.27$, $p < 0.001$).

Mean time from exposure to hospital arrival was 6.96 ± 12.94 (Range: 0.5–72) hours. Results of Kruskal Wallis test showed that there was a significant difference for time between exposure and presentation to hospital when comparing various xenobiotics [Opioids 9.18 ± 17.35 h, Alcohol 14.37 ± 22.67 h]. Mann-Whitney test showed that those exposure to alcohol and unknown

Table 3 Frequency of poisoning cases according to cause of poisoning

Poisoning agent	Accidental	Suicide	Overdose	Unknown	Test results
Acetaminophen	0(0%)	2(100%)	0(0%)	0(0%)	$\chi^2 = 219.03$ $P < 0.001$
Tramadol	0(0%)	6(66.7%)	0(0%)	3(33.3%)	
Benzodiazepines	1(2.9%)	20(58.8%)	1(2.9%)	12(35.3%)	
Tricyclic antidepressants	0(0%)	16(69.6%)	0(0%)	7(30.4%)	
Antipsychotics	0(0%)	17(85%)	0(0%)	3(15%)	
Anticonvulsant	0(0%)	3(75%)	0(0%)	1(25%)	
Beta Blocker	0(0%)	4(66.7%)	0(0%)	2(33.3%)	
Opioids	6(8.6%)	7(10%)	43(61.4%)	14(20%)	
Alcohol	0(0%)	2(50%)	2(50%)	0(0%)	
Cannabis	0(0%)	0(0%)	0(0%)	3(100%)	
Co-Poisoning	2(25%)	0(0%)	0(0%)	6(75%)	
Aluminum phosphide	0(0%)	2(100%)	0(0%)	0(0%)	
Pesticides	9(24.3%)	14(37.8%)	0(0%)	14(37.8%)	
Others	3(27.3%)	2(18.2%)	3(27.3%)	3(27.3%)	
Unknown	1(2.9%)	7(20.6%)	0(0%)	26(76.5%)	

agents had higher time of presentation to the hospital, in comparison with other agents ($p = 0.03$; Table 6).

Discussion

Poisoning remains as a significant medical complaint across the globe [8, 12–20] with various patterns of acute toxicity in different regions. South Khorasan province especially Birjand city in Iran is no exception, and there is a paucity of information regarding poisonings in this region. According to our results, the most common agents of poisoning were pharmaceutical drugs, opioids followed by pesticides.

Table 4 Poison exposure for survivors and non-survivors of poisoning admitted to Intensive Care Unit (ICU)

		Total	Survival	Non-survivors	Test result
poisoning agents	Acetaminophen	2 (0.7%)	2 (0.9%)	0 (0%)	$\chi2 = 37.08$ $P = 0.001$
	Tramadol	9 (3.4%)	8 (3.7%)	1 (1.9%)	
	Benzodiazepines	34 (12.7%)	32 (14.9%)	2 (3.8%)	
	Tricyclic antidepressants	23 (8.6%)	21 (9.8%)	2 (3.8%)	
	Antipsychotics	20 (7.5%)	20 (9.3%)	0 (0%)	
	Anticonvulsant	4 (1.5%)	4 (1.9%)	0 (0%)	
	Beta Blocker	6 (2.2%)	6 (2.8%)	0 (0%)	
	Opioids	70 (26.2%)	45 (20.9%)	25 (48.1%)	
	Alcohol	4 (1.5%)	2 (0.9%)	2 (3.8%)	
	Cannabis	3 (1.1%)	3 (1.4%)	0 (0%)	
	Co-Poisoning	8 (3.0%)	7 (3.3%)	1 (1.9%)	
	Aluminum phosphide	2 (0.7%)	2 (0.9%)	0 (0%)	
	Pesticides	37 (13.9%)	33 (15.3%)	4 (7.7%)	
	Others	11 (4.1%)	8 (3.7%)	3 (5.8%)	
	Unknown	34 (12.7%)	22 (10.2%)	12 (23.1%)	
	total	267 (100%)	215 (100%)	52(100%)	
Intubation	Yes	110.0 (41.2%)	63 (23.6%)	47 (17.6%)	$\chi2 = 64.49$ $p < 0.001$
	No	157 (58.8%)	152 (56.9%)	5 (1.9%)	
Seizure	Yes	33 (12.4%)	24 (9.0%)	9 (3.4%)	$\chi2 = 1.43$ $P = 0.17$
	No	234 (87.6%)	191 (71.4%)	43 (16.2%)	

Table 5 Comparison of median length of hospital stay among study population

Variable		Length of hospital stay (days) Median[IQR]	Test result
Poisoning agent	Acetaminophen	2.0 [1.0–2.0]	χ2 = 23.89 $P = 0.04$
	Tramadol	2.0 [1.5–3.5]	
	Benzodiazepines	2.0 [1.0–3.0]	
	Tricyclic antidepressants	2.0 [2.0–3.0]	
	Antipsychotics	2.0 [1.25–3.0]	
	Anticonvulsant	3.0 [2.0–4.0]	
	Beta Blocker	2.5 [1.0–3.0]	
	Opioids	3.0 [2.0–6.0]	
	Alcohol	1.0 [1.0–4.0]	
	Cannabis	1.0 [1.0–1.0]	
	Co-Poisoning	2.0 [2.0–18.0]	
	Aluminum phosphide	6.5 [3.0–6.5]	
	Pesticides	3.0 [2.0–5.5]	
	Others	2.0 [1.0–8.0]	
	Unknown	3.0 [2.0–7.25]	
Cause of poisoning	Casual	2.0 [1.75–9.0]	χ2 = 3.62 $P = 0.30$
	Suicide	2.0 [2.0–4.0]	
	Accidental/overdose	3.0 [2.0–5.5]	
	Unknown	3.0 [2.0–5.0]	
Route of use	Oral ingestion	3.0 [2.0–4.0]	χ2 = 1.84 $P = 0.61$
	Inhalation	3.0 [2.0–12.0]	
	Injection	3.0 [1.0–3.0]	
	Unknown	2.0 [1.0–5.0]	
Outcome	Survival	2.0 [2.0–4.0]	Z = 4.27 $p < 0.001$
	Non-survivors	5.5 [2.0–13.0]	

Table 6 Mean time from exposure to poison and arriving to hospital in various poison agents

Poisoning agent	Hours (Mean ± SD)	Median[IQR]	Test result
Acetaminophen	2.00 ± 0.00	2.00[2.00–2.00]	X2 = 5.17 $P = 0.03$
Tramadol	5.30 ± 4.46	4.00[1.25–10.00]	
Benzodiazepines	4.97 ± 4.12	3.00[2.00–10.00]	
Tricyclic antidepressants	3.54 ± 3.53	2.00[1.00–5.00]	
Antipsychotics	2.78 ± 2.62	2.00[0.75–4.50]	
Anticonvulsant	2.35 ± 2.12	2.00[2.00–2.00]	
Beta Blocker	3.00 ± 0.89	3.00[2.00–4.00]	
Opioids	9.18 ± 17.35	4.00[1.00–10.00]	
Alcohol	14.37 ± 22.67	4.50[0.62–38.00]	
Cannabis	2.98 ± 2.35	2.00[1.50–3.00]	
Co-Poisoning	5.00 ± 4.24	5.00[2.00–7.00]	
Aluminum phosphide	5.50 ± 0.71	5.00[5.00–5.00]	
Pesticides	9.04 ± 19.31	2.00[1.25–9.50]	
Others	2.00 ± 1.73	1.00[1.00–1.00]	
Unknown	19.00 ± 22.58	6.00[3.00–48.00]	

Pharmaceutical drugs were the most commonly used group of toxic substances in our patients, which is consistent with previous studies in Iran and other countries [12, 17]. This observation can be attributed to the accessibility of pharmaceutical drugs in Iran, especially in the studied region. We suspect that the availability of benzodiazapines without prescription is a major contributor to its common use amongst this population.

Opioids poisoning was the second most common agent of poisoning in this study. Several recent studies have shown that opioids poisoning is the most common cause of death annually in many regions of Iran. For instance, Farzaneh et al.[18] in the northwestern city of Ardabil, Afzali [19] in Hamadan City (west of Iran), and Ayatollahi et al. [20] in Yazd City (center of Iran) illustrated that from among xenobiotics, opioids were the most frequent cause of acute poisoning. In Iran opium and opium residue are the most common opioid. Infact Iran has the highest rate of opium addiction in the world [21]. The availability of opioids in the region due to the sharing border with Afghanistan and the sociocultural characteristics of Iran are potential contributory factors to this finding. The high rate of opioid poisoning is similar to other geographical areas as evidenced by Hamilton et al. [22] who reported that the opioids and other medications are the most common causes of acute poisoning in New York City.

Pesticides were found to be the third most common agent of poisoning. Azin et al. (2008) conducted a study in six big cities of Iran and reported similar results [23]. Most recently, poisoning with AlP is the cause of many poisoning-related deaths in Iran for which no antidotes have yet been reported [24, 25]. Mortality rate from AlP poisoning is even high in the ICU patients, and in some studies, it has been reported to be 75–100% [26]. In our study, two (0.7%) cases of AlP poisoning, both severe cases, were recorded but improved by means of certain treatments including intra-aortic balloon pump insertion. We have already reported successfully treated cases of severe AlP poisoning by this method [27].

Interestingly, three (1.4%) of the patients in our study used a compound locally called *Majoon Birjandi*, which is unique to this region of Iran [21]. It is a mixture of several hot-natured herbs mixed with some cannabis. Made in solid form in diamond-shaped molds, it is used mostly by young people to induce euphoria. No mortality in such cases was observed.

The frequency distribution of consciousness level at referral based on Glasgow Coma Scale/Score (GCS) showed that most patients had a score of than 9. In the study of Taghaddosinejad et al. [28] in Baharlou Hospital in Tehran, the frequencies of the REED coma grades 2, 3, and 4 were 49.7, 41.7, and 8.6%, respectively.

In our study, 12.4% of the patients developed seizure after poisoning, while in the study of Taghaddosinejad et al. [28] in the poisoned patients in the intensive care unit (ICU), 2% of the patients developed seizure, which was associated with the agents of poisoning, especially tramadol. In our study, seizures occurring in patients without a seizure history were related to tramadol poisoning. The relationship between tramadol poisoning and seizure has been reported [29, 30].

In our study, 41.2% of patients were intubated. This similar to Sulaj et al.'s study (2015) where 31.4% of patients underwent mechanical ventilation[31]. In the study of Ahuji et al. (2015) on 67 patients, 43 (64%) needed mechanical ventilation [32], and in Lam et al.'s study in Hong Kong, 67.9% of 265 patients were intubated [33]. Much lower intubation rates in acute poisoning patients have been reported. For example, in the studies of Exiara in Greece [34] and Ismail Demirel in Turkey [14], 4.48 and 6.2% of the patients were respectively intubated because of respiratory failure.

Mortality rate in our study was 19.5%. Similarly, Khodabandeh et al. [35] reported an approximately 27% mortality rate in the Tehran-based Loghman-Hakim Hospital ICU.

In our study, opioids and pesticides were the main causes of poisoning-related death. The overall mortality rate in the ICU in the Iranian-based hospital poison centers in Tehran, Khoramabad, Mazandaran, and are reported as 17.7, 11.6, and 14.6% respectively [36, 37].

This mortality rate is considerably high and should be therefore be thoroughly examined. In previous studies in Iran, similar rates of mortality have been reported in the ICU poisoned patients [11.6–18.6%) [38, 39]. Similar mortality rates have been reported in other developing countries [3, 40]. However, two recent studies in Germany and Hong Kong have reported mortality rates of, 0.7% and 3% respectively in the ICU poisoned patients [33, 41]. Several reasons can be presented to explain the high variation in mortality rates in different countries. One possibility is that a referral center for poisoning, as with our study setting, may have selectivity toward more severe poisonings leading to admission. Another possibility is that the criteria for admission to the ICU are widely different in different hospitals and countries [33]. Moreover, in our setting, ICU admission was limited only to obviously severe and life-threatening poisonings, while other institutions routinely admit all poisoned patients to the ICU, irrespective of the severity of their symptoms at arrival [39].

Interestingly, most of the mortality in our center was related to opioid and unknown cases. In a 6-year study in Tehran, Hassanian-Moghaddam et al. [42] reported that opioids were the most common cause of poisoning and second most common cause of death after pesticides. In another study, Torkashvand et al. [38] illustrated that 23.8 and 8.1% of the 260 poisoned cases were caused by methadone and opium, respectively. Similarly, in the study of Bjornaas [17] in Norway, opioids (48.1%) were the most common agent of poisonings leading to death . In the study of Shadnia in Tehran, Iran, opioids (40%) were reported as the most common cause of death [7]. It seems that since opioids can cause hypoxia, delay in treatment of toxicity may cause brain hypoxia and also death. Addressing opioid toxicity promptly with reversal agents and/or mechanical ventilation and save thousands of lives. Take-home naloxone programs are expanding around the world and may be applicable to patients in our study area. In these programs, those who abuse drugs, especially those addicted to opioids and their relatives are given naloxone to be administered subcutaneously or intranasally by bystanders or by the individual user after opioid overdose.

Our study had some limitations. We were unable to determine mortality rate and outcomes in poisoned patients referred to the emergency department. Therefore, we could not determine the in-hospital mortality rate in all the poisoned patients. The external validity of our study is also limited to the data from a single center, although the studied center is the main referral hospital for poisoning in the province and one of the main centers of this type in eastern Iran. Another limitation was its retrospective design. Because of the retrospective nature of this study, it is possible that some information is missed. Moreover, no data were available concerning the outcomes after hospital discharge, and death occurring after discharge may have been specifically missed.

Conclusion

In our study, the most common agents of poisoning were pharmaceutical drugs, opioids followed by pesticides; most cases were suicide attempts and the mortality rate associated with the study population was high. This study was the first study evaluating cause and pattern of poisoning cases in the South Khorasan Province in east Iran. This study has data that compliments the literature and can help to characterize the poisoning cases seen in this area.

Opioid poisoning is a major concern and most important cause of death due to poisoning in the region. Recognition of this important cause of death may lead to actions to mitigate harm such as providing naloxone for potential opioid misusers. Self-administration of naloxone can decrease time to treatment after overdose and reverse life threating toxicity before it is too late. Further measures to address poisonings, such as regulation to deal with drug trafficking and laws controlling the availability of these substances can help reduce cases of these preventable causes of death.

Abbreviations

AlP: Aluminum phosphide; CO: Carbon monoxide; ED: Emergency department; HIS: Hospital information system; ICD10: International classification of diseases, tenth revision; ICU: Intensive care unit; RR: Respiratory distress

Acknowledgements

This study was derived from the MD thesis of the FJ. The authors would like to gratefully acknowledge all of our colleagues at Medical Toxicology and Drug Abuse Research Center (MTDRC) and personnel of ICU of Birjand University of Medical Sciences who contributed greatly to this study.

Funding

This study was supported by Birjand University of medical sciences [grant number: 95/739].

Authors' contributions

OM, FJ, ARA, PN made substantial contributions to conception and design, acquisition of data, contributed to the writing of the manuscript and provided critical revision and final approval. ARA, AA, BM and PN made substantial contributions in drafting the manuscript and revising it critically for important intellectual content. ARA and EA involved in data acquisition, analysis and interpretation and have given final approval to be published. All authors have read and approved the final version of manuscript.

Competing interests

The authors declare that they have no competing interests.

Author details

[1]Medical Toxicology and Drug Abuse Research Center (MTDRC), Birjand University of Medical Sciences, Moallem Avenue, Birjand 9717853577, Iran. [2]Rocky Mountain Poison and Drug Center, Denver, CO, USA. [3]Social Determinants of Health Research Center, Birjand University of Medical Sciences, Birjand, Iran.

References

1. Moradi M, Ghaemi K, Mehrpour O. A hospital base epidemiology and pattern of acute adult poisoning across Iran: a systematic review. Electronic physician. 2016;8(9):2860–70.
2. Lee H-L, Lin H-J, Yeh S-Y, Chi C-H, Guo H-R. Etiology and outcome of patients presenting for poisoning to the emergency department in Taiwan: a prospective study. Human & experimental toxicology. 2008;27(5):373–9.
3. Eddleston M. Patterns and problems of deliberate self-poisoning in the developing world. Qjm. 2000;93(11):715–31.
4. Al-Jahdali H, Al-Johani A, Al-Hakawi A, et al. Pattern and risk factors for intentional drug overdose in Saudi Arabia. The Canadian Journal of Psychiatry. 2004;49(5):331–4.
5. Van Hoving D, Veale D, Müller G. Clinical Review: Emergency management of acute poisoning. African Journal of Emergency Medicine. 2011;1(2):69–78.
6. Orsini J, Din N, Elahi E, et al. Clinical and epidemiological characteristics of patients with acute drug intoxication admitted to ICU. Journal of community hospital internal medicine perspectives. 2017;7(4):202–7.
7. Shadnia S, Esmaily H, Sasanian G, Pajoumand A, Hassanian-Moghaddam H, Abdollahi M. Pattern of acute poisoning in Tehran-Iran in 2003. Hum. Exp. Toxicol. 2007;26(9):753–6.
8. Abdollahi M, Jalali N, Sabzevari O, Hoseini R, Ghanea T. A restrospective study of poisoning in Tehran. J. Toxicol. Clin. Toxicol. 1997;35(4):387–93.
9. Alizadeh AM, Hassanian-Moghaddam H, Shadnia S, Zamani N, Mehrpour O. Simplified acute physiology score II/acute physiology and chronic health evaluation II and prediction of the mortality and later development of complications in poisoned patients admitted to intensive care unit. Basic & clinical pharmacology & toxicology. 2014;115(3):297–300.

10. Mehrpour O, Abdollahi M. Poison treatment centers in Iran. Hum Exp Toxicol. 2012;31(3):303–4.
11. Edwards IR, Aronson JK. Adverse drug reactions: definitions, diagnosis, and management. The lancet. 2000;356(9237):1255–9.
12. Kamau MS, Kipbichii CA, Ruiru MH. Intensive care management of poisoning in a resource-limited health care setting in Western Kenya. Int J Humanit Soc Sci. 2014;4(189):189–94.
13. Yaylacı S, Genc A, Demir M, Cinemre H, Tamer A. Retrospective evaluation of patients at follow-up with acute poisoning in Intensive Care Unit. Nigerian journal of clinical practice. 2016;19(2):223–6.
14. Demİrel İ. A retrospective analysis of intoxication cases in intensive care unit of Elazığ Education and Research Hospital. Firat Tip Dergisi. 2010;15(4):184–7.
15. Klein-Schwartz W, Smith GS. Agricultural and horticultural chemical poisonings: mortality and morbidity in the United States. Ann Emerg Med. 1997;29(2):232–8.
16. Rajasuriar R, Awang R, Hashim SB, Rahmat HR. Profile of poisoning admissions in Malaysia. Hum Exp Toxicol. 2007;26(2):73–81.
17. Bjornaas MA, Teige B, Hovda KE, Ekeberg O, Heyerdahl F, Jacobsen D. Fatal poisonings in Oslo: a one-year observational study. BMC Emerg Med. 2010; 10(1):13.
18. Farzaneh E, Amani F, Etemad F. A Clinico-Epidemiologic Study on Patients with Opium Toxicity Treated at Ardabil Hospitals, Iran, 2014–2015. Asia Pac J Med Toxicol. 2016;5:111–4.
19. Afzali S. Pattern of mortality due to poisoning by drugs and chemical agents in Hamadan, Iran, 2005–2007. Qom Uni Med Sci J. 2012;2(2):15–22.
20. Ayatollahi V, Behdad S, Oliwiaie H, Hajiesmaili MR, Dehghan M, Mehrpour O. Characteristic features of patients hospitalized with Narcotic poisoning in Yazd. Iran. Iran J Toxicol. 2011;4(4):362–6.
21. Alinejad S, Zamani N, Abdollahi M, Mehrpour O. A narrative review of acute adult poisoning in Iran. Iranian journal of medical sciences. 2017;42(4):327–46.
22. Hamilton BE, Hoyert DL, Martin JA, Strobino DM, Guyer B. Annual summary of vital statistics: 2010–2011. Pediatrics. 2013;2:2012–3769.
23. Azin S, Shahidzadeh Mahani A, Abadi M, Omidvari S, Montazeri A. Substances Involved in Human Poisoning a Comparison between Intentional and Accidental Poisoning Cases. Iranian Journal of Epidemiology. 2008;4(2):7–17.
24. Mehrpour O, Keyler D, Shadnia S. Comment on Aluminum and zinc phosphide poisoning. Clinical toxicology (Philadelphia, Pa). 2009;47(8):838–9.
25. Mehrpour O, Jafarzadeh M, Abdollahi M. A systematic review of aluminium phosphide poisoning. Arh Hig Rada Toksikol. 2012;63(1):61–73.
26. Farzaneh E, Ghobadi H, Akbarifard M, Nakhaee S, Amirabadizadeh A, Akhavanakbari G,et al. Prognostic Factors in Acute Aluminium Phosphide Poisoning: A Risk-Prediction Nomogram Approach. Basic Clin Pharmacol Toxicol.2018, 123(3):347-355 2018 Mar 12. https://doi.org/10.1111/bcpt. 13005. [Epub ahead of print] .
27. Mehrpour O, Amouzeshi A, Dadpour B, et al. Successful treatment of cardiogenic shock with an intraaortic balloon pump following aluminium phosphide poisoning. Arhiv za higijenu rada i toksikologiju. 2014;65(1):121–6.
28. Taghaddosinejad F, Sheikhazadi A, Yaghmaei A, Mehrpour O, Schwake L. Epidemiology and treatment of severe poisoning in the intensive care unit: lessons from a one-year prospective observational study. J Clinic Toxicol S. 2012;S1:007.
29. Mehrpour O. Addiction and seizure ability of tramadol in high-risk patients. Indian J Anaesth. 2013;57(1):86–7.
30. Goodarzi F, Mehrpour O, Eizadi-Mood N. A study to evaluate factors associated with seizure in Tramadol poisoning in Iran. Indian Journal of Forensic Medicine & Toxicology. 2011;5(2):66–9.
31. Sulaj Z, Prifti E, Demiraj A, Strakosha A. Early Clinical Outcome of Acute Poisoning Cases Treated in Intensive Care Unit. Medical archives (Sarajevo, Bosnia and Herzegovina). 2015;69(6):400–4.
32. Ahuja H, Mathai AS, Pannu A, Arora R. Acute poisonings admitted to a tertiary level intensive care unit in northern India: patient profile and outcomes. Journal of clinical and diagnostic research: JCDR. 2015;9(10): UC01–4.
33. Lam SM, Lau AC, Yan WW. Over 8 years experience on severe acute poisoning requiring intensive care in Hong Kong. China. Hum Exp Toxicol. 2010;29(9):757–65.
34. Exiara T, Mavrakanas TA, Papazoglou L, Papazoglou D, Christakidis D, Maltezos E. A prospective study of acute poisonings in a sample of Greek patients. Cent Eur J Public Health. 2009;17(3):158–60.
35. Khodabandeh F, Emamhadi M, Mostafazadeh B. Epidemiological Assessment of acute poisoning Death–One year Survey. International Journal of Medical Toxicology and Forensic Medicine. 2012;2(3):103–9.
36. Moghadamnia AA, Abdollahi M. An epidemiological study of poisoning in northern Islamic Republic of Iran. Eastern Mediterranean health journal. 2002;8(1):88–94.
37. Akhlaghi M, Arbabi Z, Khadivi R. Pattern of acute poisoning in Shahrekord (Western Iran). Asian Journal of Epidemiology. 2009;2(1):9–12.
38. Torkashvand F, Sheikh Fathollahi M, Shamsi S, Kamali M, Rezaeian M. Evaluating the Pattern of Acute Poisoning in Cases Referred to the Emergency Department of Ali-ebn Abi Taleb Hospital of Rafsanjan from October 2013 to September 2014. Journal of Rafsanjan University of Medical Sciences. 2015;14(4):311–24.
39. Hassaniam-Moghaddam H, Baghbanian N, Kolah AA. Evaluating the factors accompanying coma in patients admitted to the poisoning ICU of Loghman-Hakim Poison Hospital. Iranian Journal of Toxicology. 2007;1(2):1.
40. Eddleston M, Haggalla S, Reginald K, et al. The hazards of gastric lavage for intentional self-poisoning in a resource poor location. Clinical toxicology. 2007;45(2):136–43.
41. Schwake L, Wollenschlager I, Stremmel W, Encke J. Adverse drug reactions and deliberate self-poisoning as cause of admission to the intensive care unit: a 1-year prospective observational cohort study. Intensive Care Med. 2009;35(2):266–74.
42. Hassanian-Moghaddam H, Zamani N, Rahimi M, Shadnia S, Pajoumand A, Sarjami S. Acute adult and adolescent poisoning in Tehran, Iran; the epidemiologic trend between 2006 and 2011. Archives of Iranian medicine. 2014;17(8):534–8.

30

Epidemiology of patients presenting to a pediatric emergency department

Nadir Ijaz[1], Matthew Strehlow[1*], N. Ewen Wang[1], Elizabeth Pirrotta[1], Areeba Tariq[2], Naseeruddin Mahmood[3] and Swaminatha Mahadevan[1]

Abstract

Background: There is little data describing pediatric emergencies in resource-poor countries, such as Pakistan. We studied the demographics, management, and outcomes of patients presenting to the highest-volume, public, pediatric emergency department (ED) in Karachi, Pakistan.

Methods: In this prospective, observational study, we approached all patients presenting to the 50-bed ED during 28 12-h study periods over four consecutive weeks (July 2013). Participants' chief complaints and medical care were documented. Patients were followed-up at 48-h and 14-days via telephone.

Results: Of 3115 participants, 1846 were triaged to the outpatient department and 1269 to the ED. Patients triaged to the ED had a median age of 2.0 years (IQR 0.5–4.0); 30% were neonates (< 28 days). Top chief complaints were fever (45.5%), diarrhea/vomiting (32.3%), respiratory (23.1%), abdominal (7.5%), and otolaryngological problems (5.8%). Temperature, pulse and respiratory rate, and blood glucose were documented for 66, 42, and 1.5% of patients, respectively. Interventions included medications (92%), IV fluids (83%), oxygen (35%), and advanced airway management (5%). Forty-five percent of patients were admitted; 11 % left against medical advice. Outcome data was available at time of ED disposition, 48-h, and 14 days for 83, 62, and 54% of patients, respectively. Of participants followed-up, 4.3% died in the ED, 11.5% within 48 h, and 19.6% within 14 days.

Conclusions: This first epidemiological study at Pakistan's largest pediatric ED reveals dramatically high mortality, particularly among neonates. Future research in developing countries should focus on characterizing reasons for high mortality through pre-ED arrival tracking, ED care quality assessment, and post-ED follow-up.

Keywords: Global health, Pediatric emergency medicine, Epidemiology, Outcomes, Pakistan

Background

Pakistan is a resource-poor country in South Asia that has recently taken significant steps to improve its national healthcare delivery. Despite its efforts, Pakistan continues to perform poorly on many international health indicators, especially with regard to its pediatric population. In 2016, its neonatal, infant, and under-five mortality rates were 46, 64, and 79 per 1000 live births, respectively, giving Pakistan the world's highest neonatal mortality rate, as well as the 11th highest infant and 20th highest under-five mortality rates [1]. One contributor to high pediatric morbidity and mortality in Pakistan is the absence of an organized emergency care system, which could account for nearly half of deaths and one-third of disability-adjusted life years (DALYs) [2].

Recent work in Pakistan has identified serious issues which hinder access to quality emergency care, including overall dissatisfaction with emergency medical services, low staff confidence in their ability to handle emergencies, and a general shortage of essential equipment and supplies [3]. While improving access to quality emergency care is recognized internationally as an important step in reducing morbidity and mortality in low- and middle-income

* Correspondence: strehlow@stanford.edu
[1]Department of Emergency Medicine, Stanford University School of Medicine, 300 Pasteur Dr, Rm M121, Alway Building MC 5119, Stanford, CA 94305, USA
Full list of author information is available at the end of the article

countries (LMICs) [4], there is a dearth of data describing the epidemiology of patients seeking emergency care in Pakistan, particularly pediatric patients.

Characterization of patients seeking emergency care services is essential to determine a country's emergency care resource needs and develop a locally appropriate emergency healthcare system [5]. The 2013 Academic Emergency Medicine consensus conference, "Global Health and Emergency Care: A Research Agenda," highlighted the lack of published data on chief complaints as a critical gap in global emergency care research [6]. We seek to bridge this gap by describing the epidemiology and outcomes of children presenting to the emergency department of Pakistan's largest government children's hospital, the National Institute of Child Health (NICH).

Methods

Study design and setting

The study was conducted in the emergency department (ED) of a public, tertiary care, pediatric hospital in Karachi, Pakistan. The 500-bed hospital houses a 50-bed ED run as a public-private partnership between the hospital and the ChildLife Foundation (CLF), a local nonprofit organization focused on quality improvement in pediatric emergency care. The facility mainly serves the surrounding urban population, with a small percentage of patients coming from rural areas in the southern provinces of Sindh and Balochistan. While there are other private hospitals in the area, it remains the sole government healthcare facility that specializes in the delivery of pediatric care in Karachi, a city of 14.9 million people [7].

Selection of participants

All patients presenting to the ED waiting room for an unscheduled visit were approached for enrollment during 28 12-h study periods spanning four consecutive weeks: two weeks of daytime (8 AM-8 PM) enrollment followed by two weeks of nighttime (8 PM-8 AM) enrollment from July 1–28, 2013. Upwards of 90% of patients consented to participate. Patients with parents/guardians who did not speak Urdu (< 3%) were excluded due to lack of translation services.

Data collection and measurements

After obtaining verbal consent, trained research assistants collected demographic and clinical data using a standardized, secure, web-based survey form in Research Electronic Data Capture (REDCap). Paper questionnaires served as backups when necessary, and any data recorded on paper was later entered into REDCap using a double data entry procedure.

An ED nurse obtained chief complaint information and vital signs in the waiting room prior to triaging patients either to the outpatient department (OPD, a separate section of the ED open 24 h per day for urgent care) or to ED treatment areas. Patient gender, age, and up to three chief complaints were recorded for all patients. If a patient was triaged to the OPD, no further information was collected and initial vital signs were not recorded.

Clinical information was obtained from ED medical records and, for admitted patients, from inpatient records. Medical records were paper-based. Vital signs were documented as "unmeasured" if not recorded by the triage nurse or during initial ED evaluation. In situations where multiple modes of transportation were needed to reach the hospital, only the final mode of transportation was recorded. Patients were classified as underweight if their weight fell below the 3rd percentile using World Health Organization (WHO) weight-for-age standards.

Patients were followed-up by examination of discharge or admission records and by telephone at 24–72 h and 14 days following their initial ED visit. If medical records were not locatable at the end of their ED course, patients were deemed lost to follow up at time of ED disposition. Patients unable to provide contact phone numbers, those who provided invalid phone numbers, and those who were contacted twice without response were deemed lost to follow-up. Some patients unable to be reached at 24–72 h were successfully contacted at 14 days. Limited disposition information was gathered at 48-h and 14-day phone follow-up for patients for whom discharge records were unavailable, and this information was used to determine their ED disposition status.

Outcomes

Measured outcomes included mortality, hospital admission, and guardian-reported functional status relative to baseline at 48-h and 14-days after initial presentation to the hospital.

Primary data analysis

Categorical demographic and clinical characteristics were assessed with frequency tabulations and chi-squared tests; for age groups and sex, odds ratios were calculated through descriptive univariate logistic regression models. Summary statistics were calculated for continuous variables, and are presented as sample medians and interquartile ranges (IQR). Two descriptive multivariate logistic regression models were constructed with primary outcomes of admission and mortality using independent variables identified as significant with p-values of less than or equal to 0.2 through univariate analysis. Predictors in the multivariate logistic regression models with p-values of less than or equal to 0.05 was deemed significant. Models controlled for gender and date of ED arrival, and model fit was evaluated with the c-statistic. The admission model of patients ages >than 28 days used 87% of available records, c = 0.77. The 14-day mortality model used 85% of available records, c = 0.82. SAS Enterprise Guide software, Version 4.3, was used for statistical analysis.

Results

Comparison of OPD and ED patients

During the 28-day study period, 3115 patients were enrolled. Forty-one percent ($n = 1269$) of these patients were triaged to the ED; the remaining 1846 patients were directed to the OPD (Fig. 1). Enrolled patients ranged in age from 0 to 13 years, with a median age of 2.0 years (IQR 0.5–4.0). ED patients were significantly younger than OPD patients, with neonates and infants more likely to be triaged to the ED in comparison to children older than 5 years (Table 1).

ED patient presentation

Only 22.0% of patients arrived at the hospital by ambulance (including both pre-hospital care and transfers from other healthcare facilities). Median patient travel time was 30 min (Table 2). Almost two-thirds of patients (64.2%) had sought medical care for their current condition prior to their arrival in the ED, with 7.3% being transferred from another health care facility, predominantly by ambulance. An additional 38.9% of patients were referred or advised to come to the hospital by an outside provider (Table 2).

Documentation of patient vital signs by medical staff was inconsistent. Temperature was recorded in two-thirds of visits, with all other vital signs charted in less than half of patients. Blood pressure was seldom charted (0.8%). Respiratory rate was the most frequent abnormal vital sign, with a quarter of patients presenting with an abnormal value (Table 2).

ED patient chief complaints

For all enrolled ED pediatric patients, the most common chief complaints (not mutually exclusive) were fever (45.5%), diarrhea/vomiting (32.3%), and respiratory problems (23.1%). For neonates, top chief complaints were respiratory problems (30.5%), perinatal complaints defined as complications at birth or referral by birth attendant (28.9%), and fever (16.2%). For patients ≥28 days, the top three complaints aligned with those for all patients: fever (50.5%), diarrhea/vomiting (35.7%), and respiratory problems (22.0%) (Fig. 2).

ED therapeutic or procedural interventions

Nearly all patients (92.2%) received medications during their visit. Antibiotics, nebulized medications, and antipyretics (including acetaminophen and non-steroidal anti-inflammatory drugs) were the most common medication types, prescribed to 43.3, 10.9, and 10.7% of patients, respectively. All other medication types (e.g. other analgesic, antimalarial) were prescribed to less than 10% of patients. The second most common intervention was intravenous (IV) access with IV hydration, which was utilized in 82.7% of patients. More than one-third of patients (35.4%) received some form of supplemental oxygen, with 4.6% of patients receiving an advanced airway intervention. Nasogastric tubes were placed in 10.3% of patients.

ED patient disposition and outcomes

Of the 1269 patients triaged to the ED, 1053 (83.0%) patients were followed-up at the time of ED disposition (Table 3). Of those patients followed up, 44.7% were admitted to either the hospital ward or ICU, 24.7% were discharged to home, 10.9% left against medical advice, and 13.9% did not have a recorded reason for leaving. Of

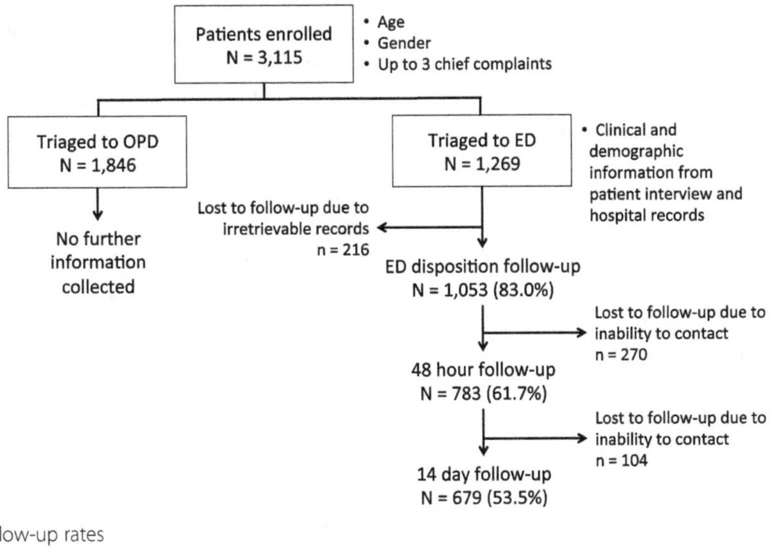

Fig. 1 Study design and follow-up rates

Table 1 Demographics of OPD and ED visits

	All visits, *N* (%)	ED visits, *N* (%)	OPD visits, *N* (%)	Odds ratio[a]
No. of visits	3115	1269 (40.7)	1846 (59.3)	–
Age, yrs., median (IQR)	2.0 (0.50–4.0)	0.83 (0.03–3.0)	2.0 (0.92–5.0)	0.90 (0.88–0.93)
Neonate (<28d)	439 (14.1)	378 (29.8)	61 (3.3)	12.7 (9.3–17.4)
Infant (28d- < 1 yr)	672 (21.6)	271 (21.4)	401 (21.7)	1.4 (1.1–1.7)
Young child (1-3 yrs)	778 (25.0)	245 (19.3)	533 (28.9)	0.9 (0.8–1.2)
Child (3-5 yrs)	470 (15.1)	123 (9.7)	347 (18.8)	0.7 (0.6–0.9)
Older child (> 5 yrs)	746 (24.0)	244 (19.3)	502 (27.2)	Reference
Sex				
Female	1303 (41.8)	514 (40.5)	789 (42.7)	Reference
Male	1808 (58.0)	754 (59.4)	1054 (57.1)	1.1 (0.9–1.3)

[a]Odds ratios compare likelihood of patient triage to ED instead of OPD using indicated reference groups

the 349 patients admitted from the ED whose hospital location was recorded, 16.3% had an ED arrival to disposition time of at least 6 h and 21.1% spent the night in the ED, defined as arriving before 12 AM and time of disposition after 7 AM. We created a multivariate model to identify predictors of admission; significance was only achieved with children older than 1 year. In this sub-analysis admission model, abnormal level of consciousness by AVPU, respiratory complaint, prior care, and care during Ramadan were associated with higher likelihood of admission, while age younger than 6 was associated with lower likelihood of admission (Additional file 1: Table S1).

Follow-up rates were 61.7% at 48 h and 53.5% at 14 days; 19.0% of ED patients lacked telephone access. Almost two-thirds of followed patients reported a return to normal functional level at 14 days (Table 3). Forty-five patients died while in the ED, comprising 4.3% of the 1053 patients followed-up at the time of ED disposition (Table 3). At the 48-h follow-up, 45 more patients had died for an overall 48-h mortality rate of 11.5%. An additional 43 patients died by 14 days for a cumulative mortality rate of 19.6%. Of patients who left against medical advice, 12.2% died within 14 days. Of patients who were discharged or left the ED and subsequently died, 60% returned to care before death. Of deaths that occurred within 48 h after ED disposition, 13% occurred at home; within 14 days, 31% occurred at home. Neonates were more likely to be admitted, leave against medical advice, and die as compared to their older counterparts. A multivariate model for predictors of cumulative mortality at 14 days identified neonate status, abnormal AVPU, respiratory complaint, underweight for age, ambulance arrival, and prior care as being associated with higher likelihood of mortality; fever complaint and care during Ramadan were protective (Additional file 2: Table S2).

Discussion

This report is the first in-depth investigation of the epidemiology of patients presenting to a pediatric emergency department in Pakistan and one of only a handful of such studies conducted to-date in developing countries [8–11]. Prior studies in Pakistan have focused primarily on the epidemiology of pediatric traumatic injuries, which account for only 3.7% of patients in our study [12]. We sought to characterize the population of all pediatric patients seeking acute care in Pakistan and found a high burden of infant visits and an alarming cumulative 14-day mortality rate, which was particularly high among neonates.

In comparison to urban pediatric emergency departments in other LMICs, our overall reported pediatric mortality rate (19.6%) was exceedingly high, with a full one-third (33.3%) of neonates having died within 14-days of their ED visit. In comparison, an Indian study reported a substantially lower in-hospital mortality rate of 12.2%, although this number does not include patients who were sent home from the ED. [13] In our study, 4.3% of children died while in the ED, a similar rate to that published in a separate study (5.7%) of Indian children between 1995 and 2000 [8]. Dramatically lower ED mortality rates have been reported in Egypt (0.9%) and Turkey (2.6%), an unexpected contrast given their similar resource and training limitations [9, 14]. Pakistan's high death rates also stand in sharp contrast to the numbers reported from countries with developed emergency care infrastructures. Studies in the United States demonstrate few deaths in the ED, with a < 0.1% mortality rate among pediatric patients [15]. To our knowledge, there are no other studies that track all patients following ED discharge to assess for delayed mortality. As the majority of deaths in our study occurred after the patient left the ED (a post-ED mortality rate of 15.3%, accounting for 66% of deaths), our study highlights a need to monitor the progression of patients following ED disposition.

Table 2 ED patient characteristics

Characteristic	No. ED visits (%)[a] (*N* = 1269)
Travel to hospital	
Mode of transport	
Taxi/rickshaw	421 (33.2)
Ambulance	279 (22.0)
Motorbike	190 (15.0)
Bus	127 (10.0)
Other[b]	114 (9.0)
Travel time, median (IQR), min	30 (20–60)
Illness timeline	
Symptom duration (before ED visit)	
Sudden (< 24 h)	481 (37.9)
Recent (1–3 days)	340 (26.8)
Subacute (4–14 days)	245 (19.3)
Chronic (> 2 weeks)	96 (7.6)
Time before seeking any medical care[c]	
< 24 h	381 (30.0)
≥ 24 h	274 (21.6)
Time of ED presentation (HH:MM)	
00:00–05:59	193 (15.2)
06:00–11:59	339 (26.7)
12:00–17:59	442 (34.8)
18:00–23:59	295 (23.3)
Prior Care	
No prior care	331 (26.1)
Referral from another provider	494 (38.9)
Returning to same hospital	123 (9.7)
Direct transfer from another provider	92 (7.3)
Vital signs[d]	
Prior care without referral	105 (8.3)
Abnormal (≤36 °C or ≥ 38 °C)	105 (8.3)
Unmeasured	430 (33.9)
Pulse	
Abnormal[e]	153 (12.1)
Unmeasured	727 (57.3)
Respiratory rate	
Abnormal[e]	327 (25.8)
Unmeasured	736 (58.0)
Blood pressure	
Abnormal[f]	Not calculated
Unmeasured	1259 (99.2)
Pain present	380 (30.0)
Prior health status	
Underweight[g]	421 (33.2)
Neonates, *n* = 378	
Preterm[h]	85 (22.5)
Low birth weight[i]	97 (25.7)
Age ≥ 28 days, *n* = 883	
No vaccinations	91 (10.3)

[a]Not all categories sum to 100% as some values are missing
[b]Other modes of transport included private car, bicycle, and walking
[c]Time lapse between onset of illness/injury episode and visit to first healthcare provider
[d]"Unmeasured" vitals were either not measured or not recorded by ED staff
[e]Abnormal pulse and respiratory rate were classified based on patient age
[f]Blood pressure was measured in too few patients (*n* = 10) to draw clinical conclusions
[g]Defined as <3rd percentile on WHO weight-for-age curves
[h]Defined as > 37 weeks gestational age, as reported by parent/guardian
[i]Defined as weight < 2500 g at birth, as reported by parent/guardian

Many factors likely contribute to the exceedingly high mortality rate we observed. First and foremost, delays in care seeking likely exacerbated delays in reaching the appropriate healthcare facility. One study of Pakistani households reported that less than half of family members with emergency medical conditions were taken to the nearest primary care facility for treatment [16]. In our study, almost two-thirds of our patients were seen by outside health care providers prior to their arrival in the ED, but only a quarter (22.0%) were transferred by ambulance from that initial medical facility. Most patients travelled to the ED via public or private vehicle, therefore benefiting from neither the speed nor the en route emergency medical treatment that ambulance transport provides. Our results, therefore, complement the findings of a prior study that described prolonged travel times to the appropriate health care facility as an important contributor to pediatric deaths in Karachi [17].

Most of our study deaths occurred following ED evaluation and disposition, suggesting the failure of ED medical staff to recognize illness severity and promptly initiate life-saving therapy [18]. One study in northern Pakistan found that misinterpretation of symptom severity by the initial providers and mis-triage at the initial medical facility led to poor outcomes in many cases of surgically treatable illnesses [19]. Despite vital signs being important markers of illness acuity and reliable predictors of death in emergency settings [20], initial vital signs were not reliably documented or reported at our study hospital. Obtaining a complete set of vital signs and implementing effective ED triage have been shown to reduce mortality in resource-poor settings [21]. Our results suggest that improved training for Pakistani medical staff on the importance of taking and documenting vital signs may lead to the proper identification of the most severely ill patients, thus reducing overall mortality.

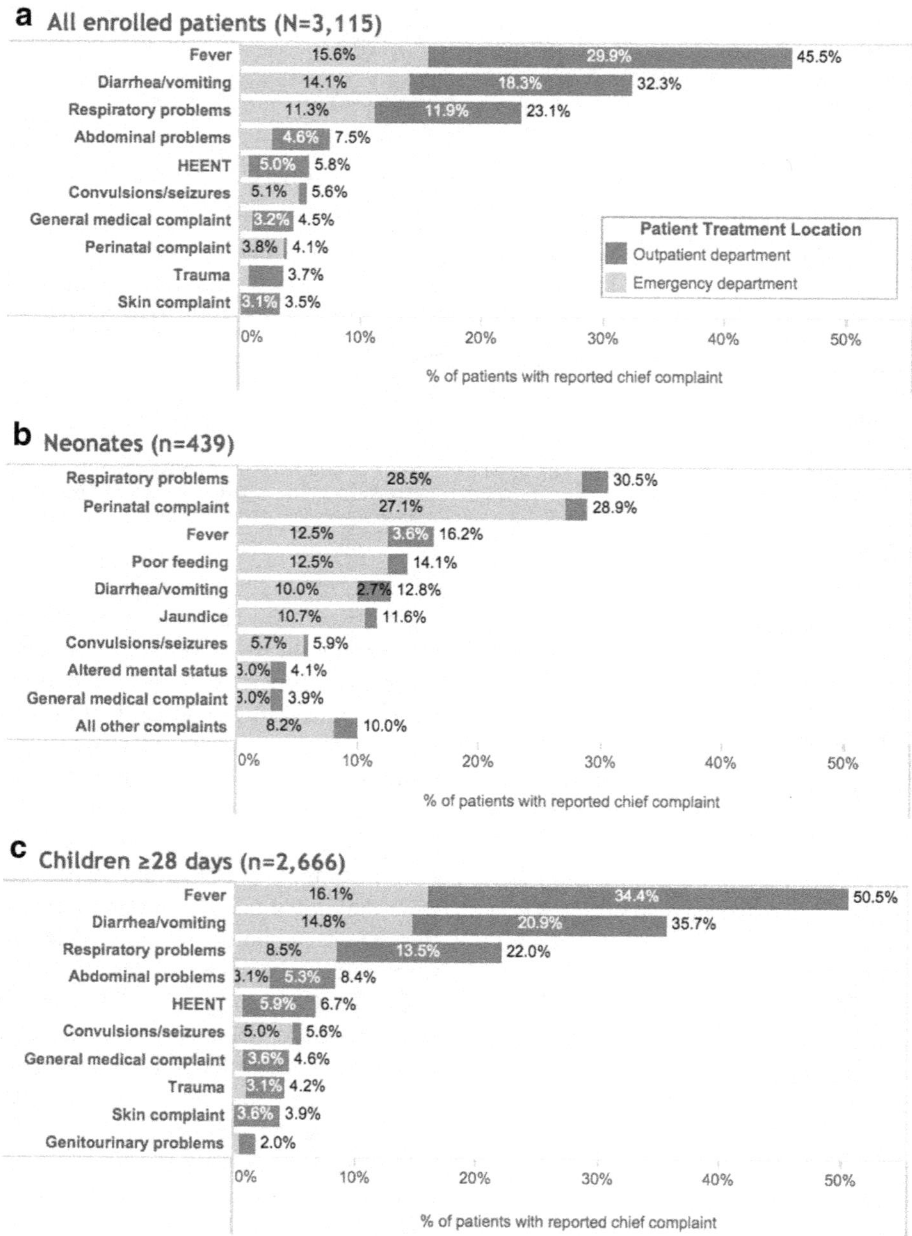

Fig. 2 Common chief complaints by location of treatment for (**a**) all enrolled patients ($N = 3115$), (**b**) neonates ($n = 439$), and (**c**) patients ≥28 days ($n = 2666$)

The observed elevated mortality rates are also likely impacted by both a lack of essential equipment and inadequate physician education regarding its use when available [22, 23]. Research has identified significant gaps in the availability of essential emergency equipment and medications, as well as the knowledge necessary for Pakistani physicians to use these resources effectively in relevant settings [22]. Remarkably, much of the frequently unavailable equipment, such as suction catheters and pediatric-sized blood pressure cuffs, consists of relatively inexpensive items capable of saving lives in emergency scenarios.

Finally, a significant percentage (10.9%) of patients left against medical advice (AMA). As one-eighth (12.2%) of these children died within 14 days of their initial presentation, clearly leaving AMA was a significant contributor to our high mortality rates. This behavior has previously been identified as a common problem in Karachi hospitals [24]. Many parents and guardians cited delays in care and inadequate communication from hospital staff about the ED process as reasons for leaving the hospital prematurely. It has been shown that leaving AMA is associated with higher mortality and readmission rates [25]. Therefore, improving patient-provider communication and the

Table 3 Patient disposition and outcomes at 48 h and 14 days with comparison of neonates and children ≥28 days

Disposition and Outcomes[a]	All ED visits N (%)	Neonatal visits N (%)	Children ≥ 28 days N (%)	Odds ratio (comparing neonates vs. children ≥ 28 days)
No. of total ED visits	1269	378	883	
ED Disposition				
Followed up at time of ED disposition[b]	1053 (83.0)	333 (88.1)	714 (80.9)	–
Admitted	471 (44.7)	194 (58.3)	272 (38.1)	3.5 (2.4–5.1)
Home	528 (50.1)	111 (33.3)	416 (58.3)	
Left against medical advice	115 (10.9)	51 (15.3)	64 (9.0)	3.9 (2.4–6.4)
Left before seen by provider	7 (0.7)	3 (0.9)	4 (0.6)	3.7 (0.8–17.0)
Discharged home by provider	260 (24.7)	44 (13.2)	215 (51.7)	Reference
Unknown reason for leaving	146 (13.9)	13 (3.9)	133 (18.6)	0.5 (0.2–0.9)
Transferred out	4 (0.4)	1 (0.4)	3 (0.4)	1.6 (0.2–16.0)
Died in ED	45 (4.3)	26 (7.8)	19 (2.7)	6.7 (3.4–13.1)
48-h follow-up				
Followed up at 48 hours[b]	783 (61.7)	252 (66.7)	526 (59.6)	–
Returned to normal function[c]	277 (35.4)	70 (27.8)	206 (39.2)	0.8 (0.5–1.1)
Still in original hospital	197 (25.2)	76 (30.2)	119 (22.6)	2.4 (1.6–3.5)
Returned to care[d]	167 (21.3)	43 (17.1)	123 (23.4)	1.1 (0.7–1.8)
Surgery by 48 h	20 (2.6)	5 (2.0)	15 (2.9)	0.8 (0.3–2.2)
Cumulative deaths by 48 h	90 (11.5)	48 (19.0)	41 (7.8)	2.8 (1.8–4.4)
14-day follow-up				
Followed up at 14 days[b]	679 (53.5)	225 (59.5)	450 (51.0)	–
Returned to normal function[c]	420 (61.9)	115 (51.1)	303 (67.3)	1.0 (0.6–1.5)
Still in original hospital	37 (5.4)	11 (4.9)	25 (5.6)	1.2 (0.6–2.4)
Returned to care[d]	257 (37.8)	80 (35.6)	177 (39.3)	1.1 (0.8–1.6)
Surgeries, 48 hours - 14 days	18 (2.7)	4 (1.8)	14 (3.1)	0.6 (0.2–2.2)
Cumulative deaths by 14 days	133 (19.6)	75 (33.3)	57 (12.7)	3.4 (2.3–5.1)

[a]Not all categories sum to 100% as some values are missing
[b]For these rows, percentages are out of the number of total ED visits
[c]"Return to normal function" is guardian's perception of recovery relative to child's baseline
[d]"Return to care" is guardian's report of returning to medical care after leaving hospital

hospital efficiency should be further studied as these factors may be contributing to families leaving AMA.

The most common chief complaints (fever, diarrhea/vomiting, and respiratory problems) reported during our study were similar, but varied in frequency, to those previously reported in other developing countries [8–11]. Respiratory (23.4%) and gastrointestinal illness (23.3%) accounted for almost half of visits to a pediatric ED in India [8]. In Egypt and Tunisia, respiratory complaints accounted for 41.7 and 39.9% of visits, respectively [9, 10]. Respiratory complaints may have been lower in our study because our data was collected during the summer months, when such illness tend to diminish. While injuries were the most common complaint for pediatric ED patients in a Malaysian study, fever (24%), breathing difficulties (16.6%), and diarrhea/vomiting (9.7%) were the next most frequent presentations [11]. The observed trend of similar chief complaints among LMICs in connection with high mortality rates suggests that focusing on these specific chief complaints in developing provider training materials and patient management protocols may be effective in reducing mortality. A recent WHO study also reports that the majority ED providers in LMICs have no specialty training in emergency medicine [26]. Additional study exploring the training local providers receive on managing chief complaints associated with high mortality would be of further benefit.

Our study documents a staggeringly high mortality rate at Pakistan's largest children's emergency department. Addressing this mortality rate, which even significantly exceeds other comparable resource-limited countries, is crucial for Pakistan to achieve its goal of improving its national healthcare delivery. Focusing training on the most common regional chief complaints may ultimately improve patient management and outcomes. Additional studies are needed to further characterize which factors – delays in seeking and accessing care, inadequate triage, gaps in physician education, lack of necessary equipment, or others – are the greatest contributors to the high mortality observed at our study site. Likewise, investigating the quality of care patients received and the appropriateness of discharge in patients who were not admitted is vital to decreasing morbidity and mortality at the National Institute of Child Health in Karachi and other similar hospitals.

Limitations

While this is the first, large-scale pediatric emergency medicine epidemiological study in Pakistan, we had relatively low 48-h and 14-day follow-up rates, largely due to poor medical record-keeping and patients' lack of phone access. Secondly, three out of four weeks of data collection occurred during the religious month of Ramadan. As a result, follow-up data collection was challenging during the hours (8–9:30 PM) when fasting had concluded for the day. Additionally, it is possible that we captured some trends unique to the month of Ramadan that are different from the remainder of the year. It is unclear what effect Ramadan would have on our data.

Conclusions

This first investigation of pediatric emergency epidemiology in Pakistan has provided a broader understanding of the most common presentations and resulting outcomes. Our study's findings can be used to inform quality improvement and policy changes in ED management, create guidelines and needs-based training materials for local healthcare providers, and serve as a baseline for measurement of future trends in health outcomes. Future work should focus on identifying high-risk patients earlier in their clinical course by improving triage, training staff to increase their competency in managing the most common chief complaints, especially neonatal complaints, improving local prenatal and neonatal care, and assessing the impact of such interventions on morbidity and mortality. Much of the knowledge gained from this study will have applicability and value to other developing nations facing similar challenges.

Abbreviations

AMA: Against medical advice; CLF: ChildLife Foundation, Pakistan; DALY: Disability-adjusted life year; ED: Emergency department; HEENT: Head, eyes, ears, nose, and throat; IV: Intravenous; LMICs: Low and middle-income countries; NICH: National Institute of Child Health, Karachi, Pakistan; OPD: Outpatient department; REDCap: Research Electronic Data Capture; WHO: World Health Organization

Acknowledgements

Authors are grateful for the contributions of the staff at the National Institute of Child Health in Karachi (M. Gowa), the ChildLife Foundation (I. Adamjee) for its technical and logistical support, research assistants (O. Adil, A. Baig, A. Khan, P. Kumar, and F. Shah) for their help in data collection, and A. Tecklenburg Strehlow for assistance reviewing and revising the manuscript.

Funding

This study was funded by the ChildLife Foundation in Karachi, Pakistan. Funding for electronic data capture via REDCap was provided by Stanford Center for Clinical Informatics (Stanford CTSA award number UL1 RR025744 from NIH/NCRR). Additional funding was provided by the Stanford Medical Scholars Program.

Authors' contributions

NI contributed to study conception and design; data collection, analysis, and interpretation; and manuscript preparation. He approved the final manuscript. MS contributed to study conception and design; data analysis and interpretation; and manuscript review. He approved the final manuscript. NEW contributed to study conception and design; data analysis and interpretation; and manuscript review. She approved the final manuscript. EP contributed to study conception and design; data analysis and interpretation; manuscript review; and preparation of figures and tables. She approved the final manuscript. AT contributed to study design, data collection and interpretation, and manuscript review. She approved the final manuscript. NM contributed to study conception and design, data interpretation, and manuscript review. He approved the final manuscript. SM contributed to study conception and design; data analysis and interpretation; and manuscript review. He approved the final manuscript.

Competing interests

The authors declare that they have no competing interests.

Author details

[1]Department of Emergency Medicine, Stanford University School of Medicine, 300 Pasteur Dr, Rm M121, Alway Building MC 5119, Stanford, CA 94305, USA. [2]Honors Program in Medical Education, Northwestern University, Evanston, IL, USA. [3]Department of Paediatrics and Child Health, Aga Khan University, Karachi, Pakistan.

References

1. UNICEF. Pakistan: Statistics. https://data.unicef.org/country/pak/. Published 2016. Accessed 30 June 2018.
2. Kobusingye OC, Hyder AA, Bishai D, Joshipura M, Hicks ER, Mock C. Emergency Medical Services: The International Bank for Reconstruction and Development/The World Bank; 2006. http://www.ncbi.nlm.nih.gov/pubmed/21250323. Accessed 19 June 2017
3. Razzak JA, Hyder AA, Akhtar T, Khan M, Khan UR. Assessing emergency medical care in low income countries: a pilot study from Pakistan. BMC Emerg Med. 2008; https://doi.org/10.1186/1471-227X-8-8.
4. Anderson PD, Suter RE, Mulligan T, et al. World Health Assembly Resolution 60.22 and its importance as a health care policy tool for improving emergency care access and availability globally. Ann Emerg Med. 2012; https://doi.org/10.1016/j.annemergmed.2011.10.018.
5. Begier EM, Sockwell D, Branch LM, et al. The national capitol region's emergency department syndromic surveillance system: do chief complaint and discharge diagnosis yield different results? Emerg Infect Dis. 2003; https://doi.org/10.3201/eid0903.020363
6. Mowafi H, Dworkis D, Bisanzo M, et al. Making recording and analysis of chief complaint a priority for global emergency care research in low-income countries. Cone DC, ed. Acad Emerg Med. 2013; doi:https://doi.org/10.1111/acem.12262.
7. Pakistan Bureau of Statistics, Government of Pakistan. Population Census 2017. Published 2017. http://www.pbscensus.gov.pk. Accessed 30 June 2018.

8. Singhi S, Jain V, Gupta G. Pediatric emergencies at a tertiary care hospital in India. J Trop Pediatr. 2003;49(4):207–11.
9. Bazaraa HM, El Houchi S, Rady HI. Profile of patients visiting the pediatric emergency service in an Egyptian university hospital. Pediatr Emerg Care. 2012; https://doi.org/10.1097/PEC.0b013e3182442eeb.
10. Matoussi N, Fitouri Z, Maaroufi N, Berriche I, Ben BS. Epidemiologic profile and management of pediatric medical emergencies at a Tunisian children's hospital. Tunis Med. 2007;85(10):843–8.
11. Goh AY, Chan TL, Abdel-Latiff ME. Paediatric utilization of a general emergency department in a developing country. Acta Paediatr. 2003;92(8): 965–9.
12. Razzak J, Luby S, Laflamme L, Chotani H. Injuries among children in Karachi, Pakistan—what, where and how. Public Health. 2004; https://doi.org/10.1016/S0033-3506(03)00147-1.
13. Santhanam I, Pai M, Kasturi K, Radhamani MP. Mortality after admission in the pediatric emergency department: a prospective study from a referral children's hospital in southern India. Pediatr Crit Care Med. 2002; https://doi.org/10.1097/01.PCC.0000031466.62825.5E.
14. Karaböcüoğlu M, Kartoğlu U, Molzan J, Uğur S, Uzel N, Neyzi O. Analysis of patients admitted to the emergency unit of a university children's hospital in Turkey. Turk J Pediatr. 1995;37(3):209–16.
15. Center for Health Statistics N. National Hospital Ambulatory Medical Care Survey: 2011 Emergency department summary tables. Centers for Disease Control and Prevention. https://www.cdc.gov/nchs/data/ahcd/nhamcs_emergency/2011_ed_web_tables.pdf. Accessed 19 June 2017.
16. Siddiqi S, Kielmann A, Khan M, et al. The effectiveness of patient referral in Pakistan. Health Policy Plan. 2001;16(2):193–8.
17. Hasan IJ, Khanum A. Health care utilization during terminal child illness in squatter settlements of Karachi. J Pak Med Assoc. 2000;50(12):405–9.
18. Han YY, Carcillo JA, Dragotta MA, et al. Early reversal of pediatric-neonatal septic shock by community physicians is associated with improved outcome. Pediatrics. 2003;112(4):793–9.
19. Ahmed M, Shah M, Luby S, Drago-Johnson P, Wali S. Survey of surgical emergencies in a rural population in the northern areas of Pakistan. Tropical Med Int Health. 1999;4(12):846–57.
20. Olson D, Davis NL, Milazi R, et al. Development of a severity of illness scoring system (inpatient triage, assessment and treatment) for resource-constrained hospitals in developing countries. Trop Med Int Heal. 2013; https://doi.org/10.1111/tmi.12137.
21. Molyneux E, Ahmad S, Robertson A. Improved triage and emergency care for children reduces inpatient mortality in a resource-constrained setting. Bull World Health Organ. 2006; doi:/S0042–96862006000400016.
22. Razzak JA, Baqir SM, Khan UR, Heller D, Bhatti J, Hyder AA. Emergency and trauma care in Pakistan: a cross-sectional study of healthcare levels. Emerg Med J. 2015; https://doi.org/10.1136/emermed-2013-202590.
23. Razzak JA, Ahmed A, Saleem AF, Nasrullah M. Perceived need for emergency medicine training in Pakistan: a survey of medical education leadership. Emerg Med Australas. 2009; https://doi.org/10.1111/j.1742-6723.2008.01139.x.
24. Fayyaz J, Khursheed M, Mir MU, Mehmood A. Missing the boat: odds for the patients who leave ED without being seen. BMC Emerg Med. 2013; https://doi.org/10.1186/1471-227X-13-1.
25. Southern WN, Nahvi S, Arnsten JH. Increased risk of mortality and readmission among patients discharged against medical advice. Am J Med. 2012; https://doi.org/10.1016/j.amjmed.2011.12.017.
26. Obermeyer Z, Abujaber S, Makar M, Stoll S, Kayden SR, Wallis LA, Reynolds TA. Emergency care in 59 low-and middle-income countries: a systematic review. Bull World Health Organ. 2015;93:577–86.

31

Socioeconomic gradients in admission to coronary or intensive care units among Australians presenting with non-traumatic chest pain in emergency departments

George Mnatzaganian[1*], Janet E Hiller[2,3], Jason Fletcher[4], Mark Putland[5], Cameron Knott[4,6,7], George Braitberg[5,8], Steve Begg[1] and Melanie Bish[1]

Abstract

Background: Socioeconomic inequalities in cardiovascular morbidity have been previously reported showing direct associations between socioeconomic disadvantage and worse health outcomes. However, disagreement remains regarding the strength of the direct associations. The main objective of this panel design was to inspect socioeconomic gradients in admission to a coronary care unit (CCU) or an intensive care unit (ICU) among adult patients presenting with non-traumatic chest pain in three acute-care public hospitals in Victoria, Australia, during 2009–2013.

Methods: Consecutive adults aged 18 or over presenting with chest pain in three emergency departments (ED) in Victoria, Australia during the five-year study period were eligible to participate. A relative index of inequality of socioeconomic status (SES) was estimated based on residential postcode socioeconomic index for areas (SEIFA) disadvantage scores. Admission to specialised care units over repeated presentations was modelled using a multivariable Generalized Estimating Equations approach that accounted for various socio-demographic and clinical variables.

Results: Non-traumatic chest pain accounted for 10% of all presentations in the emergency departments (ED). A total of 53,177 individuals presented during the study period, with 22.5% presenting more than once. Of all patients, 17,579 (33.1%) were hospitalised over time, of whom 8584 (48.8%) were treated in a specialised care unit. Female sex was independently associated with fewer admissions to CCU / ICU, whereas, a dose-response effect of socioeconomic disadvantage and admission to CCU / ICU was found, with risk of admission increasing incrementally as SES declined. Patients coming from the lowest SES locations were 27% more likely to be admitted to these units compared with those coming from the least disadvantaged locations, $p < 0.001$. Men were significantly more likely to be admitted to such units than similarly affected and aged women among those diagnosed with angina pectoris, arrhythmia, myocardial infarction, heart failure, chest pain, and general signs and symptoms.

Conclusions: This study is the first to report socioeconomic gradients in admission to CCU / ICU in patients presenting with chest pain showing a dose-response effect. Our findings suggest increased cardiovascular morbidity as socioeconomic disadvantage increases.

Keywords: Chest pain, Cardiovascular morbidity, Emergency department, Intensive care, Socioeconomic gradients

* Correspondence: G.Mnatzaganian@latrobe.edu.au
[1]La Trobe Rural Health School, College of Science, Health and Engineering, La Trobe University, PO Box 199, Bendigo, VIC 3552, Australia
Full list of author information is available at the end of the article

Background

Socioeconomic inequalities in cardiovascular morbidity and mortality have been reported in many regions including the US [1], the UK [2], Australia [3] and other Organisation for Economic Cooperation and Development (OECD) countries [4]. Cardiovascular morbidity measures such as admission rates for cardiac related conditions have generally dropped over the past two decades [5]. However, relative inequality in cardiovascular emergency admissions and cardiovascular related mortality actually increased in the most disadvantaged compared with the least disadvantaged [6]. These disparities have been attributed to a range of socioeconomic determinants of health and health behaviours, rooted in social rank as determined by education, occupational hierarchy and income [1, 4, 7, 8]. The relationship between socioeconomic status and general health, and, in particular, cardiovascular health, has been demonstrated within different races and ethnic groups [9], suggesting that cultural and ethnic dissimilarities do not explain the socioeconomic differences. These associations were also observed in countries with universal access to health care [2, 3], and when comparing those who have similar rates of smoking, obesity and alcohol use [9].

Despite the mounting evidence of direct associations between socioeconomic disadvantage and poorer health outcomes, disagreement remains regarding the strength of the evidence to support causality [10–14] with reverse causation proposed as a contributor to the relationship. For example, illness may lead to lower academic achievement or loss in income [10]. Studies investigating these relationships have predominantly followed a cross-sectional design and have not been population-based limiting their generalisability [13]. Furthermore, no study found dose-response associations between lower SES and increased cardiovascular morbidity.

Chest pain is a frequently seen symptom in emergency departments, being the most common reason for presenting in the ED among Americans over the age of 65 and contributing to approximately 6 million visits per annum under the US Medicare system [15]. Clinical management of chest pain is highly variable, often depending on the underlying causes and is considered a medical emergency until all life-threatening causes have been ruled out. Potentially life-threatening causes of chest pain include acute myocardial infarction and other acute coronary syndromes as well as aortic dissection, pneumothorax, pneumonia and pulmonary embolism. Patients presenting with chest pain who require critical care are often more likely to be severely ill and / or are at risk of imminent death [16, 17]. This study used emergency admissions following repeated non-traumatic chest pain presentations to emergency departments (ED) to explore the associations between sex, age, geographic-based socioeconomic disadvantage score and cardiovascular morbidity, expressed as admission to specialised care units.

Methods

Study population

Consecutive adults aged 18 or over presenting with chest pain (including chest heaviness, heart pain, and chest tightness) in three emergency departments in Victoria, Australia during January 2009 and December 2013 were eligible to participate in this population-based panel study. Cases were identified using the International Classification of Diseases, 10th Revision, (Australian Modification) (ICD-10-AM) code of R07. Patients presenting with chest pain due to trauma or other injury were excluded from this analysis.

All three hospitals serve different catchment populations in metropolitan Melbourne, Australia, with a combined total of more than 200,000 ED presentations per annum [18]. The hospitals differ by their bed capacity, with Hospital A being the smallest and Hospital C the largest.

Study variables

Sociodemographic and presentation-related variables together with clinical variables were collected from the ED electronic database (SYMPHONY Version 2.29). The collected information included age, sex, country of origin, residential postcode, main language spoken at home, arrival mode, arrival time, presenting symptoms, a registered nurse-allocated triage urgency score that categorised the presentation as being an emergency (triage scores of 1 or 2), urgent (triage score of 3) or semi and non-urgent (triage scores of 4 or 5) and length of stay in the ED. The final main acute diagnosis reached on discharge from the ED was also collected together with the discharge destination. Among admitted patients, three possible admission departments were recorded: CCU, ICU and medical ward. The medical ward was used to categorise all adult hospital departments that did not have intensive specialised care. The admitting ward of patients transferred to another public or private hospital was also recorded and accounted for in this analysis. All diagnoses were identified using ICD-10-AM codes.

Each individual's residential postcode was merged with the Australian Bureau of Statistics to obtain the Socio Economic Index For Areas (SEIFA) [19], estimated from the 2011 census data. SEIFA is a composite index of relative advantage or disadvantage based on geographic areas across Australia, with higher scores indicating less socioeconomic disadvantage. The SEIFA was further used to calculate a Relative Index of Inequality (RII) which is a regression-derived index summarising the magnitude of socioeconomic disadvantage while taking into account the sample size and the relative disadvantage experienced by each individual [20]. The estimated RII was further introduced as quintiles categorised according to the score's distribution in the sample.

Statistical analysis

Patient characteristics were compared by study categorical variables using Pearson Chi-square while ANOVA tests compared the means. The multivariable analyses were conducted on the first presentation [Model 1] (irrespective of study outcome) and on all repeated presentations [Model 2] during the study five-year period. A logistic regression was used to model admission to these units on the first presentation. The dose-response effect of different levels of relative index of socioeconomic inequality on admission to specialised care was tested using log likelihood ratio tests which evaluated linear trends. An insignificant p value of the log likelihood test indicated linearity.

Admission to CCU or ICU over the five-year study period was analysed using the Generalized Estimating Equations (GEE) approach [21]. An exchangeable working covariance matrix was used to account for correlation and dependence between repeated measurements on the same individual over time while accounting for: age, sex, relative index of socioeconomic inequality, country of origin, main language spoken at home, ambulance arrival mode, arrival time, presenting symptoms, nurse allocated triage urgency score, treating hospital, length of stay in the ED, and main diagnosis on discharge from the ED.

In a sub analysis, the multivariable regression was further run on only patients who were admitted to hospital. Stata statistical program (version 15, StataCorp, College Station, TX, USA) was used to conduct the analyses.

Results

Descriptive

During the study's five-year period, a total of 82,859 chest pain presentations were recorded, for a total of 54,138 individuals, being approximately 10% of all presentations in the EDs of the three hospitals combined. Of these, 961 (1.8%) were excluded because of missing information on residential postcode (Fig. 1). Of the remaining 53,177 individuals, 77.5% presented once, 14.2% presented twice, and 8.3% presented three or more times. Hospital admission rates significantly rose with increased number of presentations ($p < 0.001$); admission to a CCU or ICU similarly rose with increased presentations ($p < 0.001$) (Fig. 1). The geographic-based socioeconomic groups considerably differed on age, country of birth, spoken language at home, and presentation characteristics (Table 1). Patients coming from low SES locations tended to repeatedly present with chest pain during the five-year study period ($p < 0.001$) (Table 2). Such patients also tended to receive lower urgency triage scores on arrival to the ED. However, except for those coming from the least disadvantaged locations, crude admission rates to CCU or ICU were similar in all other sub-groups (Table 1), with no evidence for trend observed.

Of the 53,177 presenting individuals, 17,579 (33.1%) were hospitalised over time, of whom 8584 (48.8%) received specialised care. Compared to men, presenting women were more likely to be discharged home, and those admitted were less likely to be treated in a specialised care unit. Sex differences were mainly observed

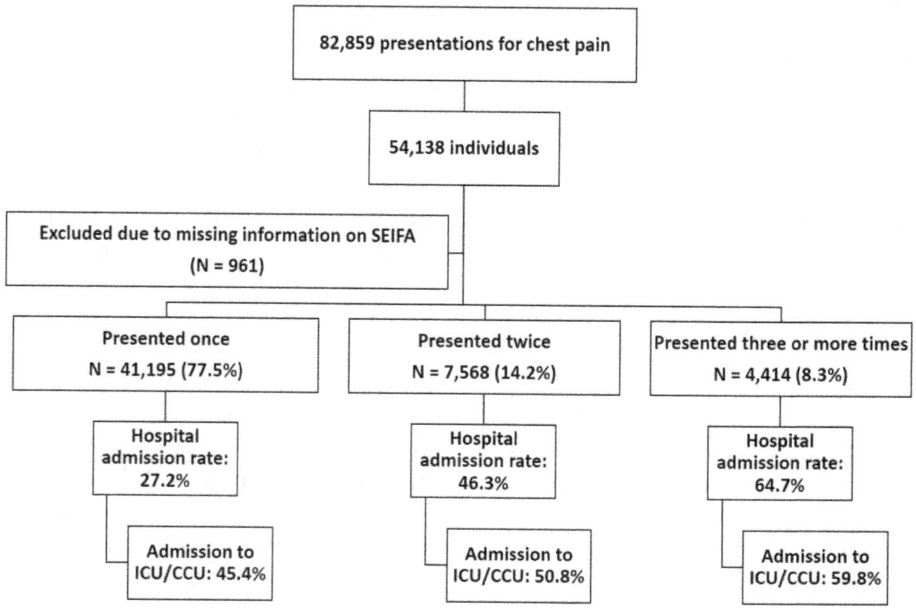

Fig. 1 Flow chart of study participants

Table 1 Patient characteristics and emergency department visit outcome on first presentation by quintiles of the relative index of inequality of socioeconomic disadvantage

	All *N* = 53,177	RII_1 Highest SES *N* = 10,815	RII_2 N = 10,666	RII_3 N = 10,994	RII_4 N = 10,831	RII_5 Lowest SES *N* = 9871	*P* value^
Median age of study sample,%							
53 years or younger	50.4	49.3	52.3	49.7	54.0	46.5	< 0.001
54 years or older	49.6	50.7	47.7	50.3	46.0	53.5	
Female sex, %	48.8	49.3	49.2	48.5	49.1	47.9	0.2
Region of birth,%							
Oceania	55.1	58.7	60.0	59.7	56.7	39.3	< 0.001
Europe / Americas	23.8	22.0	21.4	24.9	21.3	29.7	
Asia / Middle East	15.8	14.2	13.6	10.9	16.7	24.5	
All other	5.3	5.1	5.1	4.6	5.3	6.4	
English spoken at home, %	90.4	94.0	94.0	92.0	91.5	79.8	< 0.001
Arrival to ED by ambulance, %	44.0	40.3	46.8	45.8	43.7	43.4	< 0.001
Nurse Triage presentation urgency score, %							
Resuscitation / Emergency	44.6	46.2	45.2	44.8	43.9	42.9	< 0.001
Urgent	43.5	42.6	43.4	43.5	43.7	44.3	
Semi-urgent / Non-urgent	11.9	11.2	11.4	11.7	12.4	12.8	
ED visit outcome, %							
Admitted to CCU / ICU	13.2	11.8	13.4	13.8	13.7	13.4	< 0.001
Admitted to a medical ward	15.9	16.1	16.6	15.8	14.9	16.1	
Died in the ED	0.4	0.4	0.6	0.3	0.4	0.5	
Discharged home	70.5	71.8	69.4	70.1	71.0	69.9	

Abbreviations: *CCU* coronary care unit, *ED* emergency department, *ICU* intensive care unit, *RII* relative index of inequality, *SES* socio-economic status
^ Proportions were compared using chi-square tests and means were compared using one-way ANOVA tests

among those diagnosed with myocardial infarction, heart failure, angina pectoris, arrhythmia, chest pain, and general signs and symptoms. In all these diagnoses, men were significantly more likely than women to be admitted to a specialised care unit, $p < 0.001$ in each. Proportion of males admitted to specialised care units was higher than those of females shown in all age categories (Table 4 in Appendix).

Multivariable analyses

In the logistic multivariable regression [Model 1], younger age and female sex were independently associated with fewer admissions to a CCU or ICU, whereas, patients coming from low SES locations were more likely to be admitted to such units compared to those coming from the least disadvantaged locations. Likelihood ratio tests to investigate linear associations showed a dose-response effect of geographic-based socioeconomic disadvantage and admission to a specialised care unit, with risk of admission increasing incrementally as socioeconomic disadvantage increased (Likelihood-ratio Chi-square = 0.6, $p = 0.897$) (Table 3).

The GEE multivariable model [Model 2], that accounted for repeated presentations over time, showed identical results. Females were 39% less likely than males to be admitted to a specialised care bed (Adjusted-OR = 0.61, 95% CI 0.57–0.64, $p < 0.001$). Patients coming from the lowest SES locations were 27% more likely to

Table 2 Number of chest pain presentations over study five-year period by quintiles of the relative index of inequality of socioeconomic disadvantage

	All *N* = 75,105	RII_1 Highest SES *N* = 14,551	RII_2 N = 14,578	RII_3 *N* = 15,170	RII_4 *N* = 15,318	RII_5 Lowest SES N = 15,488	*P* value
Presented once	54.9	59.1	58.4	56.7	53.9	46.6	< 0.001
Presented twice	19.4	19.5	18.2	19.1	20.6	19.4	
Presented three or more times	25.8	21.4	23.4	24.2	25.5	34.0	

Table 3 Multivariable regressions[b] investigating risk of admission to a coronary care unit or intensive care unit among patients presenting with non-traumatic chest pain in emergency departments: 2009–2013

Model[a]	Covariates	Adjusted-OR	95% CI	*P* value
1	Age (continuous)	1.00	1.00–1.01	< 0.001
	Female sex	0.58	0.54–0.61	< 0.001
	Relative index of SES inequality quintiles			
	1st quintile (Highest SES)	1.00		
	2nd quintile	1.10	0.99–1.22	0.054
	3rd quintile	1.14	1.02–1.26	0.017
	4th quintile	1.24	1.12–1.36	< 0.001
	5th quintile (Lowest SES)	1.33	1.21–1.47	< 0.001
	Testing linear trends for RII: Likelihood ratio test Chi-square = 0.6, p = 0.897			
2	Age (continuous)	1.00	1.00–1.01	< 0.001
	Female sex	0.61	0.57–0.64	< 0.001
	Relative index of SES inequality quintiles			
	1st quintile (Highest SES)	1.00		
	2nd quintile	1.07	0.99–1.17	0.1
	3rd quintile	1.07	0.97–1.16	0.2
	4th quintile	1.18	1.08–1.28	< 0.001
	5th quintile (Lowest SES)	1.27	1.17–1.39	< 0.001

[a] Model 1: Logistic regression that modelled risk of admission to CCU or ICU on first presentation
Model 2: Generalized Estimating Equations regression that modelled risk of admission to CCU or ICU including all repeated presentations during study five-year period
[b] Both multivariable models were also accounted for: region of birth, language spoken at home, mode of arrival, time of arrival, hospital type, nurse triage urgency score, symptoms on arrival, length of stay in the ED, and main acute admission diagnosis

be admitted to these units compared with the least disadvantaged category, (Adjusted-OR = 1.27, 95% CI 1.17–1.39, $p < 0.001$) (Table 3). Other covariates associated with increased admission to ICU or CCU included arrival by ambulance, higher presentation urgency scores, altered consciousness on presentation, arrival time (with highest rates seen during the evening hours), and acute diagnoses such as acute myocardial infarction.

A sub-analysis that was limited to patients who were admitted to the hospital showed similar results except for age. Among admitted patients, older patients were less likely than their younger counterparts to be admitted to ICU or CCU.

Discussion

In this large population-based panel analysis that investigated emergency non-traumatic chest pain admissions, geographic-based socioeconomic disadvantage scores were independently associated with increased admissions to a coronary or intensive care unit, showing a dose-response. These associations were independent of the patient's sex, age, ethnicity, main presenting symptoms, hospital setting, urgency of presentation, length of stay in the ED, and main acute admission diagnosis. Females compared to males of the same age were less likely to be admitted to such units.

The findings of this study suggest increased chest pain severity or increased general and, in particular, cardiovascular morbidity among those coming from low SES locations. However, although this study reports dose-response effect between socioeconomic disadvantage and admission to intensive or coronary care units, and despite the mounting and consistent findings of direct associations [4, 8, 9, 11], this study was observational, and a causal relationship between socioeconomic disadvantage and worse health outcomes cannot be inferred. The relationship between socioeconomic disadvantage and health is complex and often indirect involving multiple, temporally-evolving relationships between biological, behavioural, psychological, sociological or environmental factors [22]. Residual confounding by many factors not accounted for in this study cannot be excluded [23]. The found inverse associations could possibly be explained by unmeasured factors un-accounted for in this current study. Some of such factors relate to obesity and to smoking. Individuals coming from more disadvantaged backgrounds often smoke more and are more likely to have tobacco-related comorbidities that impact cardiovascular morbidity [24]. Similarly, the relationship of obesity with heart disease, hypertension, some cancers, type 2 diabetes and stroke are well established [25]. However, the association of obesity with socioeconomic disadvantage is multifaceted. Although obesity has been rising across all social classes, research indicates that some groups are more vulnerable than others. This variation of obesity by socioeconomic classes is complex as highlighted by a study that measured prevalence of obesity by different socioeconomic groups in 67 countries [26]. These authors show that in low-income and developing economies the affluent are more likely to be obese; however, a reverse relationship is noted in rich and developed economies where obesity is more prevalent among those coming from lower socioeconomic classes.

This current study also reports significant associations relating to age and sex – findings that may have ramifications for critical care services. As the population ages, the proportion of patients in need of critical care resources will likely increase. A six-year retrospective study that investigated 57 ICUs in Australia and New Zealand reported a significant rise in admission rates among patients aged 80 years or older of nearly 6% per year [27]. A similar rise in demand for critical care by the elderly has been reported in other countries as well [28]. In the United States, over the past ten years, the number of ICU beds per adult population mainly grew in regions with the largest elderly populations [28], with approximately 55% of all intensive care beds being occupied by patients aged 65 or more with 14% of patients 85 or more dying in the ICU setting. A Dutch study, that compared 1996 with 2006, found a 33% increase in number of patients aged 75 or more that needed critical care [29]. This rise in demand for critical care has been reported in North America, Europe, Australia and other regions, but not all patients meeting critical care admission criteria are admitted to such facilities [30, 31]. A British study that investigated ICU admissions among surgical patients in 94 National Health Service hospitals between 1999 and 2004 reported that approximately 85% of the surgical patients who died during admission were never admitted to an intensive care facility [30]. An Israeli incidence study found that 55% of all critically ill hospitalised patients were treated in medical wards that had no intensive specialised care [31]. Similar to these authors who reported that older age was associated with less admissions to an ICU, our study found that among the hospitalised population, older patients were less likely than younger patients to be admitted to a critical care unit. Given higher prevalence of comorbidities and frailty in the elderly, a less favourable risk profile for adverse outcomes and mortality may render them unfit to be admitted to a specialised care unit. This prognosis-based selection bias is commonplace when the demand for these specialised beds far exceeds their availability [31].

Sex variation in hospital admission rates among those presenting to the ED with coronary syndromes has also been previously reported by many studies [32–35]. In general, women take longer than men to seek medical advice for chest pain [33], and when they do, compared to men diagnosed with similar conditions, women are less likely to be admitted to an acute care hospital and to undergo coronary revascularisation. Admitted women are also less likely to be treated in a specialised care unit. A two-year retrospective Canadian study found sex- and age-specific differences in ICU admission rates observed in over 24,000 consecutive adult ICU admissions [36]. A large three-year prospective European study showed that women admitted to critical care units were less likely than their male counterparts to receive invasive therapy and to have shorter ICU durations of stay, despite women having higher severity of illness scores than men needing admission to ICU [34]. The authors also reported a significantly higher risk adjusted in-hospital and ICU mortality among women. Age may be one explanation, as women are often older than men when diagnosed with a serious cardiac condition such as AMI. Compared to men, women also undergo fewer invasive procedures which might have lowered their chances of being admitted to an ICU or CCU as such admissions are higher following major procedures and surgeries [37, 38]. Our study and others [34, 36] show that age and acute diagnoses such as AMI cannot explain the sex differences in hospital care following a chest pain presentation in the ED.

Strengths and limitations

This study utilised a large population-based dataset that included all emergency non-traumatic chest pain presentations in three Victorian hospitals that serve uniquely different sub-populations. The study population was limited to those presenting with emergency non-traumatic chest pain. This has subsequently minimised elective admissions, such as for coronary angioplasty where the highest rates are reported in the more affluent. Compared to the latter, patients coming from socioeconomically disadvantaged backgrounds often wait longer for, and have less access to, a coronary angioplasty consistently observed in the US, UK, and Australia [5, 38]. The admitting ward of patients transferred to other hospitals was also captured in this analysis; for example, if patients coming from higher SES locations chose to be transferred to other private hospitals.

The study is limited primarily by the available data and the ability to account for comorbidities, obesity, severity of illness, actual geographic distances that the patients needed to travel to reach the ED, and health behaviours including smoking and physical exercise. Although comorbidities may affect medical outcomes [39] and influence clinical decision-making for CCU or ICU admission, the analysis found sex-specific differences in all age groups and not specifically in the older patients

Appendix

Table 4 Percent admitted to CCU or ICU by age and sex

Age categories in years	% Male admitted to CCU / ICU	% Female admitted to CCU / ICU	*P* value
24 or younger	29.0	19.1	0.09
25–29	39.8	21.8	0.008
30–34	46.7	32.5	0.018
35–39	56.3	31.6	< 0.001
40–44	51.6	37.6	< 0.001
45–49	60.8	36.9	< 0.001
50–54	59.9	46.7	< 0.001
55–59	58.6	49.4	0.001
60–64	56.9	48.5	0.001
65–69	58.0	42.3	< 0.001
70–74	51.6	41.8	< 0.001
75–79	47.6	40.5	0.003
80–84	38.9	31.2	0.001
85 or older	28.6	16.6	< 0.001
All ages together	51.6	36.7	< 0.001

Abbreviations: *CCU* coronary care unit, *ED* emergency department, *ICU* intensive care unit

who are more likely to have multiple comorbidities. Higher admission rates among patients coming from lower SES locations may indicate more morbidity and more severity of illness, as specialised care units are more likely to admit those with greater illness severity [31, 40]. CCU / ICU bed availability was not known; however, availability of beds cannot explain the risk-adjusted differences found. We had no information on patients' level of education or income and we used an ecological index to infer social status. The use of the composite variable of SEIFA could have misclassified the true socioeconomic status. The study was confined to the three participating hospitals. Finally, the effect of transfer between clinical care wards was not known as no information on inter-departmental movements was known.

Conclusions

To our knowledge, this study is the first to report dose-response relationships between geographic-based socioeconomic disadvantage and higher admission rates to specialised care units in a population-based representative sample of patients presenting with emergency chest pain. The relationship between socioeconomic disadvantage and cardiovascular morbidity is complex and multifactorial. Not every individual exposed to lower socioeconomic disadvantage develops disease and our results cannot infer causal relationships but our findings add to the accumulating evidence supporting a direct association between socioeconomic disadvantage and increased morbidity.

Abbreviations

AMI: Acute myocardial infarction; CCU: Coronary care unit; ED: Emergency department; GEE: Generalized Estimating Eqs.; ICD-10-AM: The International Classification of Diseases, 10th Revision, (Australian Modification); ICU: Intensive care unit; RII: Relative Index of Inequality; SEIFA: Socio Economic Index For Areas; SES: Socioeconomic status

Acknowledgements

The authors thank all staff members of the three emergency departments and all the patients who contributed to this study.

Funding

This study had no funding.

Authors' contributions

GM led the conceptual development of the manuscript. Subsequent study conception and design: GM, JF, GB, MP, CK, MB; Analysis of data: GM; Interpretation of findings: GM, JEH, JF, GB, MP, CK, SB, MB. All authors were involved in drafting the article and revising it critically for important intellectual content, and all authors approved the final version to be published.

Competing interests

The authors declare that they have no competing interests.

Author details

[1]La Trobe Rural Health School, College of Science, Health and Engineering, La Trobe University, PO Box 199, Bendigo, VIC 3552, Australia. [2]School of Health Sciences, Faculty of Health, Arts and Design, Swinburne University of Technology, John Street, Hawthorn, VIC, Australia. [3]School of Public Health, The University of Adelaide, North Terrace, Adelaide, SA, Australia. [4]Intensive Care Unit, Bendigo Health, Barnard Street, Bendigo, VIC, Australia. [5]Department of Emergency Medicine, Royal Melbourne Hospital, Parkville, VIC, Australia. [6]Monash Rural Health Bendigo, Monash University, Bendigo, VIC, Australia. [7]Department of Intensive Care, Austin Health, Heidelberg, VIC, Australia. [8]Centre for Integrated Critical Care Medicine, Department of Medicine and Radiology, The University of Melbourne, Parkville, VIC, Australia.

References

1. Singh GK, Siahpush M, Azuine RE, Williams SD. Increasing area deprivation and socioeconomic inequalities in heart disease, stroke, and cardiovascular

disease mortality among working age populations, United States, 1969-2011. Int J MCH AIDS. 2015;3(2):119–33.
2. Murphy NF, Simpson CR, MacIntyre K, McAlister FA, Chalmers J, McMurray JJ. Prevalence, incidence, primary care burden and medical treatment of angina in Scotland: age, sex and socioeconomic disparities: a population-based study. Heart. 2006;92(8):1047–54.
3. Korda RJ, Soga K, Joshy G, et al. Socioeconomic variation in incidence of primary and secondary major cardiovascular disease events: an Australian population-based prospective cohort study. Int J Equity Health. 2016;15(1):189.
4. Mackenbach JP, Cavelaars AE, Kunst AE, Groenhof F. Socioeconomic inequalities in cardiovascular disease mortality; an international study. Eur Heart J. 2000;21(14):1141–51.
5. Australian Institute of Health and Welfare. Australian hospital statistics 2003–04, AIHW Cat. No. HSE 37. Health Services Series No. 23. Canberra: AIHW. Available from: http://www.aihw.gov.au/publication-detail/?id=6442467720. Accessed 12 Jul 2017.
6. Mackenbach JP, Stirbu I, Roskam AJ, et al. Socioeconomic inequalities in health in 22 European countries. N Engl J Med. 2008;358(23):2468–81.
7. Wilkinson RG, Pickett KE. Income inequality and population health: a review and explanation of the evidence. Soc Sci Med. 2006;62(7):1768–84.
8. Stringhini S, Sabia S, Shipley M, et al. Association of socioeconomic position with health behaviors and mortality. JAMA. 2010;303(12):1159–66.
9. Kivimäki M, Lawlor DA, Smith GD, et al. Socioeconomic position, co-occurrence of behavior-related risk factors, and coronary heart disease: the Finnish public sector study. Am J Public Health. 2007;97(5):874–9.
10. Kawachi I, Adler NE, Dow WH. Money, schooling, and health: mechanisms and causal evidence. Ann N Y Acad Sci. 2010;1186:56–68.
11. Kaplan GA, Keil JE. Socioeconomic factors and cardiovascular disease: a review of the literature. Circulation. 1993;88(4 Pt 1):1973–98.
12. Braveman P, Egerter S, Williams DR. The social determinants of health: coming of age. Annu Rev Public Health. 2011;32:381–98.
13. Hämmig O, Bauer GF. The social gradient in work and health: a cross-sectional study exploring the relationship between working conditions and health inequalities. BMC Public Health. 2013;13(1):1170.
14. Hemingway H, Malik M, Marmot M. Social and psychosocial influences on sudden cardiac death, ventricular arrhythmia and cardiac autonomic function. Eur Heart J. 2001;22(13):1082–101.
15. Pitts SR, Niska RW, Xu J, Burt CW. National Hospital Ambulatory Medical Care Survey: 2006 emergency department summary. Natl Health Stat Report. 2008;7:1–38.
16. Mnatzaganian G, Sprung C, Zitser-Gurevich Y, et al. Effect of infections on 30-day mortality among critically ill patients hospitalized in and out of the intensive care unit. Crit Care Med. 2008;36(4):1097–104.
17. Mnatzaganian G, Galai N, Sprung C, Zitser-Gurevich Y, Mandel M, Ben-Hur D, et al. Increased risk of bloodstream and urinary infections in intensive care unit (ICU) patients compared with patients fitting ICU admission criteria treated in regular wards. J Hosp Infect. 2005;59(4):331–42.
18. Monash Health Annual Report 2016-17. http://monashhealth.org/. Last Accessed 25 Sept 2018.
19. Australian Bureau of Statistics. SEIFA: Socio-Economic Indexes for Areas. http://www.abs.gov.au/websitedbs/censushome.nsf/home/seifa Last Accessed 12 Nov 2017.
20. Mackenbach JP, Kunst AE. Measuring the magnitude of socio-economic inequalities in health: an overview of available measures illustrated with two examples from Europe. Soc Sci Med. 1997;44(6):757–71.
21. Liang KY, Zeger SL. Longitudinal data-analysis using generalized linear-models. Biometrika. 1986;73(1):13–22.
22. Moor I, Rathmann K, Stronks K, Levin K, Spallek J, Richter M. Psychosocial and behavioural factors in the explanation of socioeconomic inequalities in adolescent health: a multilevel analysis in 28 European and north American countries. J Epidemiol Community Health. 2014;68(10):912–21.
23. Mnatzaganian G, Davidson DC, Hiller JE, Ryan P. Propensity score matching and randomization. J Clin Epidemiol. 2015;68(7):760–8.
24. Hiscock R, Bauld L, Amos A, Fidler JA, Munafo M. Socioeconomic status and smoking: a review. Ann N Y Acad Sci. 2012;1248(1):107–23.
25. World Health Organization. Obesity and Overweight. Geneva, Switzerland: World Health Organization; September 2006. Fact Sheet No.311. http://www.who.int/mediacentre/factsheets/fs311/en/. Accessed 28 Nov 2017.
26. Pampel FC, Denney JT, Krueger PM. Obesity, SES, and economic development: a test of the reversal hypothesis. Soc Sci Med. 2012;74(7):1073–81.
27. Bagshaw SM, Webb SA, Delaney A, et al. Very old patients admitted to intensive care in Australia and New Zealand: a multi-Centre cohort analysis. Crit Care. 2009;13(2):R45.
28. Wallace DJ, Angus DC, Seymour CW, Barnato AE, Kahn JM. Critical care bed growth in the United States. A comparison of regional and national trends. Am J Respir Crit Care Med. 2015;191(4):410–6.
29. Blot S, Cankurtaran M, Petrovic M, et al. Epidemiology and outcome of nosocomial bloodstream infection in elderly critically ill patients: a comparison between middle-aged, old, and very old patients. Crit Care Med. 2009;37(5):1634–41.
30. Pearse RM, Harrison DA, James P, et al. Identification and characterisation of the high-risk surgical population in the United Kingdom. Crit Care. 2006;10(3):R81.
31. Simchen E, Sprung C, Galai N, et al. Survival of critically ill patients hospitalized in and out of intensive care. Crit Care Med. 2007;35(2):449–57.
32. Kaul P, Chang WC, Westerhout CM, Graham MM, Armstrong PW. Differences in admission rates and outcomes between men and women presenting to emergency departments with coronary syndromes. CMAJ. 2007;177(10):1193–9.
33. Mnatzaganian G, Braitberg G, Hiller JE, Kuhn L, Chapman R. Sex differences in in-hospital mortality following a first acute myocardial infarction: symptomatology, delayed presentation, and hospital setting. BMC Cardiovasc Disord. 2016;16(1):109.
34. Valentin A, Jordan B, Lang T, Hiesmayr M, Metnitz PGH. Gender-related differences in intensive care: a multiple-center cohort study of therapeutic interventions and outcome in critically ill patients. Crit Care Med. 2003;31(7):1901–7.
35. Merz CN, Shaw LJ, Reis SE, et al. Insights from the NHLBI-sponsored Women's ischemia syndrome evaluation (WISE) study, part II: gender differences in presentation, diagnosis, and outcome with regard to gender-based pathophysiology of atherosclerosis, macro-, and microvascular coronary disease. J Am Coll Cardiol. 2006;47(Suppl A):21–9.
36. Fowler RA, Sabur N, Li P, et al. Sex-and age-based differences in the delivery and outcomes of critical care. CMAJ. 2007;177(12):1513–9.
37. Takakuwa KM, Shofer FS, Limkakeng AT Jr, Hollander JE. Preferences for cardiac tests and procedures may partially explain sex but not race disparities. Am J Emerg Med. 2008;26(5):545–50.
38. Quatromoni J, Jones R. Inequalities in socio-economic status and invasive procedures for coronary heart disease: a comparison between the USA and the UK. Int J Clin Pract. 2008;62(12):1910–9.
39. Mnatzaganian G, Bish M, Fletcher J, Knott C, Stephenson J. Application of accelerated time models to compare performance of two comorbidity-adjusting methods with APACHE II in predicting short-term mortality among the critically ill. Methods Inf Med. 2018;57(1):81–8.
40. Simchen E, Sprung C, Galai N, et al. Survival of critically ill patients hospitalized in and out of intensive care units under paucity of intensive care unit beds. Crit Care Med. 2004;32(8):1654–61.

Permissions

All chapters in this book were first published in EM, by BioMed Central; hereby published with permission under the Creative Commons Attribution License or equivalent. Every chapter published in this book has been scrutinized by our experts. Their significance has been extensively debated. The topics covered herein carry significant findings which will fuel the growth of the discipline. They may even be implemented as practical applications or may be referred to as a beginning point for another development.

The contributors of this book come from diverse backgrounds, making this book a truly international effort. This book will bring forth new frontiers with its revolutionizing research information and detailed analysis of the nascent developments around the world.

We would like to thank all the contributing authors for lending their expertise to make the book truly unique. They have played a crucial role in the development of this book. Without their invaluable contributions this book wouldn't have been possible. They have made vital efforts to compile up to date information on the varied aspects of this subject to make this book a valuable addition to the collection of many professionals and students.

This book was conceptualized with the vision of imparting up-to-date information and advanced data in this field. To ensure the same, a matchless editorial board was set up. Every individual on the board went through rigorous rounds of assessment to prove their worth. After which they invested a large part of their time researching and compiling the most relevant data for our readers.

The editorial board has been involved in producing this book since its inception. They have spent rigorous hours researching and exploring the diverse topics which have resulted in the successful publishing of this book. They have passed on their knowledge of decades through this book. To expedite this challenging task, the publisher supported the team at every step. A small team of assistant editors was also appointed to further simplify the editing procedure and attain best results for the readers.

Apart from the editorial board, the designing team has also invested a significant amount of their time in understanding the subject and creating the most relevant covers. They scrutinized every image to scout for the most suitable representation of the subject and create an appropriate cover for the book.

The publishing team has been an ardent support to the editorial, designing and production team. Their endless efforts to recruit the best for this project, has resulted in the accomplishment of this book. They are a veteran in the field of academics and their pool of knowledge is as vast as their experience in printing. Their expertise and guidance has proved useful at every step. Their uncompromising quality standards have made this book an exceptional effort. Their encouragement from time to time has been an inspiration for everyone.

The publisher and the editorial board hope that this book will prove to be a valuable piece of knowledge for researchers, students, practitioners and scholars across the globe.

List of Contributors

Madeleine Huei Tze Kho and Hiang Chuan Chan
Emergency Medicine and Trauma Department, Sarawak General Hospital, Jalan Hospital, Kuching 93586, Sarawak, Malaysia

Keng Sheng Chew
Faculty of Medicine and Health Sciences, Universiti Malaysia Sarawak, Kota Samarahan 94300, Sarawak, Malaysia

Muhaimin Noor Azhar and Aida Bustam
Faculty of Medicine, University of Malaya, Kuala Lumpur 50603, Malaysia

Mohd Lotfi Hamzah
Emergency Medicine and Trauma Department, Hospital Sultanah Nur Zahirah, Kuala Terengganu 20400, Trengganu, Malaysia

Kee Man Chuah
Faculty of Language Studies and Communication Studies, Universiti Malaysia Sarawak, Kota Samarahan 94300, Sarawak, Malaysia

Igor Jeroukhimov, Itay Wiser, Yehuda Hershkovitz and Zahar Shapira
Trauma Unit, Assaf Harofeh Medical Center, Zerifin 7030000, Israel, affiliated with the Sackler Faculty of Medicine, Tel Aviv University, Tel Aviv, Israel

Kobi Peleg and Adi Givon
National Center for Trauma and Emergency Medicine Research, Gertner Institute for Epidemiology and Health Policy Research, Sheba Medical Center, 52621 Tel Hashomer, Israel

Ricardo Alfici
Surgical Division, Hillel Yaffe Medical Center,38100 Hadera, Israel

Boris Kessel
Trauma Unit, Hillel Yaffe Medical Center, 38100 Hadera, Israel

Femke S. Jonkers and Suze L.Lambooij
Department of Internal Medicine, Máxima Medical Centre, 5600 BM Eindhoven/Veldhoven, the Netherlands

Steffie H. A. Brouns and Joyce J. Wachelder
Department of Internal Medicine, Máxima Medical Centre, 5600 BM Eindhoven/Veldhoven, the Netherlands
Maastricht University, Department of Health Services Research, and CAPHRI School for Public Health and Primary Care, 6229 ER Maastricht, the Netherlands

Harm R. Haak
Department of Internal Medicine, Máxima Medical Centre, 5600 BM Eindhoven/Veldhoven, the Netherlands
Maastricht University, Department of Health Services Research, and CAPHRI School for Public Health and Primary Care, 6229 ER Maastricht, the Netherlands
Department of Internal Medicine, division of general medicine, section acute medicine, Maastricht University Medical Centre, 6229 HX Maastricht, the Netherlands

Jeanne P. Dieleman
Máxima Medical Centre Academy, Máxima Medical Centre, Eindhoven/Veldhoven, the Netherlands

Damien Di Rocco
Medical Student, Faculty of Medicine, University of Lausanne, Lausanne, Switzerland

Mathieu Pasquier, Pierre-Nicolas Carron and Fabrice Dami
Emergency Department, Lausanne University Hospital (CHUV), Bugnon 46, 1011 Lausanne, Switzerland

Eric Albrecht
Department of Anaesthesia, Lausanne University Hospital, Lausanne, Switzerland

Abel Negussie
Department of Social and Population Health, Yirgalem Hospital Medical College, Yirgalem, Ethiopia

Andarge Getie
Administration for Refugee and Returnee Affairs (ARRA), Addis Ababa, Ethiopia

Elias Manaye
Department of Internal Medicine, Wollo University, Dessie, Ethiopia

Tamrat Tekle
Dawro General Hospital, SNNPR, Dawro, Ethiopia

Sami Alsolamy
Emergency Medicine and Intensive Care Department, College of Medicine, King Saud Bin Abdulaziz University for Health Sciences, King Abdulaziz Medical City, Riyadh, Kingdom of Saudi Arabia

Atheer Al-Sabhan and Najla Alassim
Emergency Medicine Department, King Abdulaziz Medical City, Riyadh, Kingdom of Saudi Arabia

Musharaf Sadat
Intensive Care Department, King Abdulaziz Medical City, Riyadh, Kingdom of Saudi Arabia

Yaseen M Arabi
Intensive Care Department, King Abdulaziz Medical City, Riyadh, Kingdom of Saudi Arabia
King Saud Bin Abdulaziz University for Health Sciences, King Abdullah International Medical Research Center, Riyadh, Kingdom of Saudi Arabia
College of Medicine, King Saud Bin Abdulaziz University for Health Sciences, Riyadh, Kingdom of Saudi Arabia
Respiratory Services, King Abdulaziz Medical City, Riyadh, Kingdom of Saudi Arabia

Eman Al Qasim
King Saud Bin Abdulaziz University for Health Sciences, King Abdullah International Medical Research Center, Riyadh, Kingdom of Saudi Arabia

Hani Tamim
King Saud Bin Abdulaziz University for Health Sciences, King Abdullah International Medical Research Center, Riyadh, Kingdom of Saudi Arabia
Department of Internal Medicine, American University of Beirut- Medical Center, Beirut, Lebanon

David Fitzpatrick
Faculty of Health Sciences and Sport, University of Stirling, Stirling FK9 4LA, Scotland

Douglas Maxwell
Royal Alexandra Hospital Paisley, NHS Greater Glasgow and Clyde, Corsebar Rd, Paisley, Glasgow PA2 9PN, Scotland

Alan Craigie
Scottish Ambulance Service, 28 Laverockhall St, G21 4AB, Glasgow, Scotland

Muna Al Jalaf, Hanan Fadali, Rasha Alanee and Firas Najjar
Department of Emergency Medicine, Rashid Hospital and Trauma Centre,Dubai Health Authority, Dubai, UAE

Zulfa Al Deesi and Rania M.Seliem
Laboratory Medicine Department, Rashid Hospital and Trauma Centre, Dubai Health Authority, Dubai, UAE

Eric J. Nilles
Department of Emergency Medicine, Brigham & Women's Hospital, Boston, USA
Harvard Medical School, Boston, USA

Jack J. M. Ligtenberg
Emergency Department, Internal Medicine, University Medical Center Groningen (UMCG), Hanzeplein 1, 9700, RB, Groningen, The Netherlands
Internist acute medicine, Emergency physician, Emergency Department, University Medical Center Groningen, Groningen, The Netherlands

Anna S. M. Dobbe
BSc of Medicine, Faculty of Medicine, University of Groningen, Groningen, The Netherlands

Renate Stolmeijer
Emergency physician, Emergency Department, University Medical Center Groningen, Groningen, The Netherlands

Jan C. ter Maaten
Internist acute medicine, Emergency physician, Emergency Department, University Medical Center Groningen, Groningen, The Netherlands

Paul I. Musey Jr, Cassandra A. Hall and Jeffrey A. Kline
Department of Emergency Medicine, Indiana University School of Medicine, Indianapolis, IN 46202, USA

John A. Lee
Department of Emergency Medicine, Indiana University School of Medicine, Indianapolis, IN 46202, USA
University of Virginia School of Medicine, Charlottesville, Virginia 22908, USA

Sophie Hardy
Emergency Department, St George's Hospital, Tooting, London, UK

Sabina Fattah
The Norwegian Air Ambulance Foundation, Drøbak, Norway
Anaesthesia and Critical Care Research Group, Faculty of Health Sciences, University of Tromsø, Tromsø, Norway

Marius Rehn
The Norwegian Air Ambulance Foundation, Drøbak, Norway
Department of Health Studies, University of Stavanger, Stavanger, Fig. 4 Triage categories for each incident (category numbers marked as "unknown" on the report are not entered) Norway
Division of Emergencies and Critical Care. Department of Anaesthesia, Oslo University Hospital, Oslo, Norway

Torben Wisborg
Anaesthesia and Critical Care Research Group, Faculty of Health Sciences, University of Tromsø, Tromsø, Norway
Hammerfest Hospital, Department of Anaesthesiology and Intensive Care, Finnmark Health Trust, Hammerfest, Norway
Norwegian National Advisory Unit on Trauma, Division of Emergencies and Critical Care, Oslo University Hospital, Oslo, Norway

Lasse Raatiniemi
Hammerfest Hospital, Department of Anaesthesiology and Intensive Care, Finnmark Health Trust, Hammerfest, Norway
Centre for Pre-Hospital Emergency Care/ FinnHEMS 50, Oulu University Hospital, Oulu, Finland
Anaesthesia Research Group, MRC, University of Oulu, Oulu, Finland

Trine Staff
Paramedic Sciences, Oslo and Akershus University College, Oslo, Norway

Warren M. Perry and Rubayet Hossain
Emergency Medicine Department, Yale School of Medicine, 464 Congress Avenue, Suite #260, New Haven, CT 06450, USA
Emergency Department, Yale New Haven Hospital, 20 York Street, New Haven, CT 06510, USA

Richard A. Taylor
Emergency Medicine Department, Yale School of Medicine, 464 Congress Avenue, Suite #260, New Haven, CT 06450, USA
Emergency Department, Yale New Haven Hospital, 20 York Street, New Haven, CT 06510, USA
Yale School of Medicine, Yale New Haven Hospital, 464 Congress Avenue, Suite #260, New Haven, CT 06450, USA

Liliana Pinto
Ordem dos Médicos de Moçambique (Mozambique Medical Council), Maputo, Mozambique

Adriana Lein
Duke Global Health Institute, Duke University, 310 Trent Drive, Durham, North Carolina 27710, USA

Catherine A. Staton
Duke Global Health Institute, Duke University, 310 Trent Drive, Durham, North Carolina 27710, USA
Division of Emergency Medicine, Department of Surgery, Duke University Medical Center, 2301 Erwin Road, Durham, North Carolina 27710, USA
Division of Global Neurosurgery and Neurology, Department of Neurosurgery, Duke University Medical Center, 2301 Erwin Road, Durham, North Carolina 27710, USA

Raquel Mahoque
World Health Organization, Rua Pereira Marinho 280, CP 377 Maputo, Mozambique

David W. Wright
Emory Department of Emergency Medicine, 531 Asbury Circle, Annex Building, Suite N340, Atlanta, GA 30322, USA

Scott M. Sasser
Department of Emergency Medicine, Greenville Health System, University of South Carolina School of Medicine Greenville, Greenville, SC 29605, USA

Yonas Abebe and Tolesa Dida
Department of Emergency and Critical Care Nursing, St. Paul's Hospital Millennium Medical College, Addis Ababa, Ethiopia

Engida Yisma
School of Allied Health Sciences, College of Health Sciences, Addis Ababa University, Addis Ababa, Ethiopia
Robinson Research Institute, School of Medicine, The University of Adelaide, Adelaide, Australia

David M. Silvestri
National Clinician Scholars Program and Department of Emergency Medicine, Yale School of Medicine, New Haven, USA

Mohamed Amine Msolli, Kaouther Beltaief, Wahid Bouida, Mohamed Habib Grissa, Hamdi Boubaker and Semir Nouira
Emergency Department, FattoumaBourguiba University Hospital Monastir, 5000 Monastir, Tunisia
Research Laboratory (LR12SP18), University of Monastir, 5000 Monastir, Tunisia

Nahla Jerbi
Emergency Department, Mahdia University Hospital, 5100 Mahdia, Tunisia
Research Laboratory (LR12SP18), University of Monastir, 5000 Monastir, Tunisia

Riadh Boukef
Emergency Department, Sahloul University Hospital, 4011 Sousse, Tunisia
Research Laboratory (LR12SP18), University of Monastir, 5000 Monastir, Tunisia

Martin Høhrmann Hangaard
Upper GI Section, Department of Surgery, Odense University Hospital, Sdr. Boulevard 29, DK-5000 Odense C, Denmark

Brian Malling
Department of Diagnostic Radiology, Rigshospitalet, Blegdamsvej 9, DK-2100 København Ø, Denmark

Christian Backer Mogensen
Emergency Department, Hospital of Southern Jutland, Kresten Philipsensvej 15, DK-6200 Aabenraa, Denmark

Rayan El Sibai and Rana Bachir
Department of Emergency Medicine, American University of Beirut Medical Center, Riad El Solh, Beirut 1107 2020, Lebanon

Mazen El Sayed
Department of Emergency Medicine, American University of Beirut Medical Center, Riad El Solh, Beirut 1107 2020, Lebanon
Emergency Medical Services and Prehospital Care Program, American University of Beirut Medical Center, Beirut, Lebanon

Mary Matthews, Peter Richman, Scott Krall, Kimberly Leeson and Albert L Gest
Department of Emergency Medicine, CHRISTUS HEALTH/Texas A&M Residency in Emergency Medicine, Corpus Christi, TX 78404, USA

K Tom Xu
Department of Emergency Medicine Texas Tech College of Medicine, Lubbock, TX, USA

Osbert Blow
Department of Acute Care Surgery, Trauma & Surgical Critical Care, CHRISTUS Spohn Hospital, Corpus Christi, TX, USA

Natalie Baier, Susanne Felgner and Cornelia Henschke
Institute of Health Care Management, Berlin Centre of Health Economics Research (BerlinHECOR), Technische Universität Berlin, Straße des 17. Juni 135 (H80), 10623 Berlin, Germany

Karsten Roth
Institute of Health Care Management, Berlin Centre of Health Economics Research (BerlinHECOR), Technische Universität Berlin, Straße des 17. Juni 135 (H80), 10623 Berlin, Germany
ASB Köln e.V, Sülzburgstraße 146, 050937 Köln, Germany

Naohiko Imai, Kiyomi Osako, Nagayuki Kaneshiro and Yugo Shibagaki
Division of Nephrology and Hypertension, Department of Internal Medicine, St. Marianna University School of Medicine, 2-16-1 Sugao, Miyamae-ku, Kawasaki, Kanagawa, Japan

Mohammed-Najeeb Mahama and Ahmed Nuhu Zakariah
National Ambulance Service, Accra, Ghana

Ernest Kenu and Delia Akosua Bandoh
Ghana Field Epidemiology and Laboratory Training Program, Department of Epidemiology, School of Public Health, University of Ghana, Accra, Ghana

Waheeb Nasr Naser
King Khalid Hospital Najran, King Abdul-Aziz Road, Najran, Kingdom of Saudi Arabia

Huda Ba Saleem
Faculty of Medicine and Health Sciences, Aden University, Aden, Yemen

Judith E. van Zanden, Susanne Wagenaar, Jan C. ter Maaten and Jack J. M. Ligtenberg
Department of Emergency Medicine, University of Groningen, University Medical Center Groningen, Groningen, The Netherlands.

Jozine M. ter Maaten
Department of Cardiology, University of Groningen, University Medical Center Groningen, Groningen, The Netherlands

Federico Franchi, Chiara De Fazio, Jean-Louis Vincent, Jacques Creteur and Fabio Silvio Taccone
Department of Intensive Care, Erasme Hospital, Université libre de Bruxelles, Brussels, Belgium

Antonella Cotoia
Department of Intensive Care, Erasme Hospital, Université libre de Bruxelles, Brussels, Belgium
Department of Anaesthesiology and Intensive Care, University of Foggia, Foggia, Italy

Samiha Jarrah
Faculty of Nursing, Applied Science Private University, Amman, Jordan

Mohannad Eid AbuRuz
Faculty of Nursing, Applied Science Private University, Amman, Jordan. Amman, Jordan

Mahfuz Judeh
Applied Science Private University, Amman, Jordan

Nolan Mann, Kellen Welch, Andrew Martin, Michael Subichin, Lauren E. Birmingham, Tiffany D. Marchand and Richard L. George
Summa Health System- Department of Surgery, Akron Campus, Akron, OH, USA

Katherine Wietecha
Summa Health System- Department of Surgery, Division of Trauma Akron Campus, Akron Ohio, USA Northeast Ohio Medical University, Rootstown, OH, USA

Charles Morin
Service de Médecine Polyvalente, Centre Hospitalier du Mans, 194 Avenue Rubillard, 72000 Le Mans, France

Jacques Choukroun
Service des Urgences Adultes, Centre Hospitalier du Mans, 194 Avenue rubillard, 72000 Le Mans, France

Jean-Christophe Callahan
Service de Réanimation Polyvalente, Centre Hospitalier du Mans, 194 Avenue Rubillard, 72000 Le Mans, France

Pham Thi Ngoc Thao, Ton Thanh Tra and Nguyen Truong Son
Cho Ray Hospital, 201B Nguyen Chi Thanh Street, District 5, Ho Chi Minh City, Vietnam

Koji Wada
International University of Health and Welfare, Tokyo, Japan

Ayob Akbari, Firoozeh Jahani, Alireza Amirabadizadeh and Borhan Mansouri
Medical Toxicology and Drug Abuse Research Center (MTDRC), Birjand University of Medical Sciences, Moallem Avenue, Birjand 9717853577, Iran

Omid Mehrpour
Medical Toxicology and Drug Abuse Research Center (MTDRC), Birjand University of Medical Sciences, Moallem Avenue, Birjand 9717853577, Iran
Rocky Mountain Poison and Drug Center, Denver, CO, USA

Patrick C. Ng
Rocky Mountain Poison and Drug Center, Denver, CO, USA

Elaheh Allahyari
Social Determinants of Health Research Center, Birjand University of Medical Sciences, Birjand, Iran

Nadir Ijaz, Matthew Strehlow, N. Ewen Wang, Elizabeth Pirrotta and Swaminatha Mahadevan
Department of Emergency Medicine, Stanford University School of Medicine, 300 Pasteur Dr, Rm M121, Alway Building MC 5119, Stanford, CA 94305, USA

Areeba Tariq
Honors Program in Medical Education, Northwestern University, Evanston, IL, USA

Naseeruddin Mahmood
Department of Paediatrics and Child Health, Aga Khan University, Karachi, Pakistan

George Mnatzaganian, Steve Begg and Melanie Bish
La Trobe Rural Health School, College of Science, Health and Engineering, La Trobe University, Bendigo, VIC 3552, Australia

Janet E Hiller
School of Health Sciences, Faculty of Health, Arts and Design, Swinburne University of Technology, John Street, Hawthorn, VIC, Australia
School of Public Health, The University of Adelaide, North Terrace, Adelaide, SA, Australia

Jason Fletcher
Intensive Care Unit, Bendigo Health, Barnard Street, Bendigo, VIC, Australia.

Cameron Knott
Intensive Care Unit, Bendigo Health, Barnard Street, Bendigo, VIC, Australia
Monash Rural Health Bendigo, Monash University, Bendigo, VIC, Australia
Department of Intensive Care, Austin Health, Heidelberg, VIC, Australia

Mark Putland
Department of Emergency Medicine, Royal Melbourne Hospital, Parkville, VIC, Australia

George Braitberg
Department of Emergency Medicine, Royal Melbourne Hospital, Parkville, VIC, Australia
Centre for Integrated Critical Care Medicine, Department of Medicine and Radiology, The University of Melbourne, Parkville, VIC, Australia

Index

N

O

P

R

S

T

V

www.ingramcontent.com/pod-product-compliance
Lightning Source LLC
LaVergne TN
LVHW080709210926
848485LV00003B/439
9781632428769